Cardiac Amyloidosis

Eyal Herzog
Editor

Cardiac Amyloidosis

Springer

Editor
Eyal Herzog
Department of Cardiology
Hadassah Medical Center
Jerusalem, Israel

ISBN 978-3-031-88341-5 ISBN 978-3-031-88342-2 (eBook)
https://doi.org/10.1007/978-3-031-88342-2

This Springer imprint is published by the registered company Springer Nature Switzerland AG
The registered company address is: Gewerbestrasse 11, 6330 Cham, Switzerland

Contents

Management of Cardiac Amyloidosis

Clinical Cases of Patients Using the "Cardiac Amyloidosis" Pathway

About the Editor

Prof. Eyal Herzog is the Director of the Department of Cardiology at Hadassah Medical Center, The Hebrew University of Jerusalem, in Jerusalem, Israel.

In his prior positions he was a professor of Medicine at the Icahn School of Medicine at Mount Sinai Medical Center in New York where he was the director of Critical Care Cardiology and Echocardiography for over two decades at Mount Sinai, St. Luke's Hospital.

Over the past three decades, Dr. Herzog has developed highly respected methods for improving cardiovascular healthcare through the application of novel algorithmic pathways that simplify the diagnosis, treatment, and management of cardiovascular disease.

Dr. Herzog is internationally recognized for his leadership in Critical Care Cardiology and Echocardiography. He had authored numerous textbooks, including the "The Cardiac Care Survival Guide" and "Herzog's CCU book," that have become bestsellers in the United States and around the globe.

Dr. Herzog is an outstanding teacher. He has been awarded "Teacher of the year" and "Physician of the year" prizes many times by the Department of Medicine and the Division of Cardiology at Mount Sinai.

Diagnosis of Cardiac Amyloidosis

Pathway for the Diagnosis and Management of Cardiac Amyloidosis

Eyal Herzog, David Leibowitz, Moshe E. Gatt, Tali Koren, Batel Nissan, and Arthur Pollak

Abstract The systemic amyloidoses are a broad spectrum of diseases that result from misfolding of proteins that aggregate into amyloid fibrils. In cardiac amyloidosis, amyloid fibrils accumulate in the interstitial space between cardiac myocytes causing cellular injury and impairing compliance. Current data suggest that cardiac amyloidosis is more common than previously thought. Advances in cardiac imaging, diagnostic strategies, and therapies have improved the recognition and treatment of cardiac amyloidosis. A position statement for the diagnosis and treatment of cardiac amyloidosis has been published in 2021 by the European Society of Cardiology and an expert consensus decision pathway was published in 2023 by the American College of Cardiology. These are excellent documents but quite lengthy and complex. For this reason, our team developed a novel and simple pathway to help health care providers diagnose and treat patients with cardiac amyloidosis. Our pathway has four sections. It starts with a section titled: "suspicion" in which we provide simple clues or "red flags" that are associated with the cardiac amyloidosis phenotype. It is followed by a section titled: "diagnosis", where we present in a simplified 2 × 2 format the laboratory and imaging tests that must be performed for an accurate diagnosis. In the section titled: "treatment" we describe the four pillars in the management of patients with cardiac amyloidosis which include: heart failure treatments, management of arrhythmias, treatment of significant aortic stenosis and appropriate selection of disease modifying therapies. Our algorithm ends with our simplified recommendation for follow up.

Keywords Cardiac amyloidosis · Heart failure · Tafamidis · Transthyretin protein · Pathway

E. Herzog (✉) · D. Leibowitz · T. Koren · B. Nissan · A. Pollak
Department of Cardiology, Hadassah Medical Center, Hebrew University of Jerusalem, Jerusalem, Israel
e-mail: eyalherzog10@gmail.com

M. E. Gatt
Department of Hematology, Hadassah Medical Center, Hebrew University of Jerusalem, Jerusalem, Israel

E. Herzog (ed.), *Cardiac Amyloidosis*, https://doi.org/10.1007/978-3-031-88342-2_1

Introduction

The systemic amyloidoses are a broad spectrum of diseases that result from misfolding of proteins that aggregate into amyloid fibrils. In cardiac amyloidosis (CA), amyloid fibrils accumulate in the interstitial space between cardiac myocytes causing cellular injury and impairing myocardial function. Advanced cardiac amyloidosis is physiologically characterized as a restrictive cardiomyopathy (CM).

The nomenclature for systemic amyloidosis includes an "A" for amyloid followed by an abbreviation of the protein that misfolds. The 2 most common types are AL amyloidosis, where the amyloid fibrils are composed of monoclonal immunoglobulin light chains, and ATTR amyloidosis, where the amyloid fibrils are composed of the transthyretin protein and can occur in the context of familial mutational variant (ATTRv) cardiac amyloidosis or wild-type TTR (ATTRwt) cardiac amyloidosis. While the familial type is rare, it may be diagnosed at a young adult age and the severity of the disease is correlated with the type of autosomal dominant mutation found. Neuropathy is common. In contrast, ATTRwt, formerly called senile TTR as it is most common in elderly patients, is relatively common. Interestingly, 90% of patients are male.

Although considered in the past as a rare disease, recent data suggest that wild type ATTR cardiac amyloidosis is more common than previously thought. Recent advances in cardiac imaging, diagnostic strategies, and therapies have improved the recognition and treatment of cardiac amyloidosis.

A position statement for the diagnosis and treatment of cardiac amyloidosis has been published in 2021 by the European Society of Cardiology (ESC) [1] and an expert consensus decision pathway was published in 2023 by the American College of Cardiology (ACC) [2]. These are excellent documents that are very detailed and comprehensive but quite lengthy and complex. For this reason, our team developed a novel and simple pathway to help health care providers diagnose and treat patients with cardiac amyloidosis (Fig. 1).

Description of the Pathway for the Diagnosis and Management of Cardiac Amyloidosis

Our pathway for the diagnosis and management of cardiac amyloidosis (CA) is shown in Fig. 1.

Diagnosis of cardiac amyloidosis includes two phases: a suspicion phase and a definite diagnosis phase. The latter phase also includes appropriate typing of the amyloid, which is critical to guide specific treatment.

Our pathway starts with a section titled: "suspicion" (Fig. 2) in which we provide simple clues or "red flags" that are associated with the cardiac amyloidosis phenotype. It is followed by a section titled: "diagnosis" (Fig. 3), where we present the laboratory

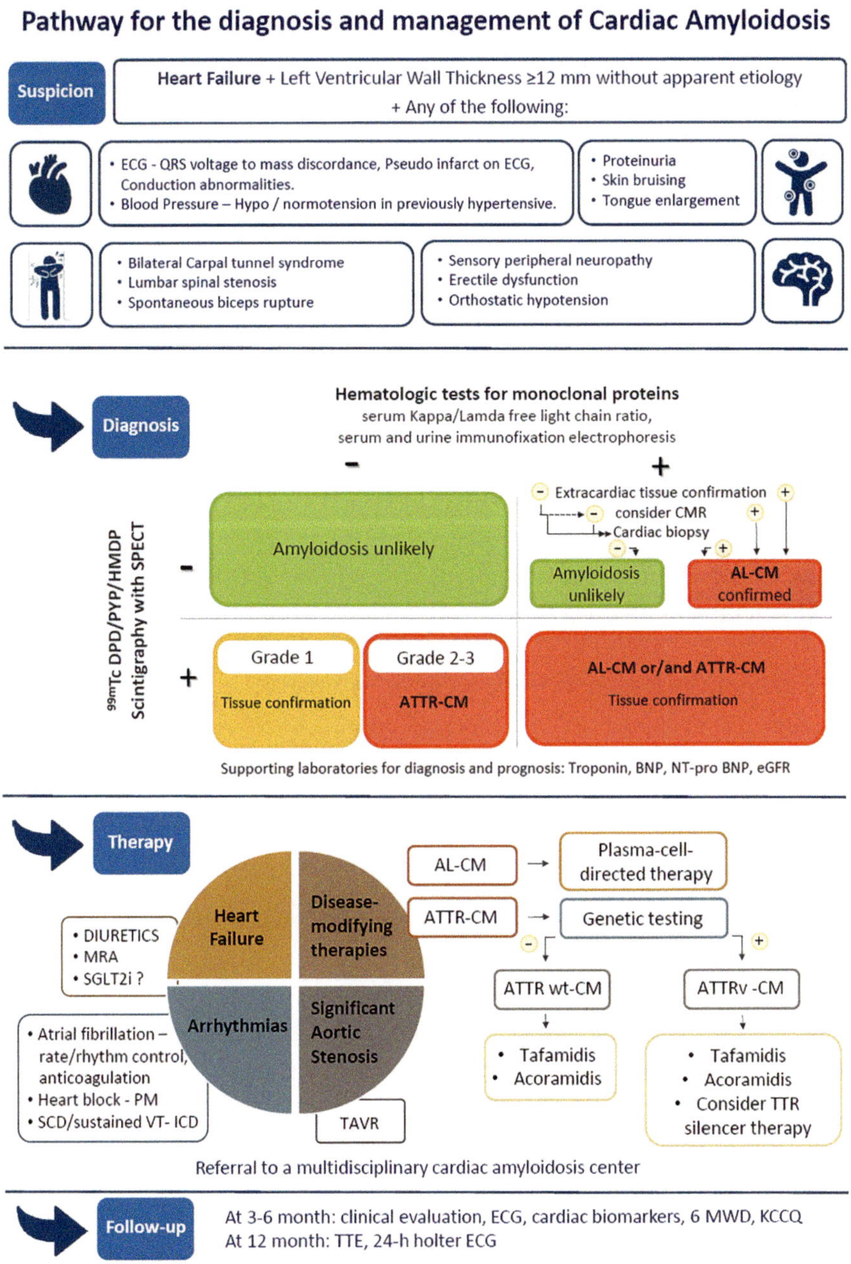

Fig. 1 Pathway for the diagnosis and management of cardiac amyloidosis

and imaging tests that must be performed for an accurate diagnosis, but should not be performed without an appropriate index of suspicion. Once cardiac amyloidosis is confirmed, an early initiation of therapy can prevent further amyloid deposition in the heart and further end organ damage. In the section titled: "treatment" (Fig. 4) we describe the four pillars in the management of patients with cardiac amyloidosis which include: heart failure treatments, management of arrhythmias, treatment of significant aortic stenosis and appropriate selection of disease modifying therapies. Our algorithm ends with our simplified recommendation for follow up (Fig. 5).

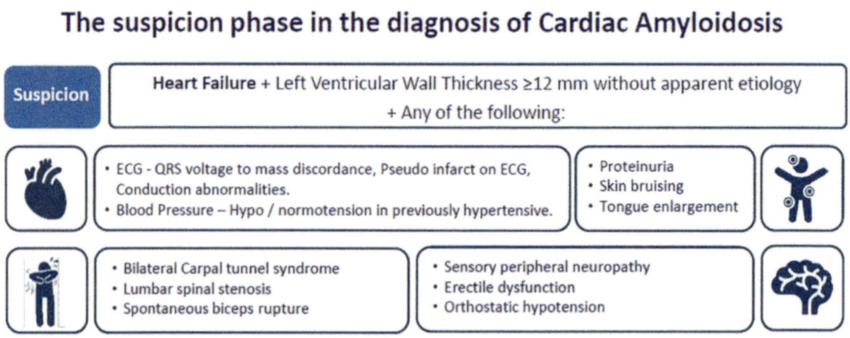

Fig. 2 The suspicion phase in the diagnosis of cardiac amyloidosis

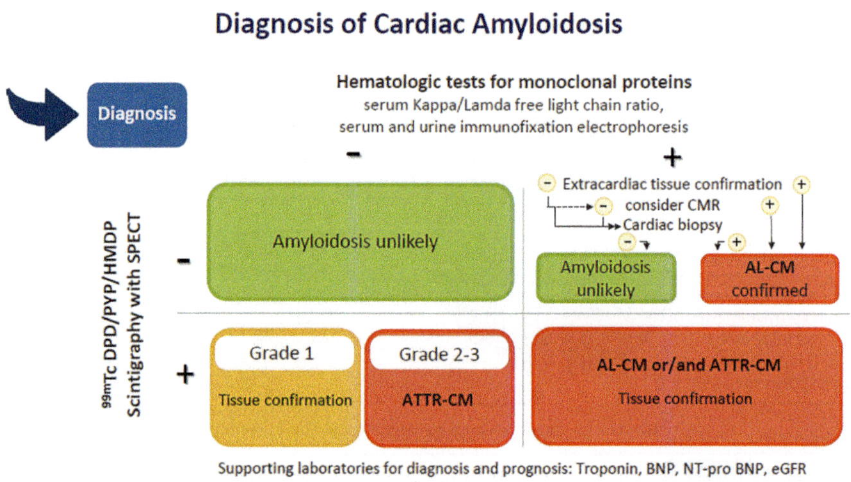

Fig. 3 Diagnosis of cardiac amyloidosis

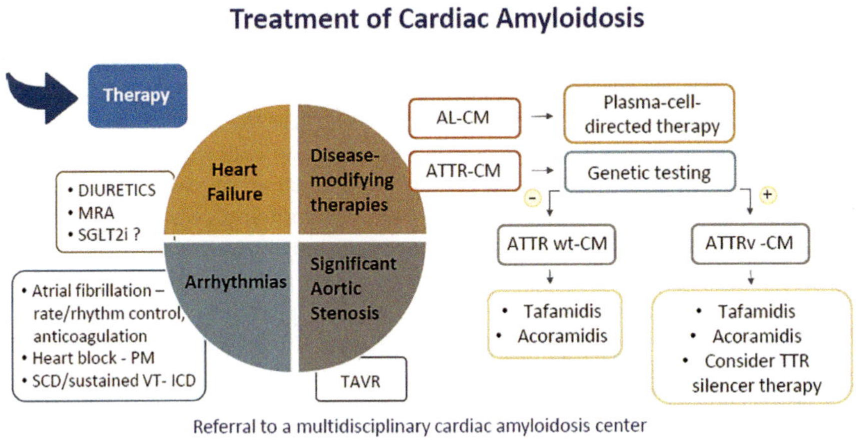

Fig. 4 Treatment of cardiac amyloidosis

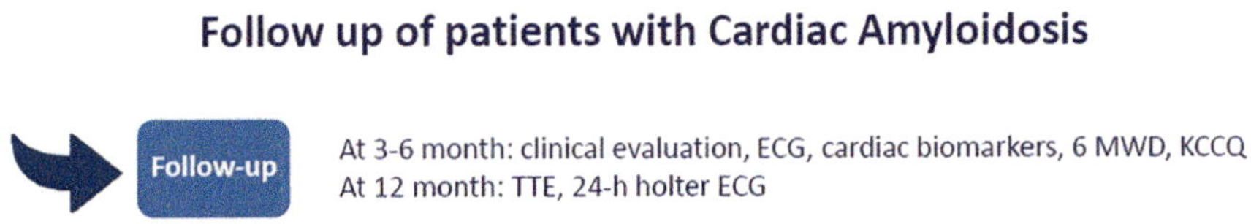
Follow up of patients with Cardiac Amyloidosis
Follow-up
At 3-6 month: clinical evaluation, ECG, cardiac biomarkers, 6 MWD, KCCQ
At 12 month: TTE, 24-h holter ECG

Fig. 5 Follow up of patients with cardiac amyloidosis

The Suspicion Phase in the Diagnosis of Cardiac Amyloidosis (Fig. 2)

The cardiac amyloidosis diagnostic process begins with a detailed clinical history and physical examination, electrocardiogram (ECG), and transthoracic echocardiogram (TTE). Cardiac amyloidosis clinical clues or "red flags" can be broadly divided into cardiac features and extracardiac manifestations.

An important clinical feature that can differentiate between AL and ATTR is the rate of symptoms and symptom deterioration. While AL is a fast and relatively aggressive disease with rapidly progressing cardiac dysfunction, ATTR is relatively indolent with cardiac dysfunction that develops over many years.

With regards to the cardiac features, discordance between QRS voltage on ECG and wall thickness seen on echocardiogram is a well-recognized finding suggestive of CA. When increased wall thickness is caused by myocyte hypertrophy, for example in hypertension, increased voltage on the ECG is seen. However, when increased wall thickness is caused by deposition within the myocardium of abnormal amyloid proteins, decreased voltage on the ECG may be noted. Low QRS voltage on ECG by commonly applied criteria is only present in about 30% of patients with cardiac amyloidosis, and thus its absence does not exclude the diagnosis. Another electrocardiographic feature of CA is the appearance of a pseudoinfarct pattern on the ECG. Echocardiographic diagnostic clues include increased left ventricular wall thickness (above the sex-specific upper limit of normal and typically $\geq$ 1.2 cm), increased wall thickness of other cardiac chambers such as the right ventricle, restrictive filling pattern on mitral Doppler, decreased mitral annular systolic velocity (s'), biatrial enlargement, and decreased global longitudinal strain with relative apical sparing ("cherry-on-top" pattern). CA may be an important cause of heart failure with preserved ejection fraction and may be associated with aortic stenosis.

The extracardiac manifestations we have included in our algorithm include the typical musculoskeletal manifestations of bilateral carpal tunnel syndrome, lumbar spinal stenosis, and spontaneous biceps rupture, as well as the neurological features of autonomic dysfunction, sensory peripheral neuropathy, orthostatic hypotension, and erectile dysfunction. These features are seen in both AL and ATTR. However, AL amyloidosis may involve almost every organ except the central nervous system. Most commonly amyloid sedimentation in the renal glomeruli causes albuminuria which may progress to nephrotic range proteinuria. In patients with obvious causes for glomerulopathy, such as a history of diabetes and hypertensive, the absence of concurrent retinal changes should raise the suspicion for amyloidosis. Gastrointestinal complaints (diarrhea, constipation) and elevated liver function tests (mainly alkaline phosphatase and gamma-glutamyl transferase (GGT)) may provide other clues for a systemic disease. The classical pathognomonic tongue enlargement and periorbital petechias appear in only 10–15% of patients.

In the top section of our algorithm titled "suspicion" we have adopted the ESC recommendation in which a patient with heart failure must have left ventricular wall thickness $\geq$ 12 mm (without an apparent etiology) in addition to at least one of the other cardiac or extracardiac manifestations (seen in Fig. 2) in order to proceed to the next phase of diagnostic testing and imaging.

Diagnosis of Cardiac Amyloidosis (Fig. 3)

Once cardiac amyloidosis is suspected, a definitive diagnosis should be obtained. As most cases of cardiac amyloidosis are either AL or ATTR, we adopted the ESC recommendation and propose a diagnostic algorithm focusing on identifying these subtypes by the initial use of Technetium-based compounds pyrophosphate (Tc-PYP) or diphosphono-1,2-ropanodicarboxylic acid (Tc-DPD) or hydroxymethylene diphosphonate (HMDP) scintigraphy coupled with assessment for monoclonal proteins by measuring serum Kappa/Lambda free light chains ratio and performing serum/urine immunofixation electrophoresis.

The results of these tests could lead to four scenarios as seen in Fig. 3 and is shown in this figure in a typical 2 $\times$ 2 format:

(1) Scintigraphy does not show any cardiac uptake (grade 0) and assessments for monoclonal proteins are negative. There is a very low probability of

cardiac amyloidosis and ATTR and AL amyloidosis are unlikely. An alternative diagnosis should be considered.

(2) Scintigraphy shows cardiac uptake and assessments for monoclonal proteins are negative. If cardiac uptake is Grade 2 or 3, ATTR cardiac amyloidosis can be diagnosed. As is seen in our therapy section of our algorithm genetic testing is recommended in these patients to differentiate between ATTRv and ATTRwt forms. If cardiac uptake is Grade 1, we recommend to consider tissue confirmation for diagnosis.

(3) Scintigraphy does not show cardiac uptake and at least one of the monoclonal protein tests is abnormal. Based on the ESC recommendations:

Light-chain amyloidosis must be ruled out promptly and cardiac magnetic resonance (CMR) can be used to confirm cardiac involvement. If CMR findings do not support cardiac amyloidosis, the diagnosis is very unlikely. In the case that CMR findings are supportive or inconclusive, cardiac or extracardiac histological demonstration of amyloid deposits is required to diagnose AL cardiac amyloidosis. Cardiac or other clinically affected organ biopsy is recommended to avoid time delay to diagnosis and consultation with a haematologist is warranted. If CMR cannot be performed promptly, consider performing biopsy directly.

An alternative approach recommended by our team is to first perform extracardiac tissue confirmation. If the biopsy is positive for AL then the diagnosis of AL CM is confirmed. If the extracardiac biopsy is negative the next step in the evaluation should be a cardiac biopsy for final diagnosis. CMR is optional if resources are available to support the diagnosis.

(4) Scintigraphy shows cardiac uptake and at least one of the monoclonal protein tests is abnormal. Transthyretin amyloidosis with concomitant MGUS (or any haematological disorder that produces FLC), AL amyloidosis, or coexistence of both AL and ATTR amyloidosis are possible in this scenario. Diagnosis of cardiac amyloidosis, in this case, requires histology with amyloid typing, e.g. from an accessible organ, and, if needed via endomyocardial biopsy.

Graphically in our algorithm (seen in Fig. 3) we have used a color code of green, yellow, and red (as in a traffic light) to indicate diagnostic status. The green color presents patients who are unlikely to have a diagnosis of cardiac amyloidosis. The yellow color presents patients with a potential diagnosis of cardiac amyloidosis and the red color presents patients with a confirmed diagnosis of cardiac amyloidosis.

There are additional supporting laboratories that we recommend to perform for diagnosis and prognosis and they include the biomarkers of troponin, BNP or NT-pro BNP as well as measurement of eGFR.

Treatment of Cardiac Amyloidosis (Fig. 4)

There are four pillars in the treatment of cardiac amyloidosis as seen in Fig. 4:

1. Heart failure therapy
2. Management of arrhythmias
3. Management of significant aortic stenosis
4. Use of disease modifying therapies.

1. **Heart failure management**

Expert consensus documents caution against the use of standard HF guideline–directed medical therapy in cardiac amyloidosis [3]. For example, beta blockers should be used with caution in patients with cardiac amyloidosis; even at low doses, they may be poorly tolerated. Angiotensin receptor–neprilysin inhibitors, angiotensin-converting enzyme inhibitors, and angiotensin receptor blockers may be poorly tolerated due to vasodilation, particularly in patients with underlying autonomic orthostatic hypotension.

Conversely, regarding mineralocorticoid antagonists, a retrospective analysis of the TOPCAT (Treatment of Preserved Cardiac Function Heart Failure With an Aldosterone Antagonist) trial with a cohort enriched for amyloidosis based on echocardiographic features observed benefit with spironolactone, with a reduction in the combined endpoint of cardiovascular death, HF hospitalization, or aborted cardiac arrest [4].

Lastly, although recent trials have shown benefit of sodium glucose cotransporter inhibitors for HFpEF [5] and there is theoretical benefit, there is insufficient evidence regarding their efficacy in cardiac amyloidosis.

Volume management is the mainstay of therapy in cardiac amyloidosis, with many patients presenting with predominant right-sided HF symptoms. Loop diuretic agents and sequential nephron blockade with mineralocorticoid receptor antagonists should be considered. Diuretics should be used with caution to avoid intravascular volume depletion and renal injury.

2. **Management of arrhythmias**

A. Atrial fibrillation (AF):

The reported prevalence of AF in cardiac amyloidosis is variable but may be as high as 56% in AL amyloidosis and 70% in ATTR-CM [6]. The risk for intracardiac thrombus may be as high as 33% in cardiac amyloidosis and can be present even in patients receiving chronic anticoagulation. Given the high risk of atrial thrombus in CA, consensus statements and guidelines recommend anticoagulation when AF is present, regardless of the CHA2DS2-VASc risk score. Additionally, transesophageal echocardiography to evaluate for left atrial appendage thrombus is mandatory before cardioversion, regardless of the duration of anticoagulation before the procedure.

Rhythm control can be considered if the patient remains symptomatic despite attempts at rate control, and amiodarone is generally well tolerated as a first-line agent.

B. Conduction disease:

Conduction disease is prevalent in patients with cardiac amyloidosis, frequently involving the His-Purkinje system in both AL-CM and ATTR-CM. There should be close monitoring for the need for a permanent pacemaker and appropriate referral to electrophysiology. In cases of pacemaker dependence or a high degree of anticipated pacing, cardiac resynchronization therapy may be considered.

C. Ventricular Tachycardia (VT) and Sudden Cardiac Death (SCD):

Nonsustained ventricular arrhythmias are very common in both AL-CM and ATTR-CM, but it is not clear if they are predictors of subsequent sudden cardiac death. Current guidelines state that there is insufficient data to provide recommendations beyond standard indications for use of implantable cardioverter defibrillators as primary prevention in cardiac amyloidosis.

3. **Significant Aortic Stenosis**

Concurrent aortic stenosis (AS) is a recognized comorbidity in cardiac amyloidosis, particularly in ATTRwt [7]. Up to 16% of patients with AS undergoing transcatheter aortic valve replacement may have ATTR-CM. Emerging data suggests that aortic valve intervention confers both symptom palliation and survival benefit relative to medical management in patients with cardiac amyloidosis. We recommend that patients with cardiac amyloidosis and significant aortic stenosis should be referred to a structural interventional cardiologist.

4. **Use of disease modifying therapies**

As of early 2025, tafamidis [8] and acoramidis [9] are approved by the U.S. Food and Drug Administration (FDA) for treatment of ATTR cardiac amyloidosis. They act as a TTR stabilizer slowing the dissociation of TTR and thus fibril formation and cardiac deposition. The FDA-approved dosages are tafamidis 61 mg or tafamidis meglumine 80 mg.

In the ATTR-ACT (Safety and Efficacy of Tafamidis in Patients With Transthyretin Cardiomyopathy) study, tafamidis compared with placebo demonstrated reductions in all-cause mortality and cardiovascular-related hospitalizations [8]. Tafamidis has a favorable side-effect profile. In ATTR-ACT, adverse events were mild to moderate in severity, and permanent discontinuation occurred more frequently in the placebo group. The major driver for starting treatment is whether a patient will meaningfully benefit (clinically relevant disease without competing life-limiting comorbidity) and whether it is affordable.

In a phase III, multicenter, double blind, placebo-controlled trial, 632 patients with ATTRwt or ATTRv cardiomyopathy were randomized in a 2:1 ratio to receive acoramidis hydrochloride or matching placebo for 30 months [9].

Acoramidis was associated with improve in the four-step primary hierarchical analysis included: death from any cause, cardiovascular-related hospitalization, NT-proBNP, and 6-min walk distance. For the 6-min walk distance, KCCQOS score, and TTR serum level, there were significant between-group differences, but not for death from any cause. This may be attributed to the trial's lower death rate.

The overall incidence of adverse events or serious adverse events during treatment period was similar in the acoramidis group and the placebo group [9].

The agents patisiran (small interfering RNA therapeutic) [10] and inotersen (an antisense oligonucleotide therapeutic) [11] are registered for treatment of neuropathy.

The recent HELIOS-B trial evaluated the cardiac efficacy and safety of vutrisiran (a small interfering RNA compound) in patients with ATTR-CM [12]. The study demonstrated that vutrisiran significantly reduced the risk of these outcomes compared to placebo. At baseline, 40% of the cohort was also receiving tafamidis. Additionally, patients treated with vutrisiran experienced less decline in their 6-min walk test performance, and showed a smaller reduction in their Kansas City Cardiomyopathy Questionnaire Overall Summary (KCCQ-OS) score. Adverse events were similar between the vutrisiran and placebo groups. In the context of this study, vutrisiran provides another alternative in the treatment of ATTR-CM and might offer better clinical benefits specially for patients with mixed phenotype who have both ATTR-CM and ATTR-PN.

Treatment of AL Amyloidosis

Because AL amyloidosis results from a clonal plasma cell disorder, the primary treatment uses chemotherapy and/or immunotherapy to target the aberrant plasma cells, eradicate the underlying clone, and decrease amyloid precursor protein production, thereby halting and ameliorating organ damage and causing regression of tissue amyloid deposits. A key to the significance of the free light chain (FLC) reduction is the understanding that the FLC themselves are toxic to the organs involved. Thus, the goal of treatment of AL amyloidosis is to eradicate the pathological plasma cells and remove the affected light chain from the circulation. Prognosis of both overall survival and organ responses (i.e. reduction of proBNP level and amelioration of NYHA stage and 6 min walk cardiac function) directly correlates with the ability to reduce FLC levels to the minimum possible.

The significance of early detection and timely treatment cannot be overemphasized. Advanced stage cardiac involvement (MAYO stage 3 as defined by elevated both proBNP and troponin levels) confers worse prognosis, and stage 3b patients (i.e. a proBNP level of more than 8500 pg/L) have an extremely grave prognosis that cannot be ameliorated even with treatment.

Management of AL amyloidosis is derived from anti–plasma-cell multiple myeloma therapies. First line treatment with immunotherapy consisting of the anti CD38 antibody daratumumab combined with bortezomib (a proteasome inhibitor), cyclophosphamide and dexamethasone has become the standard of care and the first approved treatment regimen for AL amyloidosis. Other plasma cell directed agents may be utilized in frail patients who may not endure aggressive treatment modalities such as autologous stem cell transplantation and other common anti-myeloma agents such as immunomodulators (i.e. thalidomide and lenalidomide) that pose difficulties for these patients.

During the initial treatment with chemo-immunotherapy, especially high dose steroids, fluid accumulation and heart failure symptoms may ensue, and patients should be meticulously monitored. Even in those patients achieving a complete hematological remission (i.e. FLC normalization), clinical improvement may ensue only after a few months of continued treatment.

Anti-amyloid specific antibodies to remove the sedimented amyloid from the affected heart show great promise and clinical trials are ongoing.

Follow-Up of Patients with Cardiac Amyloidosis (Fig. 5)

As recommended by the ESC [1] statement and the ACC [2] expert position documents, all patients with a diagnosis of cardiac amyloidosis should be referred to a multispecialty cardiac amyloidosis center.

Although no studies have yet addressed the optimal follow-up scheme in patients with cardiac amyloidosis, a common scheme proposed by the ESC [1] and adopted by our team, consists of 3 to 6-month visits with ECG and complete blood tests (including NT-pro BNP and troponin), and yearly echocardiogram and 24-h Holter ECG.

The ESC document also suggests to consider every 6-months to perform a 6 min walking distance (6MWD) test and to complete a Kansas City Cardiomyopathy Questionnaire (KCCQ).

Summary

The care for patients with cardiac amyloidosis is evolving, and that evolution is reflected in our novel and simplified algorithm for the diagnosis and management of patients with CA.

Abbreviations for Figs. 1, 2, 3, 4 and 5

AL-CM	Amyloid monoclonal immunoglobulin light chain cardiomyopathy;
ATTR-CM	Amyloid transthyretin cardiomyopathy;
ATTRv-CM	Variant transthyretin amyloid cardiomyopathy;
ATTRwt-CM	Wild-type transthyretin amyloid cardiomyopathy;
BNP	B-type natriuretic peptide,
CMR	Cardiac magnetic resonance;
DPD	Diphosphono-1,2-propanodicarboxylic acid;
ECG	Electrocardiogram;
HMDP	Hydroxymethylene diphosphonate;
ICD	Implantable cardioverter defibrillator;
KCCQ	Kansas City Cardiomyopathy Questionnaire;

MRA	Mineralocorticoid receptor antagonists;
NT-pro BNP	N-terminal pro–B-type natriuretic peptide;
PPM	Permanent pacemaker;
PYP	Pyrophosphate;
SCD	Sudden cardiac death;
SGLT2i	Sodium glucose cotransporter 2 inhibitor;
SPECT	Single-photon emission computed tomography;
TAVR	Transaortic valve replacement;
TTE	Transthoracic echocardiography;
TTR	Transthyretin;
VT	Ventricular tachycardia

References

1. Garcia-Pavia P, Rapezzi C, Adler Y, Arad M, Basso C, Brucato A, Burazor I, Caforio ALP, Damy T, Eriksson U, Fontana M, Gillmore JD, Gonzalez-Lopez E, Grogan M, Heymans S, Imazio M, Kindermann I, Kristen AV, Maurer MS, Merlini G, Pantazis A, Pankuweit S, Rigopoulos AG, Linhart A. Diagnosis and treatment of cardiac amyloidosis: a position statement of the ESC working group on myocardial and pericardial diseases. Eur Heart J. 2021;42(16):1554–68. https://doi.org/10.1093/eurheartj/ehab072.
2. Kittleson MM, Ruberg FL, Ambardekar AV, Brannagan TH, Cheng RK, Clarke JO, Dember LM, Frantz JG, Hershberger RE, Maurer MS, Nativi-Nicolau J, Sanchorawala V, Sheikh FH. 2023 **ACC** expert consensus decision pathway on comprehensive multidisciplinary care for the patient with cardiac amyloidosis: a report of the American College of Cardiology solution set oversight committee. J Am Coll Cardiol. 2023;81(11):1076–126. https://doi.org/10.1016/j.jacc.2022.11.022. Epub 2023 Jan 23.
3. Heidenreich PA, Bozkurt B, Aguilar D, et al. 2022 AHA/ACC/HFSA guideline for the management of heart failure: a report of the American College of Cardiology/American Heart Association joint committee on clinical practice guidelines. J Am Coll Cardiol. 2022;79:e263–421.
4. Sperry BW, Hanna M, Shah SJ, et al. Spironolactone in patients with an echocardiographic HFpEF phenotype suggestive of cardiac amyloidosis: results from TOPCAT. J Am Coll Cardiol HF. 2021;9:795–802.
5. Anker SD, Butler J, Filippatos G, et al. Empagliflozin in heart failure with a preserved ejection fraction. N Engl J Med. 2021;385:1451–61.
6. Giancaterino S, Urey MA, Darden D, et al. Management of arrhythmias in cardiac amyloidosis. J Am Coll Cardiol EP. 2020;6:351–61.
7. Nitsche C, Scully PR, Patel KP, et al. Prevalence and outcomes of concomitant aortic stenosis and cardiac amyloidosis. J Am Coll Cardiol. 2021;77:128–39.
8. Maurer MS, Schwartz JH, Gundapaneni B, et al. Tafamidis treatment for patients with transthyretin amyloid cardiomyopathy. N Engl J Med. 2018;379:1007–16.
9. Gillmore JD, Judge DP, Cappelli F, Fontana M, Garcia-Pavia P, Gibbs S, Grogan M, Hanna M, Hoffman J, Masri A, Maurer MS, Nativi-Nicolau J, Obici L, Poulsen SH, Rockhold F, Shah KB, Soman P, Garg J, Chiswell K, Xu H, Cao X, Lystig T, Sinha U, Fox JC. ATTRibute-CM investigator. Efficacy and safety of acoramidis in transthyretin amyloid cardiomyopathy. N Engl J Med. 2024 Jan 11;390(2):132–42. https://doi.org/10.1056/NEJMoa2305434.
10. Adams D, Gonzalez-Duarte A, O'Riordan WD, et al. Patisiran, an RNAi therapeutic, for hereditary transthyretin amyloidosis. N Engl J Med. 2018;379:11–21.

11. Benson MD, Waddington-Cruz M, Berk JL, et al. Inotersen treatment for patients with hereditary transthyretin amyloidosis. N Engl J Med. 2018;379:22–31.
12. Fontana M, Berk JL, Gillmore JD, et al. Vutrisiran in Patients with Transthyretin Amyloidosis with Cardiomyopathy. N Engl J Med. 2024 Aug 30. NEJMoa2409134.

Cardiac Amyloidosis—History, Pathophysiology and Epidemiology

Yaron Hellman and Ido Livneh

Abstract Amyloidosis has a special place in the history of medicine, involving numerous physicians and researchers from multiple disciplines throughout the medical field due to its initial enigmatic nature and systemic involvement. Many developments occurred during the last 2 centuries, hand in hand with advancements in the understanding of protein synthesis and folding, metachromatic staining, polarized microscopy, amyloid extraction, electrophoresis, electron microscopy, and genomics. Amyloidosis is basically a disorder of protein misfolding, forming beta sheets which in turn compose protofilaments winding around each other to form the amyloid fibril. Amyloidosis occurs when amyloid fibrils form aggregates and deposit in various tissues, causing organ dysfunction. In some instances, the circulating amyloid precursor oligomers also exert a toxic effect. The current classification of amyloidosis is based upon the precursor misfolded proteins. The two most common forms that cause cardiac amyloidosis are AL and ATTR amyloidosis. AL amyloidosis occurs when excessive amyloidogenic light chains are produced by plasma cells. ATTR amyloidosis is the result of either mutant transthyretin misfolding (ATTRv) or wild type transthyretin (ATTRwt). Age related protein oxidative modifications and failure of proteostasis and repair mechanisms contribute to the dissociation and aggregation of normal TTR (wild type) into amyloid fibrils. Similar to light chains, the misfolded TTR monomers and dimers also have a toxic cardiac effect. Cardiac amyloid deposition results in myocardial diastolic and systolic dysfunction. Furthermore, amyloid also involves the cardiac valves, the conduction system, coronary arteries and even the pericardium. If untreated, patients develop heart failure and eventually cardiogenic shock and death due to the very limited stroke volume in advanced cardiac amyloidosis. Currently, diagnosis and therapy for both forms of amyloid have drastically improved due to a better understanding of light chain and ATTR pathogenesis. The non-biopsy diagnostic algorithm incorporating free light chain measurement and scintigraphy allowed for improved recognition of ATTR

Y. Hellman (✉)
Department of Cardiology, Rambam Health Care Campus, Haifa, Israel
e-mail: yaronhellman@gmail.com

I. Livneh
Institute of Pathology and Cytology, Rambam Health Care Campus, Haifa, Israel

E. Herzog (ed.), *Cardiac Amyloidosis*, https://doi.org/10.1007/978-3-031-88342-2_2

amyloidosis in the elderly and heart failure population. Endomyocardial biopsy and genetic testing are warranted in order to diagnose the less frequent forms of amyloidosis (AA in inflammation, Abeta-2 microglobulin in long term dialysis, and the rare ApoA-I, ApoA-II, ApoA-IV, and Agel amyloidosis).

Keywords Cardiac Amyloidosis · Amyloidosis history · Congo Red · Amyloid formation · Amyloid cardiotoxicity · AL amyloidosis · Transthyretin amyloidosis · AA amyloidosis · Dialysis related amyloidosis

Definition

Amyloidosis is a group of disorders due to abnormal protein conformation and metabolism resulting in the extracellular deposition of fibrillar material (the "amyloid fibril") [1].

In cardiac amyloidosis, organ dysfunction occurs following disruption of tissue structure by the amyloid deposits as well as direct cytotoxic effects from the protein aggregates or precursors. This leads to progressive heart failure and eventual death [2].

In this chapter, we will discuss amyloid history, cardiac amyloidosis pathophysiology, pathology and epidemiology.

History

Patients with amyloidosis were probably described as early as 1639, with the description of an autopsy of a young man with ascites, jaundice and epistaxis who had an abscess in the liver and a large spleen filled with white stones. This case was reported by Nicolaus Fontanus along with another patient described by Bartholin in an extensive pathology book by Theophili Boneti (Sepulchretum sive Anatomia Practica) published in 1679 [3].

During the late 1700s and early 1800s, several reports of enlarged livers with grey, gelatinous and "lardaceous" substance were published. George Budd (known more for his work with Hans Chiari—"Budd-Chiari syndrome") concluded that the infiltrating substance was albuminous and not fatty. He also noted kidney involvement with the same infiltrating substance.

The origin of the term amyloid is the Latin word for starch—amylum (in Greek—amylon). Matthias Schleiden and Julius Vogel, German botanists, invented this term in 1838 when they studied a "starch-like" plant material. The plant constituent could acquire the known property of starch, turning blue with the addition of iodine, only after the addition of sulfuric acid [4, 5]. This material was later recognized as cellulose. In humans, "amyloid" was first used by Rudolf Virchow in 1854 when he described small round deposits in the brain—"corpora amylacea". These structures stained with pale blue after the application of iodine, and then turned violet with subsequent sulfuric acid treatment [4]. This reaction led Virchow to believe that the substance within the deposits resembles cellulose and has a "starch-like" component.

Later, Virchow applied the iodine sulfuric acid test to other tissues infiltrated with amyloid. The French and British schools preferred the names "lardaceous" (bacon like appearance—French school) and "waxy" (homogenous material—British school). Another common term referring to the previously described spleens was "sago spleens" (a nodular appearance similar to sago starch grains) [6].

In 1859, prominent German chemist August Kekulé reported a high proportion of nitrogen in organs infiltrated with amyloid—assuming "amyloid" actually represented "albumoid" compounds (similar to Budd's observation). Virchow never agreed with Kekulé, criticizing his methods of analyzing tissue at the time [6]. In contrast to Virchow, Kekulé's observation on high nitrogen contents of amyloid were accepted by several scientists, including Samuel Wilks, a renowned British physician. Wilks published many cases of "lardaceous disease"—including a patient with heart failure and nephrotic syndrome [7]. In addition to contributing to the study of amyloidosis, Samuel Wilks was the first to use the eponym Hodgkin's disease (which echoes till this day as Hodgkin's and non-Hodgkin's lymphoma), as well as describe inflammatory bowel disease (70 years before Crohn) and systemic embolism associated with endocarditis. He was an integral part of a committee appointed by the Royal Society of London, which determined that the term "lardaceous disease" should be accepted, despite high nitrogen content and albumin like origin [8]. It is not clear why the term amyloidosis prevailed, but this is probably related to Virchow's standing as a pathologist ("father of modern pathology") and to the common use of the iodine stain at the time [7].

Interestingly, the corpora amylacea initially identified by Virchow are indeed composed of carbohydrate. Currently, corpora amylacea (present in the CNS, prostate, lungs and other organs) are considered "waste containers". These waste containers, actively created by specific cells, sequester or retain waste products or foreign products, and are then secreted into the external medium or interstitial spaces. Their composition is mostly carbohydrate, although sometimes protein is a major constituent, occasionally even staining with Congo red. In order to avoid ambiguity with amyloid, corpora amylacea were proposed to be renamed wasteosomes [8].

The discovery and use of metachromatic stains (including methyl violet) improved the detection and localization of amyloid in various tissues. When applying these stains, the original color of the dye changes to another color after binding to certain tissues, thus increasing contrast. The first description of amyloid in the cardiac tissue is reportedly the one by Soyka in 1876 who used this new method. Metachromatic stains challenged Virchow's iodine sulfuric acid test for decades, but eventually were replaced by Congo red [1, 7].

Congo Red

In 1884, the Congo red dye was developed by Paul Bottiger, during his attempts to synthesize a pH indicator. He sold his patent to the AGFA dye company, which marketed the dye as "Congo red". The origin of the name was in fact an advertising strategy—marketing truly existed throughout human history. The dye is synthetic, not dependent on a specific geographical location. The term African Congo, was an exotic "hot topic" during the Berlin West Africa conference held at the time, and therefore incorporated into the dye's name [9].

Amyloid staining with Congo Red was discovered by the German physician Hans Hermann Bennhold (1893–1976). He was investigating Congo red as a clinical test involving blood volume and as a possible indicator of liver function. He measured serial blood concentrations after injecting the dye solution into patients. An autopsy on a patient who died 20 h after the injection demonstrated red areas in frozen sections of the liver, spleen and kidneys. These sections correlated with amyloid deposition stained by methyl violet (the conventional amyloid staining at the time). He then found that Congo red blood clearance was more rapid in patients with amyloidosis. Bennhold's intravenous Congo red test became a standard clinical investigation for amyloidosis until the late 1960s [5].

The use of Congo red as a histological staining method increased following a report in 1927 of Paul Divry, a Belgian psychiatrist studying degenerative changes in aging brains. He and his student, Marcel Florkin (who became a prominent biochemist) first noted the birefringence of amyloid viewed under polarized light. However, they did not mention the exact colors observed with the Congo red staining and polarized light. In 1945, a German pathologist working in Istanbul, Paul Ladewig, reported that Congo red-stained amyloid changed twice from yellow to green during 360° rotation of a slide. A few years later, the physician Hans-Peter Missmahl, who worked with Bennhold, published reports describing mainly green polarization. After this was referenced in major English language publications in the 1960s and 1970s, the term "apple-green" birefringence was popularized [5]. Interestingly, in 160 scientific papers on staining of amyloids in tissue sections with Congo red, only 31% of the illustrations showed a pure green color [10]. In fact, combinations of yellow and even blue colors are seen in practice more often than a pure green color (Fig. 1). Nevertheless, Congo red staining ("Congophillia") was established as a strong amyloid criterion.

Further Characterization of Amyloid as a Protein

In 1959 Cohen and Calkines examined a variety of amyloid specimens with electron microscopy. These included sections from a rabbit with Casein induced amyloidosis (now known as AA), and patients with "Primary amyloidosis" (a mixture of AL and possible TTR) and "visceral amyloidosis" (also AA). In all of these sections,

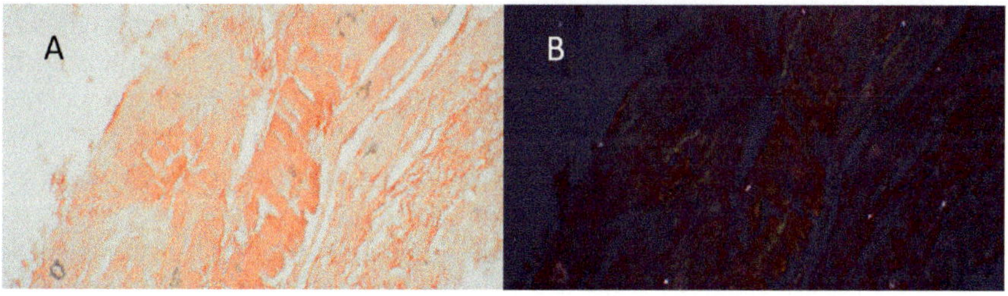

Fig. 1 Congo red staining of myocardium with ATTR cardiac amyloidosis. **a** Light microscopy. **b** Polarized light microscopy. Image courtesy of Dr. Ido Livneh, Department of Pathology, Rambam Health Care Campus. Used with permission

a similar fibrillar submicroscopic structure was present: bundles of straight, rigid fibrils ranging in width (average 75 to 100 Å) and in length (1000 to 16,000 Å). This fibrillar morphology was adopted as the second criterion by which amyloid was defined [4].

A decade later, X-ray diffraction was applied to the study of amyloid submicroscopic structure. These pivotal reports first described the generic beta pleated sheet protein conformation and defined the general structure of amyloid [3, 11] (Fig. 2).

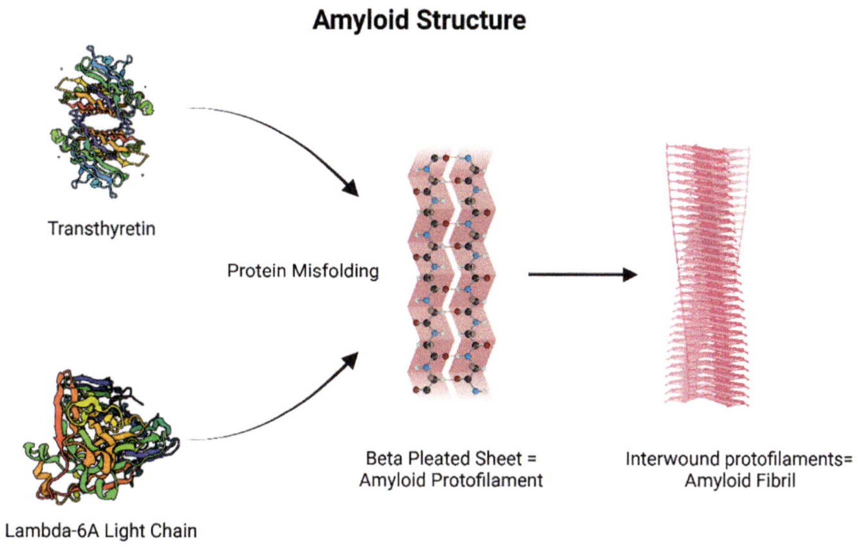

Fig. 2 Amyloid structure. Transthyretin (Protein Data Bank code 4TLT) and Lambda-6A light chain (Protein Data Bank code 6MG4), which are examples of amyloidogenic precursor proteins, can misfold into the beta sheet secondary structure forming a protofilament. The interwinding of several protofilaments form an amyloid fibril. Created in BioRender. Hellman, Y. (2025) https://BioRender.com/l66q372

A major breakthrough was the Pras water extraction method, which allowed extraction of homogenates from amyloid laden tissue, followed by separation of the amyloid fibrils by suspension in water. These protein fibrils exhibited congophillia and "green" birefringence [12]. Once the amyloid protein was isolated, the amino acid sequence could be determined. This was the beginning of the biochemical era of amyloid studies.

At the second International Symposium on Amyloidosis, held in Helsinki, Finland in 1974, the chemical nature of the first two amyloid fibril proteins were identified and it was at this symposium the foundation of modern amyloid fibril classification was established [11].

The current classification includes 42 amyloid fibril proteins (Table 1) [13].

Current Amyloid Nomenclature

The structural proteins in or derived from amyloid fibrils are named after their precursors in abbreviated form preceded by the letter A for amyloid. Therefore, immunoglobulin light chain amyloid protein is named AL and transthyretin amyloid protein ATTR (Table 1). The protein can be specified further, e.g. ATTRv for variant, ATTRV30M for a specific mutation or ATTRwt for the wild-type form. The Nomenclature Committee recommends the use of mature proteins in numbering of amino acid residues, i.e. without leader sequences. Numbering of the full precursor may be included as well but then in parenthesis after the mature protein, e.g. TTRV30M (p. TTRV50M). In addition, the nomenclature committee emphasized that the abbreviations are for the proteins, not the diseases. For the latter, the protein name followed by 'amyloidosis' should be used (e.g. ATTR amyloidosis or AL amyloidosis). Clinically useful specifications may be allowed, such as ATTR cardiomyopathy or AL neuropathy. For the sake of uniformity, it was recommended that the variant state should be stated after the name, such as ATTRwt, or ATTRv.

In ATTR, it is preferred that v should be used for variant, not m (mutant) or h (hereditary), the latter since it may be mistaken for 'human'. However, hATTR term remains in the literature and in certain legal situations where the hereditary term is necessary [13].

Overview of Protein Folding

The basic underlying mechanism of amyloid formation is the misfolding of proteins followed by aggregation and formation of fibrils.

Protein folding is a tightly regulated process since a correct three-dimensional conformation of the protein or peptide is necessary for proper physiological function.

Table 1 Amyloid fibril proteins and precursors in humans

Fibril protein	Precursor protein	Target organs
AL	Immunoglobulin light chain	All organs, usually except CNS
AH	Immunoglobulin heavy chain	All organs except CNS
AA	(Apo) Serum amyloid A	All organs except CNS
ATTR	Transthyretin, wild type	Heart mainly in males, PNS, ligaments, tenosynovium
ATTR	Transthyretin, variants	PNS, ANS, heart, eye, kidneys, leptomeninges
Aβ2M	β2-microglobulin, wild type	Musculoskeletal system
Aβ2M	β2-microglobulin, variants	ANS, tongue, heart
AApoAI	Apolipoprotein A I, variants	Heart, liver, kidney, PNS, testis, larynx, skin
AApoAII	Apolipoprotein A II, variants	Kidney
AApoAIV	Apolipoprotein A IV, wild type	Kidney medulla and systemic
AApoCII	Apolipoprotein C II, variants	Kidney
AApoCI	Apolipoprotein C I, variants	Kidney
AGel	Gelsolin, variants	Kidney
Alys	Lysozyme, variants	Kidney
ALEC2	Leukocyte chemotactic factor-2	Kidney, primarily
AFib	Fibrinogen A, variants	Kidney, primarily
AGys	Cystatin C, variants	PNS, skin
ABri	ABriPP, variants	CNS
ADan	ADanPP, variants	CNS
Aβ	Aβ protein precursor, wild type	CNS
Aβ	Aβ protein precursor, variant	CNS
AαSyn	α-Synuclein	CNS
ATau	Tau	CNS
APRPrP	Prion protein, wild type	CJD, fatal insomnia
APRPrP	Prion protein variants	CJD, GSS syndrome, fatal insomnia
APRPrP	Prion protein variant	PNS
ATMEM106B	Transmembrane 106B (TMEM106B)	Frontotemporal lobar degeneration diseases
ACal	Procalcitonin	C-cell thyroid tumors
AIAPP	Islet amyloid polypeptide	Islets of Langerhans, insulinomas
AANP	Atrial natriuretic peptide	Cardiac atria
APro	Prolactin	Pituitary prolactinomas, aging pituitary
ASom	Prosomatostatin	Somatostatinomas

(continued)

Table 1 (continued)

Fibril protein	Precursor protein	Target organs
AGluc	Glucagon	Glucagonomas
APTH	Parathyroid hormone	Parathyroid tumors, aging parathyroid glands
AIns	Insulin	Iatrogenic, local injection
AEnf	Enfurvitide	Iatrogenic, local injection
AGLP1	Glucagon-like peptide 1 analog	Iatrogenic, local injection
AIL1RAP	Interleukin-1 receptor antagonist protein	Iatrogenic, local injection
ASPC	Lung surfactant protein	Lung
ACor	Corneodesmosin	Cornified epithelia, hair follicles
AMed	Lactadherin (MFG-E8)	Aging aorta, media, elastic arteries
AKer	Kerato-epithelin	Cornea, hereditary

Adapted from Buxbaum et al. [13]

In general, polypeptide chains are synthesized in the ribosomes and endoplasmic reticulum of the cell followed by a rapid sequence of intracellular folding and conformational modifications [14]. This requires the use of multiple chaperones and catalysts in order to achieve the appropriate native structure. A molecular chaperone is defined as any protein that interacts with, stabilizes or helps another protein to acquire its functionally active conformation, without being present in its final structure [15]. Evolution and natural selection allowed for the optimal amino acid sequence yielding only a small number of conformations to be sampled for the most thermodynamically stable structure. According to this "folding energy landscape theory," the process follows a funnel-like pathway, and the conformational intermediates progressively merge into a final species. Some polypeptides can acquire a relatively stable "misfolded state" at a minimum of energy similar to the native protein [16]. Chaperones increase the efficiency of the folding process (often requiring energy/ATP) by reducing the probability of competing reactions. In addition to protection from misfolding, some molecular chaperones can rescue misfolded and even aggregated proteins, allowing for a second chance to fold correctly. The remaining misfolded proteins are normally retained by the endoplasmic reticulum, dislocated to the cytoplasm, and degraded by the proteasome [17].

Amyloid Formation

Partial unfolding of the native state of the protein is a pre-requisite for amyloid formation. The dynamic balance favoring folded proteins versus misfolded proteins can be disrupted in several ways, resulting in the amyloidogenic precursor proteins. A single amino acid replacement and conformational change is the mechanism in the hereditary amyloidosis—ATTRv—mutations in the transthyretin gene. Some proteins have an intrinsic tendency towards pathological conformations when proteostasis (a general term for the whole process of protein regulation) is impaired with aging (normal transthyretin in senile amyloidosis—ATTRwt). Another mechanism is persistently high concentrations of the misfolded protein in the serum (beta-2 microglobulin in dialysis patients). In addition to the amyloidogenic potential of the precursor protein, other factors play a role in amyloid deposition. The protein must reach a critical concentration in order to achieve fibril formation. This process is enhanced by local environmental factors and interaction with the extracellular matrix, including: glycosaminoglycans and collagen, shear forces, endoproteases, and metals that modulate aggregation and oligomer formation [16].

Amyloid Structure

The misfolded amyloid precursor proteins converge into a cross-beta super-secondary structure—the beta pleated sheet that has been well characterized by x-ray diffraction. The original conformation of the precursor protein can no longer be distinguished at this stage. These contiguous beta sheet polypeptide chains constitute a protofilament. Several (1–4 or more) protofilaments are wound around one another to form an amyloid fibril, with a distinct diameter of 7.5 to 10 nm visible on transmission electron microscopy. Protofilaments are bound to each other in a parallel fashion via their sidechains. This ultrastructure of the fibril allows the regular intercalation of Congo red dye—providing the characteristic staining and green birefringence under polarized light, a diagnostic property of amyloid (Fig. 2). The amyloid fibrils are the basic structure of amyloid [13, 16].

Amyloid Signature Proteins

In addition to the amyloid fibril, amyloid deposits include components of the extracellular matrix, such as lamin, entactin, collagen, and additional proteins (e.g. apolipoproteins) [14]. Notably, amyloid deposits also contain Serum Amyloid P-component (SAP), a glycoprotein that belongs to the pentraxin family and binds amyloid independently of the protein of origin. It undergoes reversible calcium-dependent binding and comprises up to 15% of the mass of amyloid deposits. SAP is highly protected against proteolysis and thus provides the amyloid fibrils with resistance to degradation [18]. Proteoglycans are also common in amyloid deposits and contribute extensively to the carbohydrate composition of natural amyloid. Specifically, Heparan sulfate proteoglycans (HSPG) localize with previously mentioned components of the extracellular matrix (lamin, collagen) facilitating adhesion and orientation of the first nuclei of aggregated amyloid. Despite being a common component of all amyloid deposits, proteoglycans show a degree of chemical and structural heterogeneity and may play a role in the localization of amyloid deposits in tissues. These proteins (SAP, HSPG, apolipoproteins) are designated as "amyloid signature proteins"—used as additional proof of amyloid when performing mass spectrometry analysis of tissue samples [13, 16].

Amyloid Deposition

Amyloid deposition (and aggregation) in target organs is a complex process [14]. Classic kinetic models are based on the concept of nucleation dependent polymerization. Initially, conditions do not favor aggregation, and this period corresponds to a "lag phase" consisting of amyloid protein monomers and oligomers preceding amyloid fibril formation. The duration of each phase of fibril formation is protein-specific and defines the rate at which amyloid deposition occurs (Fig. 3). Once a nucleus has been generated, the conditions change to favor aggregation with monomers contacting the growing polymer at multiple sites. Additional "seeds" can continue to capture and catalyze the conversion of precursors into misfolded aggregates of amyloid even at low concentrations [19]. Currently, some studies suggest additional processes occur in a parallel fashion—including fragmentation and elongation of fibrils, as well as secondary nucleation (nuclei catalyzed by existing fibril surfaces). Finally, previously discussed protein chaperones (controlling proper protein folding) play a significant role in suppressing amyloid fibril formation during phases of nucleation and elongation [20].

Tissue Specificity

Overall, the organ distribution of amyloid is quite diverse, with the target organs depending on the specific amyloid precursor protein (another advantage of the current amyloid classification scheme). Beta-2 microglobulin aggregation occurs mainly in joints. AL amyloidosis can involve virtually any organ except the central nervous system. This also may vary according to the specific pathological light chain produced. In ATTR amyloidosis the organs involved are mainly the peripheral nervous system and cardiac tissue, also varying according to the misfolded protein amino acid sequence. Lastly, amyloid deposition in specific tissues depends on the convergence of several factors including high local protein concentrations, low pH, and the presence of fibril seeds [16].

Amyloidosis is defined as a disease caused by amyloid fibrils or during the process of their formation [11]. The organs affected establish the prognosis. Even when amyloidosis already involves the cardiovascular system, disease progression over time and its severity depends on the type of amyloid fibril.

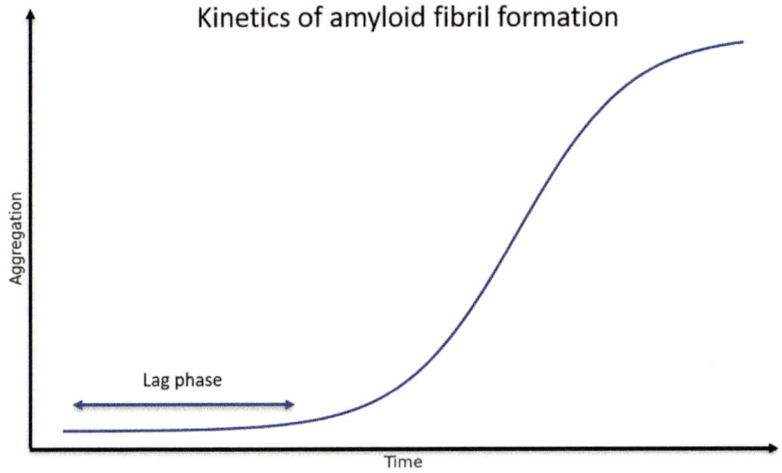

Fig. 3 Kinetics of amyloid fibril formation. This graph depicts amyloid fibril formation with nucleation dependent polymerization. Initially, conditions are unfavorable for aggregation—this corresponds to a "lag phase", with circulating monomers and oligomers. Once nuclei are established, aggregation occurs exponentially at multiple sites. Additional "seeds" and existing amyloid catalyze this process

Cardiac Pathophysiology in General

Cardiac involvement in amyloidosis includes the myocardium (ventricles and atria), as well as the pericardium, endocardium, valves, conduction system, vasculature and the autonomic nervous system.

Myocardial Involvement

Ventricular dysfunction is typically thought to occur as a result of extracellular amyloid deposition in the myocardium and distortion of the normal architecture. This ultimately results in cellular injury, tissue damage, and finally organ dysfunction. Once large deposits of amyloid are present, biventricular thickening occurs with reduced compliance and a restrictive physiology—high ventricular filling pressures are required to maintain an adequate stroke volume. At first, the clinical presentation is apparently isolated diastolic dysfunction. As the amyloid deposition process progresses, stroke volume is relatively low, leading to severe heart failure with the worst hemodynamic phenotype—"cold and wet". In addition, both the loss of atrial contractility and development of right ventricular dysfunction decrease preload and cardiac output even further [14].

Left and right ventricular systolic dysfunction occur as well. Initially, this may be evident only in longitudinal strain, preceding the decrease in ejection fraction.

Recent studies have suggested that RV dysfunction is not necessarily a consequence of left heart failure, and may represent direct involvement with amyloid toxicity and/or infiltration. Right ventricular dysfunction can occur even before left sided involvement. Therefore, right ventricular dysfunction (assessed by RVEF, strain) is an important marker of prognosis and occasionally enable an earlier diagnosis of cardiac involvement [21].

In the past, myocardial dysfunction was attributed mainly to amyloid fibril deposition. During the last 2 decades, the importance of direct small monomer and oligomer toxicity has been recognized. Circulating free light chains are probably responsible for the more aggressive trajectory of AL amyloidosis when compared to ATTR amyloidosis. The light chains increase cardiomyocyte reactive oxygen species leading to increased oxidative stress and apoptosis. The oxidative stress can impair calcium handling as well, thus directly inhibiting cardiomyocyte contraction and relaxation. These pathways lead to increased BNP transcription. The role of light chain toxicity is demonstrated by current chemotherapy effectively reducing circulating free light chains and translating into reduced BNP levels, despite unaltered amyloid deposition in the myocardium. In TTR amyloidosis, tissue dysfunction also precedes TTR fibril deposition, suggesting TTR monomer and oligomer toxicity. This may be due to interactions with membrane proteins and cholesterol [14].

In a study examining endomyocardial biopsies and autopsies of patients with AL amyloidosis, expression of Atrial Natriuretic Peptide (ANP) and B type Natriuretic Peptide (BNP) and their genes was augmented in the ventricular myocytes. Interestingly, the myocytes neighboring amyloid deposits tended to show more intense staining for natriuretic peptides. Therefore, both regional mechanical stress by amyloid deposits and hemodynamic stress by diastolic dysfunction (in addition to the direct toxic effect of light chains) may be responsible for the markedly increased expression of the natriuretic peptides in patients with cardiac amyloidosis [22].

Atrial Dysfunction

Similar to RV dysfunction, atrial dysfunction is not only a result of left ventricular failure. Amyloid directly accumulates in the atria. This has been demonstrated in several pathological studies demonstrating ATTR amyloid, AL amyloid and isolated atrial amyloidosis—ANP amyloid. Atrial amyloidosis has 3 main effects—hemodynamic, atrial arrhythmia, and thrombogenic risk. The loss of "atrial kick" reduces diastolic filling and preload, as previously mentioned. In addition, a "stiff left atrium" contributes to elevated pulmonary venous pressure resulting in pulmonary congestion [23]. The substrate for atrial fibrillation and arrhythmia is formed once amyloid fibrils accumulate between the atrial cardiomyocytes and disrupt electrical conduction. Finally, the "electromechanical dissociation" or "atrial standstill" in amyloidosis is one of the rare causes of LA thrombus during sinus rhythm, as well as thrombi in locations within the atria that are not the left atrial appendage [24].

Conduction System

Multiple mechanisms are responsible for arrhythmia and conduction system disease in cardiac amyloidosis. Amyloid deposition within the conduction system and the destruction of normal tissue architecture disrupts electrical transmission. As previously mentioned, both light chains and TTR oligomers exhibit direct cytotoxicity through oxidative stress, inflammation and additional mechanisms. This results in fibrosis, a substrate for arrhythmogenic potential. Direct fibril and oligomer cytotoxicity also cause dysregulation of intracellular calcium signaling with action potential prolongation. Lastly, several non-myocardial factors may contribute to arrhythmogenesis, including: neurotoxicity with cardiac sympathetic denervation, autonomic failure and coronary micro-vascular ischemia [25, 26].

Sinus node dysfunction occurs in cardiac amyloidosis with a prevalence of 7% in one small study. However, AV conduction disease is much more common, ranging from first degree AV block to advanced AV block requiring a pacemaker. Conduction disease progresses over time, demonstrated in several studies including patients with increased pacemaker dependance and pacing during follow up. Pacemakers are more common in ATTR amyloid than AL, although this may be confounded by advanced age [25].

Ventricular Arrhythmia

The most common ventricular arrythmia in cardiac amyloidosis is ventricular tachycardia. In some cases, the presentation is sudden cardiac death due to deterioration into VF. Despite severe amyloid infiltration is ATTR, AL amyloidosis is associated with higher rates of SCD (~33% of patients) in the first 3 months of diagnosis [8]. One explanation offered is the more heterogenous spread of conduction and repolarization differences. Chemotherapy and dexamethasone are also associated with ventricular arrhythmias in AL amyloidosis, with the underlying mechanism not entirely understood (possible cardiotoxicity and fluid retention). Sudden cardiac death can also be due to AV block and bradycardia, as well as PEA or asystole secondary to myocardial dysfunction and electromechanical dissociation. In fact, these are considered a more common cause of sudden cardiac death than ventricular arrhythmia in cardiac amyloidosis [25, 26].

Sinus Tachycardia

Due to the low end-diastolic volume and the reduced stroke volume, patients with amyloidosis present a higher heart rate in order to compensate for their low cardiac output. Since this is a compensatory mechanism, at least initially, treatment with beta blockers (and other agents) may result in hemodynamic compromise, cardiogenic shock and even death. Poor tolerance to beta blockers may persist even after medical stabilization.

Valvular Involvement

In the past, valvular thickening and infiltration has been described in amyloidosis based on case reports and series of autopsies and explanted valves. In an autopsy case series of hereditary ATTR amyloidosis with polyneuropathy, all 12 patients had valvular amyloid deposits—with a majority classified as moderate to abundant [27]. Valvular thickening was also demonstrated in a large cohort of AL amyloidosis patients during their diagnostic transthoracic echocardiogram. The prevalence of left heart valve thickening approached 50% and predicted a worse prognosis [28].

In the current era of TAVI and non-invasive diagnosis of TTR senile amyloidosis by nuclear studies, it is estimated that up to 15% of patients with AS and up to 30% of those with low-flow low-gradient AS have CA. The association between ATTR cardiac amyloidosis and aortic stenosis has several possible explanations. First, wild type TTR amyloidosis and calcific aortic stenosis occur in the same age group. Second, increased shear stress in aortic stenosis may promote plasminogen activation to plasmin which in turn cleaves the TTR tetramer into a more amyloidogenic precursor. The relationship between amyloid and calcification is bidirectional—oxidation and calcification cause valvular amyloid deposition, and amyloid deposition leads to inflammation and calcification. In contrast to ATTR amyloidosis, AL amyloidosis is not as closely associated with aortic valve stenosis, probably due to the more aggressive course and different age group affected [29].

Mitral valvular involvement consists of amyloid deposition and distortion of its components—leaflets, chorda and annulus. In addition to leaflet thickening and retraction, mitral annulus geometry is altered, the commissures are stretched, and chordae tendinae are thickened and shortened. This results in mitral valve regurgitation, which is particularly challenging for the non-compliant left atrium [29].

The morphology of the tricuspid valve leaflets is usually altered in TTR amyloidosis. However, similar to HFpEF patients, the tricuspid valve regurgitation in cardiac amyloidosis is often due to annular dilatation (atrial fibrillation) and RV dysfunction and dilation. Tricuspid regurgitation has an impact on ATTRwt cardiac amyloidosis rather than AL amyloidosis, again due to the different age group and more aggressive trajectory of AL [29].

Pericardial Involvement

A pericardial effusion can be present in up to 30% of amyloidosis patients. Although not as common, the occurrence of pericardial tamponade and constriction have also been described. The pathophysiology of pericardial effusion in amyloidosis is multifactorial. An increase in right ventricular filling pressures followed by increased venous and capillary hydrostatic pressure causes fluid transudation across the pericardium, similar to pleural effusions. In addition, renal failure with fluid retention as well as hypoalbuminemia (nephrotic syndrome, malnutrition) contribute to the imbalance of hydrostatic pressure versus oncotic pressure. Non-Starling mechanisms include direct amyloid infiltration and cytotoxic effects contributing to inflammation and increased capillary permeability [30]. Finally, amyloidosis associated bleeding diathesis contributes to hemorrhagic pericardial effusions. This tendency towards bleeding (e.g. the infamous periorbital "amyloid purpura") is explained by vascular fragility secondary to amyloid deposition and an acquired hemostatic impairment associated with light chains (in AL amyloidosis) [31]. Pericardial effusion is associated with a worse prognosis independently of other prognostic factors [30].

Coronary Arteries

Coronary vascular involvement in amyloidosis involves mainly intramyocardial arteries, veins, and capillaries. Amyloid deposition also occurs in the vasa vasorum of the epicardial coronary arteries. The microvascular amyloid infiltration and obstruction may explain angina and troponin elevation with patent epicardial arteries in patients with amyloidosis. Vascular involvement is far more frequent in AL amyloidosis compared to ATTR, acting as a relevant prognostic factor as well [1]. Coronary small vessel involvement has also been well described in Aβ2M cardiac amyloidosis [32].

Autonomic Nervous System

Autonomic neuropathy is common, and has been reported both in AL amyloidosis and ATTR amyloidosis (ATTRV and ATTRwt) [33]. Cardiovascular consequences include orthostatic hypotension, decreased heart rate variability, systemic hypotension and increased flow mediated vasodilation. The strong tendency towards hypotension usually limits the use of standard systolic heart failure medications (vasodilators), while some patients may even require vasoconstrictor therapy, such as midodrine.

Vasodilation

In an attempt to understand vasodilation in AL amyloidosis, a comprehensive study of flow mediated vasodilation was undertaken. When compared to controls, AL amyloidosis patients demonstrated increased flow mediated vasodilation along with increased exhaled NO and plasma cGMP levels. These findings suggest a mechanism of autonomic dysfunction and sympathetic denervation (rather than endothelial dysfunction). In fact increased flow mediated vasodilation in AL amyloidosis was associated with a worse prognosis [34]. Another possible mechanism of inappropriate vasodilation may be the markedly increased natriuretic peptide production in cardiac amyloidosis (which are potent vasodilators).

Cardiac Amyloidosis Epidemiology and Amyloid Subtype Specific Pathophysiology

Cardiac amyloidosis is limited to only a few amyloid precursor proteins. AL and ATTR amyloidosis are the most common causes of cardiac amyloidosis. Less frequently, AA amyloidosis and Aβ2M amyloidosis may manifest with clinical cardiac involvement. Rarer forms, such as apolipoprotein A-I, apolipoprotein A-II, apolipoprotein A-IV, gelsolin and lysozyme have also been described. Isolated atrial amyloidosis is limited to the atria with the precursor protein ANP [35]. The epidemiology of cardiac amyloidosis reflects the prevalence and incidence of these diseases.

AL Amyloidosis

Historical Background

The first case of multiple myeloma was probably reported in the year 1844, describing a 39 years old woman with fatigue and bone pain associated with multiple fractures. The patient died four years after her initial presentation, and autopsy findings included marrow replacement by aberrant cells [3].

A particularly well-known case was that of the patient Thomas McBean, who also suffered from fatigue and bone pain—sternal pain, as well as peripheral edema. He was referred by his primary care physician to Dr. William MacIntyre for consultation. Due to the possible diagnosis of "nephrosis" (nephrotic syndrome), Dr. MacIntyre attempted to isolate albumin from the urine. This was done at the time by heating the urine just below boiling point and observing precipitation. Addition of Nitric acid also precipitated albumin. In this case, the urine had a delayed precipitation, which redissolved after reheating (unlike albumin). Dr. Thomas Watson, the patient's primary care physician, also examined the urine and noted the same phenomenon. Both physicians sent urine samples to Dr. Henry Bence Jones, the chemical pathologist at St. George's hospital in London. Apparently, sending duplicate tests of the same patient to the lab occurred also in the nineteenth century. Bence Jones analyzed the urine and determined that the protein was different from albumin—he erroneously assumed that the protein was oxidized albumin ("deutoxide of albumin") [36]. His findings of this specific proteinuria were reported in 1848 [37].

The first report of myeloma associated with amyloidosis was by H. Weber, in 1867. He reported an autopsy of a patient with non-traumatic fractures of the sternum filled with a greyish red substance containing many small nucleated cells, along with a hypertrophied heart and amyloid in both the kidneys and spleen [7].

Only in 1900 James Homer Wright identified these malignant cells of multiple myeloma as plasma cells (the same Wright mainly known for "Wright's stain" and "Homer Wright pseudo-rosettes of neuroblastoma") [38].

Magnus-Levy was the first to describe the Bence Jones protein excreted in the urine of myeloma patients as "the mother substance" of amyloidosis. By the mid-twentieth century, it was evident that one form of amyloidosis was the consequence of a clonal plasma cell disorder [7].

In 1962, Edelman and Gally proved that serum monoclonal light chains ("L chains") from a patient with IgG myeloma shared the same amino acid composition and electrophoretic properties as the patient's Bence Jones protein, establishing that Bence Jones protein is derived from the clonal paraprotein ("myeloma protein") [39]. Gerald Edelman was eventually awarded the Nobel prize along with Rodney Porter for their groundbreaking work on the chemical structure of antibodies.

In 1971, Glenner and colleagues demonstrated in vitro that monoclonal immunoglobulin light chains from myeloma patients could form amyloid fibrils under experimental conditions [40]. This finalized the link between multiple myeloma, light chains, Bence Jones protein and amyloidosis.

AL Amyloidosis Specific Pathophysiology

AL amyloidosis is a disease where monoclonal Free Light Chains (FLCs) produced by abnormal plasma cells in the bone marrow form amyloid fibrils that are deposited in tissues. Human Ig is a heterotetrameric glycoprotein composed of two heavy chains (HCs) and two light chains (LCs). Each single LC is composed of two domains: a variable domain (VL) involved in antigen binding and a constant domain (CL) (Fig. 4). Light chains belong to either the Lambda (λ) or Kappa (κ) family and exhibit great diversity due to the random recombination of multiple gene segments. This is necessary for their role as antibodies against a wide range of antigens [41].

Amyloid fibril formation is the result of both excess light chains (quantitative abnormalities) as well as destabilization of the native light chain structure (qualitative abnormalities). Although plasma cell clone proliferation is required for the production of amyloidogenic light chains, amyloidogenic plasma cell clones are not

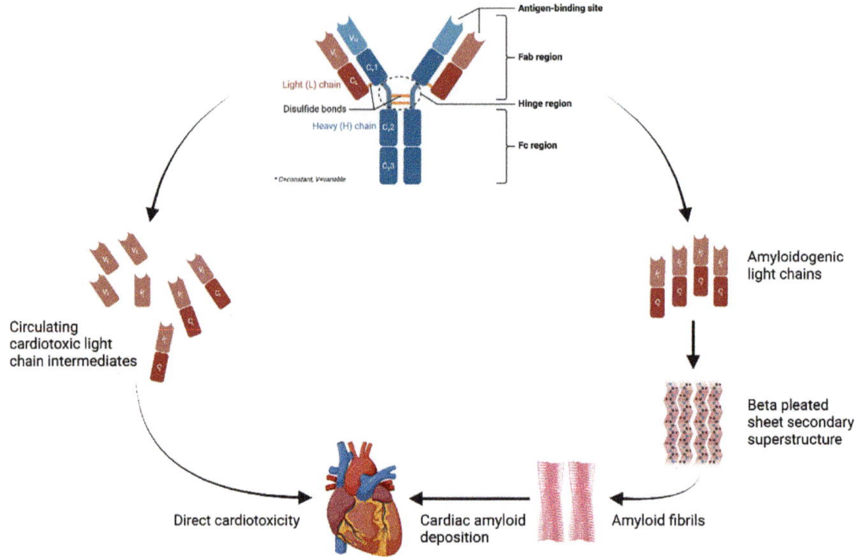

Fig. 4 Cardiac AL amyloidosis light chain toxicity and amyloid deposition. Created in BioRender. Hellman, Y. (2025) https://BioRender.com/t87g488

necessarily abundant in the bone marrow of AL patients. Overproduction of light chains can occur with less cells [41]. This is the reason that not all AL amyloidosis patients satisfy the 10% plasma cell requirement for myeloma.

In addition, not all light chains are equally amyloidogenic. AL amyloidosis is typically associated with lambda immunoglobulin light chains in 75 to 80% of cases and kappa light chains in the remaining 20 to 25%. AH amyloidosis (immunoglobulin heavy chains) and AH/AL amyloidosis (immunoglobulin heavy and light chains) are much less common. The chromosomal translocation t(11;14), which brings together the immunoglobulin heavy-chain locus (IgH) and the oncogene cyclin D1, is characteristic of AL amyloidosis, occurring in approximately 50% of cases [2]. Fortunately, this translocation is actually a marker of possible response to Venetoclax, an oral, small-molecule B cell lymphoma 2 (BCL-2) inhibitor that induces cellular apoptosis [42].

The overrepresentation of the Lambda light chains suggests that there is a gene sequence closely related to amyloid formation in this region. Indeed, some germline genes are expressed in a limited manner in AL, including the IGVL6-57 (Vλ6a), IGVL3-01 (Vλ3r), and IGVL2-14 segments of the Lambda chain variable region. This may also determine tissue specificity of the amyloid deposition. LC with the VL region derived from the rearrangement of the Vλ6a (IGVL6-57) segment is predominant in AL patients with renal disease and IGVL1-44 is associated with dominant cardiac involvement [41].

As noted previously in the discussion of myocardial involvement in amyloidosis, AL circulating light chains have a role in myocardial damage even without infiltration (Fig. 4). Light chains from patients with severe cardiac AL amyloidosis induced diastolic dysfunction when infused in an isolated mouse heart model. When this was performed with controls, including light chains from patients without AL amyloidosis, cardiac function was unaffected [43]. In another study, AL light chains provoked oxidative stress, cellular dysfunction, and apoptosis in isolated adult cardiomyocytes through activation of p38 mitogen-activated protein kinase (MAPK) [44].

AL Amyloidosis Epidemiology

Risk factors for AL amyloidosis include preexisting monoclonal gammopathy and myeloma. Among patients with monoclonal gammopathy of unknown significance (MGUS) in a large study, the relative risk of developing AL amyloidosis was 8.8. AL amyloidosis is diagnosed in as many as 10 to 15% of patients with myeloma, and 38% of patients with myeloma have Congo red–positive deposits in subcutaneous fat aspirates or bone marrow–biopsies (or both). The increase in serum free light chain levels probably precedes the development of AL amyloidosis by more than 4 years.

The estimated global incidence of AL amyloidosis is estimated as 10 cases per 1 million population. A real-world study based on a U.S. health care claims database showed a significant increase in the prevalence of AL amyloidosis, from 15.5 cases per 1 million population in 2007 to 40.5 cases per 1 million population in 2015, whereas the incidence rate remained steady, ranging from 9.7 to 14.0 cases per 1 million person-years [2].

ATTR Amyloidosis

Transthyretin-related amyloidosis consists of 2 disease forms: Hereditary disease arising from misfolding of a mutated or variant TTR (ATTRh or ATTRv also known as familial amyloid cardiomyopathy or familial amyloidotic polyneuropathy [FAP]) and a sporadic, nongenetic disease caused by mis-aggregation of wild-type transthyretin (ATTRwt also known as senile systemic amyloidosis [SSA]) [45].

Historical Background

Hereditary Amyloidosis

In 1952 a cluster of patients with neurological deficits and amyloidosis were reported from Portugal [46]. The patients suffered from peripheral motor weakness and peripheral sensory deficits, as well as gastrointestinal and sexual dysfunction. Histopathologic examination revealed amyloid deposition, and a familial, autosomal dominant pattern of inheritance. Similar reports of familial amyloidosis originated from Japan and Scandinavia. Eventually, hereditary amyloidosis was identified in many populations, with clinical syndromes that presented as neurological and/or cardiac disease [7].

Rukavina in 1956 reviewed 154 cases of "primary amyloidosis". Approximately 50% of the patients gathered from previous reports in the literature had cardiac involvement. A local hereditary form, in a family of 66 with more than half afflicted, was described [47]. In 1962 a severe form of cardiac amyloidosis was described in a Danish family [48].

In 1978 an extensive analysis of the amyloid isolated from the original Portuguese family was performed by Costa et al. Immunoelectrophoretic analysis, using FAP antiserum, detected a component in normal and FAP serum with an electrophoretic mobility identical to that of prealbumin (known today as transthyretin—TTR) [49].

This was performed again by Benson et al. in 1981—this time in a family with cardiomyopathy and nephropathy in addition to the polyneuropathy. Once more, the findings suggested that an abnormal serum prealbumin may be the precursor of the fibril protein in this type of heredo-familial amyloidosis [50].

Senile Systemic Amyloidosis

Senile Systemic Amyloidosis (Previously known as age related cardiac amyloidosis or senile cardiac amyloidosis) has been known for years and differentiated from other forms of amyloidosis.

Soyka first described age-related cardiac amyloidosis in 1876, followed by many case reports and case series published over the next 100 years [45]. In 1965, an autopsy study by Pomerance revealed a prevalence of senile cardiac amyloidosis of 10% in patients over 80 and 50% in patients over 90 years of age. Among the 21 patients, heart failure was present in 50% of the patients, and this was directly attributed to amyloidosis in 25%. The cause of this amyloid deposition remained obscure at the time [51].

The infamous digitalis toxicity was also noted in the cohort described by Pomerance. Retrospectively, this may also be the result of administering digitalis in large doses to elderly patients. The previous (and initial) report of digitalis sensitivity included 2 patients with AL amyloidosis—one patient with "primary amyloidosis" and the other with "amyloidosis secondary to plasmacytoma". Although both patients were relatively young (58 and 66), they were with very advanced heart failure and extremely sick, treated with doses which are currently considered toxic [52]. In the early 1980s, the digitalis toxicity concept was strengthened by an in vitro model. Digoxin was mixed with isolated amyloid fibrils and with amyloidotic heart homogenates—a relatively high affinity binding was noted, suggesting a mechanism for toxicity [53]. Currently, digoxin use may be feasible, when administered at a low dose and with close renal and serum digoxin level monitoring [54].

In 1981, following the hereditary amyloid studies by Costa and Benson implicating prealbumin (TTR) as the primary constituent of the amyloid protein, Cornwell, Westermark and colleagues examined this possibility in patients with senile cardiac amyloidosis. They noticed a partial homology between the amino acid sequences of human prealbumin and the protein isolated from senile cardiac amyloidosis. In a landmark study, using anti-human prealbumin antibodies and immunofluorescence, the final link between prealbumin and senile cardiac amyloidosis was established [55]. A decade later, the same group demonstrated that the TTR molecule in senile systemic amyloidosis has a normal primary structure (without mutations) [56].

Transthyretin

The history of transthyretin originates from the fields of thyroidology and plasma protein electrophoresis [57]. In the 1950s gel electrophoresis was performed on human serum and demonstrated two bands migrating ahead of albumin toward the anode. The faster migrating band was simply called "prealbumin". Jacob Robbins and his team, utilizing electrophoresis in search of thyroid hormone binding proteins, located thyroxine between α1- and α2-globulin. This protein was named thyroxine-binding globulin—TBG [57]. However, a different pattern was seen in cerebrospinal fluid (CSF)—there was a prominent prealbumin protein band carrying thyroxine. When a different buffer was used in the serum protein electrophoresis (in a group led by Sidney Ingbar), less blocking of thyroxine binding occurred, and a prominent peak of prealbumin-bound thyroxine appeared [58].

By 1960 it was evident that TBG was the principal transporter of serum thyroxine and triiodothyronine, whereas albumin and prealbumin (termed thyroxine-binding prealbumin (TBPA)) were minor carriers. Even though the concentration of TBG in serum was much lower than the concentration of TBPA, TBG carried most of the hormone because of its extremely high association constant for thyroxine. Ingbar was quoted, "TBG is the savings account for thyroxine and TBPA is the checking account" [57].

During the late 1960s and early 1970s, DeWitt Goodman and P. A. Peterson discovered an additional transport function of TBPA. It formed a complex with another protein about one-third its size that bound vitamin A, the retinol-binding protein (RBP). Due to this dual transport function, a proper name was required. In 1980, a compromise was reached by the Joint Commission of Biochemical nomenclature—transthyretin (with 3 votes in favor and 1 against this hybrid term—combination of *trans*port, *thy*roxine and *retin*ol) [57].

Human transthyretin (TTR) is a 127-amino acid (AAs) protein encoded by a single-copy gene mapped to chromosome 18q11.2-q12.1 [59]. The TTR gene product is a homotetrameric plasma protein produced primarily in the liver, with additional production and secretion by the choroid plexus and by retinal epithelia. TTR has a molecular mass of 55 kDa with each of the four identical monomers weighing approximately 14 kDa. Each monomer consists of eight β-strands structures and one short α-helix. These eight β-strands are connected by loops and are arranged in two groups of twisted β-sheets. Two TTR monomers are arranged into dimers by hydrogen binding, providing an extensive contact region which allows for the layer-by-layer packing of beta sheets (unfortunately, also an ideal precursor for amyloid formation). Two dimers then form a globular TTR tetramer through hydrophobic bonds. The two hydrophobic channels formed by the dimer-dimer interface can accommodate one T4 molecule each, including halogen binding sites for the 4 iodine atoms. Only one site is occupied by T4 due to negative co-operativity between the two sites (there is a 100-fold difference between the binding constants for the first and second T4 molecule). T4 itself assists in the connection between the 2 dimers, contributing to the TTR tetramer stabilization. Several stabilizers, such as tafamadis, employ this property of the T4 binding pocket, and prevent TTR dissociation into the amyloidogenic monomers. In contrast to T4 which is bound to the interior of the TTR tetramer, Retinol Binding Protein (RBP) binds on its external surface (Fig. 5). Despite two possible RBP binding sites per TTR dimer, only two RBP molecules can be bound to the TTR tetramer due to steric hindrance. Similar to T4, the binding of the first RBP molecule decreases the affinity of the TTR tetramer for the second RBP molecule. RBP bound to Retinol (holo-RBP) also increases TTR stability when bound to the TTR complex [59].

TTR Amyloidosis Specific Pathophysiology

Amyloid aggregation of TTR occurs when the balance between normal native homotetrameric structure and its monomer/dimer constituents is disturbed—TTR destabilization and dissociation [60]. The exposed hydrophobic surfaces and beta sheet structures of the TTR monomers reorganize into amyloid aggregates [14]. At the present, this dissociation of the TTR tetramer into monomers is considered the rate limiting step in TTR amyloid formation [60]. Of important note, similar to AL amyloidosis, prefibrillar protein aggregates and TTR monomers also contribute to organ toxicity [45]. Nerve biopsy studies in patients with FAP demonstrated Congo red negative prefibrillar aggregates of TTR with biochemical evidence of cellular toxicity. The cytotoxicity of TTR monomers and oligomers was also demonstrated in neural origin tissue cultures [61].

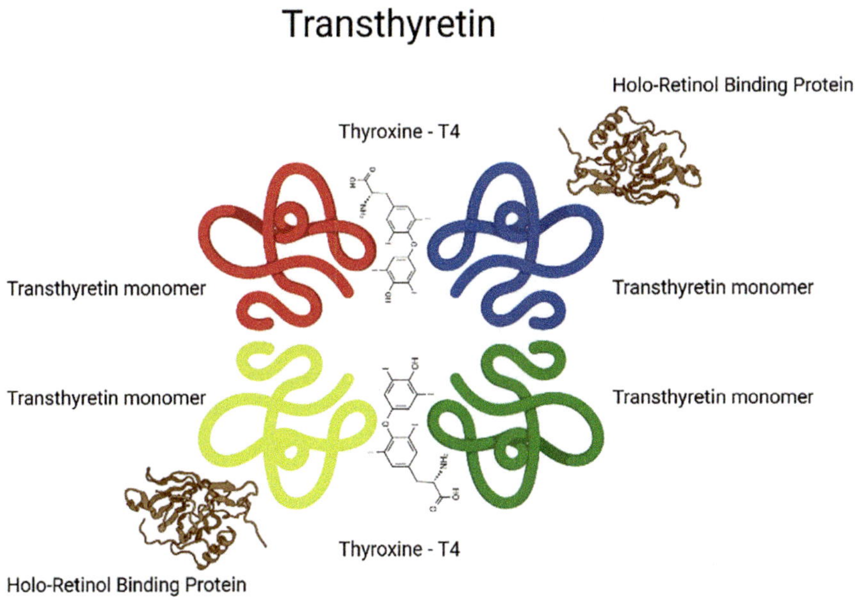

Fig. 5 A simplified model of Transthyretin—the 4 monomers assembled as the transthyretin tetramer with 2 binding sites for Holo-retinol binding protein—Retinol binding protein (protein data bank code 1RBP) bound to Retinol, and 2 binding sites for T4. Typically, only one binding site for T4 and Holo-RBP is occupied. Created in BioRender. Hellman, Y. (2025) https://BioRender.com/f67r346

ATTRwt Amyloidosis

In ATTRwt, age-related protein oxidative modifications and failure of proteostatic machinery and repair mechanisms may contribute to the dissociation and aggregation of **normal** TTR into amyloid fibrils [14]. This process is still incompletely understood. Proteostasis, the process by which cells regulate their protein content, is composed of the normal protein folding mechanisms described earlier as well as quality control mechanisms. Among the pathways deciding upon the fate of misfolded proteins are stress-responsive pathways such as the unfolded protein response (UPR), and proteolytic pathways such as the ubiquitin–proteasome (UPS), autophagosome-lysosome systems, and endoplasmic reticulum-associated degradation (ERAD). These components ultimately decide the fate of misfolded proteins and dictate whether they will be refolded or eliminated. Currently, impairment of proteostasis is considered one of the key mechanisms in cardiac aging and heart failure [62].

Interestingly, TTR amyloid is produced in the liver, but does not accumulate in this organ. On the other hand, although TTR is not produced by cardiac cells, extensive deposition occurs in the heart. This and the effect of aging were addressed in a study of a transgenic mice model expressing human TTR followed until older age (24 months).

The livers of older mice without cardiac deposition of TTR demonstrated increased chaperone and proteostatic activity when compared to the mice that did develop cardiac TTR deposition [63]. This phenomenon was named "hepatic chaperoning at a distance"—when this is impaired, cardiac TTR deposition may occur. TTR does not accumulate in the liver since it may have enough UPS and ERAD mechanisms to avoid TTR accumulation.

Recently, a peptide probe developed for TTR fibril detection revealed the presence of large TTR aggregates in the plasma of ATTR amyloidosis patients (ATTRwt and ATTRv) [64]. These findings suggest that aggregation-prone intermediates could be generated at a distance from target organs and deposit only when favorable conditions for amyloid deposition are met in specific tissues [65]. The possibility of these aggregates resulting from "shedding" of existing amyloid into the circulation is low due to the known stability of amyloid in tissues (which is classically resistant to various acids, bases and denaturing agents).

ATTRv Amyloidosis

In ATTRv, different mutations lead to unstable tetramers with an increased tendency to dissociate into the constituent monomers, which in turn lead to misfolding and amyloid formation. DNA sequencing in the last 4 decades uncovered many TTR mutations associated with amyloidosis.

There are over 140 different genotypes resulting in ATTRv. The most common TTR variants include:

(1) Val30Met mutation—the syndrome of Familial Amyloid Polyneuropathy (termed FAP) is most commonly caused by Val30Met. After initial recognition of this mutation, two phenotypes were noted—early onset and late onset. In Portugal and endemic areas of Japan, most ATTR Val30Met amyloidosis patients develop the disease between the ages of 30 and 40 (early onset) with high penetrance. In Sweden, patients with ATTR Val30Met develop disease in ages over 50 years (late onset) with low penetrance. Late onset disease typically presents with concomitant cardiomyopathy and is more prevalent in males—similar to ATTRwt. The disease prevalence is 1 in 100,000 individuals in nonendemic areas such as the United States, compared with 1 in 538 individuals affected in endemic areas of Portugal. Penetrance can also vary geographically with 22% at age 60 years in Sweden, compared with 80% at 50 years in Portugal [60].

(2) the Thr60Ala mutation—this mutation is a frequent cause of amyloid neuropathy and cardiomyopathy, affecting 1% of the population in northwest Ireland (County Donegal). Although cardiac involvement is reported in nearly 100% of T60A patients in the UK referred with neuropathy, the US experience is more heterogeneous [45]. This mutation is the second most common mutation causing ATTRv Cardiomyopathy in the US [60].

(3) Val122Ile mutation (also known as p.V142I—including the "leader sequence"). This mutation is mostly seen in the African-American population in the US with a genopositivity rate of 3–4% within this population, and is the most common cause of ATTRv cardiomyopathy in the US. From the phenotype standpoint, it causes a late-onset restrictive cardiomyopathy with neurological involvement being less prominent [60]. The V122I founder appears to have originated in West Africa, an area presumed to include most ancestors of African Americans [66]. An analysis of stored samples from the Beta-Blocker Evaluation in Survival Trial (BEST), demonstrated that 10% of African Americans with heart failure over the age of 60 carried the V122I Allele. Interestingly, this trial enrolled patients with systolic dysfunction (left ventricular ejection fraction under 35%), a cardiac profile more frequently observed in V122I than in other TTR mutations [67]. Another challenge with this specific mutation is the differentiation from hypertensive heart disease, also prevalent in the elderly African American population.

TTR Cardiac Amyloidosis Epidemiology—Autopsy Studies

When senile amyloidosis was finally attributed to TTR amyloid, the post mortem study by Pomerance was repeated by Cornwell et al. in 1983, this time with the addition of TTR immunohistochemical staining. Among 85 consecutive autopsies in patients $\geq$ 80 years of age, TTR amyloid was demonstrated in the atria or left ventricle of 21 hearts, a 25% prevalence in this elderly population. However, histologically significant cardiac TTR amyloid involvement occurred only in 8% to 16% [68]. In 2008, an autopsy prospective study was performed in Finnish octogenarians and identified TTR amyloid deposits in 25% of hearts from 256 autopsies [69]. Significant cardiac amyloid deposition occurred in only 5.5% of the study population. A pooled assessment of these autopsy studies and others in unselected elderly individuals found a global prevalence of 21% with a high degree of heterogeneity [70].

Amyloidosis in Heart Failure

Patients with Heart Failure and Preserved Ejection Fraction (HFpEF) are an important subgroup where an etiology of ATTR amyloidosis should be considered. An autopsy study of patients with an antemortem diagnosis of HFPEF (without known amyloid) revealed an ATTRwt cardiomyopathy prevalence of 17% [71]. A recent prospective endomyocardial biopsy (and right heart catheterization) study of 108 patients with HFpEF yielded 15 patients with cardiac amyloidosis—a prevalence of 14% [72]. 7 of these patients had ATTRwt, 4 patients with ATTRv, 3 patients with AL amyloidosis and 1 patient with AA amyloidosis. Of note, 7 of the 15 cases would not have been suspected to have amyloidosis based on recently published screening guidelines (1 AL, 1 AA, and 5 ATTR).

Non-invasive Diagnosis and Epidemiology of ATTR Cardiac Amyloidosis

The major breakthrough in the understanding of cardiac amyloidosis epidemiology in general and specifically in ATTR cardiomyopathy, occurred during the last 2 decades with the development of non-invasive diagnosis. Several factors contributed to this advancement. First, amyloidosis turned out to be a treatable disease—TTR stabilizers and other therapies became available for ATTR amyloidosis and in AL amyloidosis immunotherapy transformed the field (along with multiple myeloma). Second, the introduction in 2001 of a new assay to quantify both free Kappa and Lambda light chains in the serum has literally revolutionized the diagnosis of monoclonal gammopathies (FreeliteTM, the Binding Site Ltd., UK) [73]. The assay is able to recognize a hidden antigen located on the inside of light chain (not when it is part of the whole immunoglobulin)—significantly improving the sensitivity of sFLC (Free Light Chains) measurement. This FLC assay (and others that followed) allowed for a simplified detection and follow up of AL amyloidosis patients. Third, nuclear bone scintigraphy evolved from a coincidental hint at a diagnosis of cardiac amyloidosis during a routine bone scan to a major diagnostic tool in ATTR cardiac amyloidosis. Finally, upon entering the TAVR era, elderly patients with heart failure and aortic stenosis have available echocardiograms. Some of these patients are now diagnosed with concomitant ATTRwt amyloidosis. In addition to the susceptibility of elderly patients to ATTRwt amyloidosis, aortic stenosis and TTR amyloid may share common pathophysiological pathways as previously discussed.

After the initial case report in 1981 [74] and additional reports of technetium-labeled bisphosphonates localizing amyloid, several studies systematically evaluated this modality as a means of diagnosis in cardiac amyloidosis. The isotopes 99mTc-labeled 3,3-diphosphono-1,2-propanodicarboxylic acid (DPD), pyrophosphate (PYP), and 99mTc-labeled hydroxymethylene diphosphonate (HMDP) were both sensitive and specific for imaging cardiac ATTR. Despite lower specificity, bone scintigraphy can differentiate between cardiac TTR amyloidosis and AL amyloidosis in most cases [75]. However, in some patients, AL amyloidosis can also cause significant cardiac radiotracer uptake. Furthermore, an old myocardial infarction with calcification can also result in localized cardiac radiotracer uptake.

In order to establish a non-invasive algorithm for the diagnosis of cardiac amyloidosis, a large collaborative study combining both nuclear findings and monoclonal protein measurements was conducted in a pooled analysis of patients referred to amyloidosis centers (with available biopsy proven amyloidosis as a gold standard) [76]. Since it is absolutely essential to avoid misdiagnosis of cardiac ATTR amyloidosis in a patient who actually has cardiac AL amyloidosis (requiring chemotherapy), the primary aim of the proposed diagnostic criteria was to achieve a very high diagnostic specificity. A specificity of 100% was achieved by the combination of grade 2 or 3 cardiac uptake on a radionuclide scan and the absence of a detectable monoclonal protein.

Following the diagnosis of cardiac ATTR, genotyping is recommended in order to differentiate between ATTRwt and ATTRv. This initial "non biopsy" diagnostic algorithm for cardiac amyloidosis proposed by Gilmore et al. is currently endorsed by both the ESC and ACC guidelines. In patients with borderline findings and/or conflicting results, further investigation with CMR imaging and endomyocardial biopsy should be considered.

The mechanism of these nuclear tracers' affinity to cardiac amyloid tissue remains unclear, as well as the preferential binding of ATTR rather than AL cardiac amyloid. One hypothesis is that 99mTc-PYP may bind the calcium within the amyloid fibrils. Perhaps varying degrees of calcium and serum amyloid protein (SAP—one of the amyloid signature proteins—which is calcium dependent) establish the different levels of tissue enhancement accordingly. Another hypothesis explaining the mechanism of myocardial enhancement in ATTR is that the intensity of 99mTc-PYP binding relates to the duration over which amyloid deposition has occurred in the affected tissue. In AL patients, fibrils accumulate over shorter time periods than in ATTR patients typically characterized by a longer disease course. Finally, the degree of amyloid infiltration in the myocardium also may influence the radiotracer uptake [75].

Non-invasive diagnosis of ATTR amyloidosis paved the way to a better understanding of ATTR amyloidosis epidemiology.

The Nuclear Era

In studies involving patients undergoing bone scintigraphy for all reasons (other than suspected cardiac amyloidosis), a meta-analysis revealed a prevalence of 1% of patients with myocardial uptake [70]. The prevalence increased with age and a higher likelihood was noted in men rather than women across all age categories. In one of these studies, which included patients referred for oncologic and rheumatologic reasons, contact was established with the patients who had myocardial uptake. Further diagnostic workup was offered to these patients (ECG, echocardiography, genetic testing and biopsy), which uncovered one patient with ATTRv cardiac amyloidosis and 5 patients with biopsy proven ATTRwt cardiac amyloidosis [77].

Several studies employed the diagnostic algorithm in the HFpEF population. Similar to the histological findings by Hahn, the prevalence of cardiac amyloidosis was around 12% on average. 75% of HFpEF cardiac amyloidosis were men. In the HFmrEF (midrange) and HFrEF population, prevalence is around 10% [70]. Therefore, cardiac ATTR amyloidosis can actually present in diverse echocardiographic phenotypes (not only HFpEF) [78].

A common symptom of amyloidosis is carpal tunnel syndrome and in elderly patients is considered a "red flag". In patients over 60 years old undergoing bilateral carpal tunnel syndrome surgery, with LV thickening, and without occupational risk factors, the prevalence was 14% in one study [79]. In a more general population over 60 years old, undergoing carpal tunnel surgery, a prevalence of 8% was found in 10 out of 120 patients after consent for further workup followed by selection per echocardiographic, ECG and biomarker "red flags". These patients had less cardiac involvement when compared to matched contemporary patients with ATTRwt diagnosed through routine clinical practice. Hence, the disease is diagnosed in an early stage, which may allow for earlier therapy and perhaps postponing the onset of clinical heart failure [80]. A tenosynovial biopsy-based study yielded a histologic prevalence of 10% staining with Congo red and the diagnosis of amyloidosis [81]. Of note, AL amyloidosis was responsible for the cardiac amyloidosis in several patients participating in these studies.

Aortic Stenosis and the TAVI Era

Several studies examined the prevalence and characteristics of cardiac amyloidosis in patients with severe AS referred to surgery or percutaneous replacement. A pooled assessment found a prevalence of 8% (95% CI 5%–13%) [70]. A recent analysis of patients referred to TAVI found exactly this prevalence of 8%, mostly ATTRwt amyloidosis with one AL patient [82]. Indeed, mortality was worse in patients with cardiac amyloidosis and severe AS when compared to lone AS. However, TAVI improved survival and was superior to medical therapy in these patients. Therefore, TAVI is not futile in the cardiac amyloidosis with AS population and should not be withheld. Low gradient aortic stenosis may occur in cardiac amyloidosis due to the low stroke volume, so the threshold for cardiac amyloidosis workup should be considered also in patients with allegedly non-severe AS. Since routine screening of older AS patients with bone scintigraphy is not practical, this should be performed according to clinical assessment including risk factors such as carpal tunnel syndrome, biomarkers (troponin, NT-pro-BNP), echocardiographic markers and ECG.

In general, the prevalence of ATTRwt cardiac amyloidosis increases with advancing age, and virtually all patients are over 60 years old when diagnosed. ATTRwt cardiac amyloidosis is a remarkably sex-specific disease with a 25 to 50:1 male to female ratio. Projections of population growth over the next 20 years predict that ATTRwt cardiac amyloidosis will become the most common form of cardiac amyloidosis [45].

AA Amyloidosis

AA amyloidosis was probably first reported by Carl Rokitansky in 1842, who described hepatomegaly with hepatic infiltration by a grayish gelatinous material in an autopsy series of patients with tuberculosis or syphilis. During the following years, the relationship between chronic inflammatory diseases and the development of amyloidosis in some of these cases was established. The original Reimann classification of amyloidosis in 1935 addressed this type as "secondary" amyloidosis [3].

In 1971, Benditt and colleagues demonstrated a specific amino acid sequence at the N terminus of secondary amyloid. Several laboratories identified similar protein sequences with size varying around 76 amino acids, all with the same N-terminus. Antibodies against this amyloid protein identified a 104 amino acid precursor protein, which was then was named Serum Amyloid A—the first non-immunoglobulin protein identified as an amyloid precursor protein [83].

Serum Amyloid A proteins are a family of apolipoproteins produced by the liver along with other tissues (including macrophages, kidney, lung, adipocytes, and mammary glands) and are part of the acute phase reaction (similar to CRP). Apart from its role in the complex regulation of the acute phase inflammatory response, the nature and basis for other SAA functions have been poorly defined.

In terms of amyloid fibril formation, the ≈76 residue fragment is the most common constituent of pathologic deposits, although both longer and shorter peptides can be found as well. It is likely that the critical β sheet region for AA fibril formation is relatively short. The responsible proteases yielding these fragments have not yet been clearly identified. The reasons promoting SAA misfolding into amyloid fibrils include: a critical concentration of SAA for a prolonged period, variations in the SAA cleavage site by different proteases, polymorphisms within the SAA1 gene, and local tissue factors (pH, SAP component) [83].

The incidence of AA amyloidosis has been reported as one to two cases per million person-years. Sustained inflammation increases the risk of AA amyloidosis, therefore chronic infections (hidradenitis suppurativa, HIV, TB, syphilis) and inflammatory diseases (rheumatoid arthritis, inflammatory bowel disease) are the prevailing causes. Periodic fever syndromes, including familial Mediterranean fever (FMF) are also a major cause of AA amyloidosis [84]. Up to 20% of cases were idiopathic in one report (9 out of 43 patients with AA amyloidosis), although the underlying disease revealed itself during follow up in 2 cases [85].

AA amyloidosis manifests in multiple organs including the kidneys, gastrointestinal tract, liver, peripheral nerves, heart, blood vessels, lungs, skin, and soft tissue. Nephrotic syndrome and renal failure are the most common organ involvement, followed by the GI tract and liver. Cardiac involvement is infrequent. In a landmark long term AA amyloidosis cohort follow up study, heart failure attributable to amyloidosis was present only in 1 patient. Findings consistent with cardiac infiltration were present in only 2 of 224 patients who underwent echocardiography [86]. In a smaller retrospective cohort study, 3 patients out of 43 (7%) were diagnosed with cardiac involvement—1 via endomyocardial biopsy, 1 via MRI and 1 at autopsy [85]. An earlier study of 44 biopsy proven AA amyloidosis patients demonstrated echocardiographic findings consistent with cardiac involvement in 4.5% (2/44) of the patients. Although the echocardiographic parameters were impressive (ventricular septum in the 2 cm range), the patients were relatively without heart failure symptoms and eventually died of renal failure associated sepsis. Therefore, the authors suggested that perhaps cardiac deposition of AA amyloid fibrils is significantly different than the effect of AL amyloidosis fibrils [87]. In contrast, in the previously mentioned endomyocardial biopsy study of 108 patients with HFpEF conducted by Hahn and colleagues, 1 patient was diagnosed with AA amyloidosis [72]. In summary, AA cardiac amyloidosis is relatively uncommon, usually preceded by renal involvement. However, in the proper clinical setting, especially with an uncontrolled inflammatory disease or established AA amyloidosis, cardiac involvement should be assessed.

Dialysis Related Amyloidosis (DRA)–Beta-2 Microglobulin (Aβ2M) Amyloidosis

In patients undergoing long term dialysis, accumulation of beta-2 microglobulin results in the systemic deposition of amyloid fibrils—especially in the osteoarticular system (joints, carpal tunnel syndrome). Cardiac involvement may also occur [88]. In an autopsy study of 18 hemodialysis patients, beta-2 microglobulin amyloid was demonstrated in the cardiac tissue in 7/18 patients (39%). The main factor determining the extent of cardiac involvement was the duration of dialysis (years). Aβ2M amyloid was found in the left ventricle primarily in the walls of small coronary vessels, which may partially explain the non-atherosclerotic ischemic heart disease in long term dialysis patients. Extensive deposits of Aβ2M amyloid were noted in the atria, surrounding atrophied myocytes. This may result in atrial arrhythmia and mechanical dysfunction with a "stiff left atrium" as previously discussed [89]. Case reports and previous autopsy reports have also described Aβ2M amyloid within the left ventricle. In one of these reports, 2 long term hemodialysis patients (over 20 years) developed fatal congestive heart failure caused by extensive cardiac Aβ2M amyloid deposition. At autopsy, the distribution of amyloid was widely disseminated throughout the left ventricle, with positive immunohistochemical staining for anti-human beta2-microglobulin antibody [90]. Therefore, cardiac Aβ2M amyloidosis should be considered in patients receiving long term dialysis, especially when other manifestations of DRA are present.

Currently, newer dialysis technologies (high-flow dialysis membranes) reduce beta-2 microglobulin levels in chronic dialysis patients. These technologies, as well as renal transplantation, may decrease the incidence of this disease [88].

Remaining Types of Cardiac Amyloidosis

Aside from AL, ATTR, AA and Aβ2M amyloidosis, the rare forms including Apo-AI, ApoA-IV are increasingly recognized [91]. Although treatment is supportive, they should be differentiated from the other forms in order to avoid misdiagnosis. In these specific forms of amyloidosis, prognosis is generally better than AL amyloidosis with slow progression of disease. Other rare amyloid forms are ApoA-II, gelsolin (AGel) and lysozyme (ALys) [35]. Some of these rare forms are genetic variants, in which correct identification can have an impact on family members as well. Diagnosis is challenging in the rare forms of amyloidosis, typically requiring multimodality imaging (echocardiography, nuclear scintigraphy and MRI) and ultimately an endomyocardial biopsy [92].

Conclusion

Cardiac amyloidosis is not as rare as it was perceived in the past. In the last few decades, great progress has been made in the mechanistic insights and understanding of amyloid formation with its different precursor proteins. AL amyloidosis and multiple myeloma underwent a revolution in diagnosis and therapy with the advent of free light chain assays and targeted therapy with Daratumimab and Venetoclax, finally controlling amyloidogenic light chains. The identification of transthyretin as the cause of ATTRwt and ATTRv amyloidosis enabled development of appropriate pharmacotherapy, including TTR stabilizers and knockdown therapy with anti-sense oligonucleotides and small interfering RNA (siRNA). The algorithm for a non-biopsy diagnosis of ATTR cardiac amyloidosis utilizing scintigraphy and free light chains allowed for a better understanding of ATTRwt amyloidosis prevalence among the elderly and heart failure population. Further understanding of the sequence of events leading to ATTR amyloid deposition, including circulating intermediates, may identify possible biomarkers of ATTR amyloidosis disease activity and response to therapy. In the future, genome editing with CRISPR technology may provide a long lasting and effective therapy for patients with ATTRv or other variant amyloid precursor proteins (e.g. ApoA-I).

References

1. De Gaspari M, Finato N, Basso C. Cardiac amyloidosis: the pathologist's point of view. Vessel Plus. 2022;6:57. https://doi.org/10.20517/2574-1209.2022.05.
2. Sanchorawala V. Systemic light chain amyloidosis. N Engl J Med. 2024;390(24):2295–307. https://doi.org/10.1056/NEJMra2304088.
3. Harrison JS, Cohen Y, Ioffe I, Bulvik S. An historical overview of the amyloidoses. In: Amyloidosis—history and perspectives. IntechOpen; 2021. Available from: https://www.intechopen.com/chapters/76848.

4. Sipe JD, Cohen AS. Review: History of the Amyloid Fibril. J Struct Biol. 2000;130(2–3):88–98. https://doi.org/10.1006/jsbi.2000.4221.
5. Howie AJ. Origins of a pervasive, erroneous idea: the "green birefringence" of Congo red-stained amyloid. Int J Exp Pathol. 2019;100(3):208–21. https://doi.org/10.1111/iep.12330.
6. Tanskanen M. "Amyloid"—historical aspects. In: Amyloidosis. IntechOpen; 2013. https://doi.org/10.5772/53423. Available from: https://www.intechopen.com/chapters/44870&#8203.
7. Kyle RA. Amyloidosis: a convoluted story. Br J Haematol. 2001;114(3):529–38. https://doi.org/10.1046/j.1365-2141.2001.02999.
8. Stone MJ. Samuel Wilks: the "grand old man" of British medicine. Proc (Bayl Univ Med Cent). 2010;23(3):263–5. https://doi.org/10.1080/08998280.2010.11928684.
9. Steensma DP. "Congo" red: out of Africa? Arch Pathol Lab Med. 2001;125(2):250–2. https://doi.org/10.5858/2001-125-0250-CR.
10. Yakupova EI, Bobyleva LG, Vikhlyantsev IM, Bobylev AG. Congo Red and amyloids: history and relationship. Biosci Rep. 2019;39(1):1–22. https://doi.org/10.1042/BSR20181415.
11. Benson MD, Buxbaum JN, Eisenberg DS, Merlini G, Saraiva MJM, Sekijima Y, Sipe JD, Westermark P. Amyloid nomenclature 2020: update and recommendations by the International Society of Amyloidosis (ISA) nomenclature committee. Amyloid. 2020;27(4):217–22. https://doi.org/10.1080/13506129.2020.1835263.
12. Pras M, Schubert M, Zucker-Franklin D, Rimon A, Franklin EC. The characterization of soluble amyloid prepared in water. J Clin Invest. 1968;47(4):924–33. https://doi.org/10.1172/JCI105781.
13. Buxbaum JN, Dispenzieri A, Eisenberg DS, Fändrich M, Merlini G, Saraiva MJM, Sekijima Y, Westermark P. Amyloid nomenclature 2022: update, novel proteins, and recommendations by the International Society of Amyloidosis (ISA) nomenclature committee. Amyloid. 2022;29(4):213–9. https://doi.org/10.1080/13506129.2022.2147636.
14. Griffin JM, Rosenblum H, Maurer MS. Pathophysiology and therapeutic approaches to cardiac amyloidosis. Circ Res. 2021;128(10):1554–75. https://doi.org/10.1161/CIRCRESAHA.121.31818.
15. Hartl FU, Bracher A, Hayer-Hartl M. Molecular chaperones in protein folding and proteostasis. Nature. 2011;475(7356):324–32. https://doi.org/10.1038/nature10317.
16. Merlini G, Bellotti V. Molecular mechanisms of amyloidosis. N Engl J Med. 2003;349(6):583–96. https://doi.org/10.1056/NEJMra023144.
17. Dobson CM. Protein folding and misfolding. Nature. 2003;426(6968):884–90. https://doi.org/10.1038/nature02261.
18. Tennent GA, Lovat LB, Pepys MB. Serum amyloid P component prevents proteolysis of the amyloid fibrils of Alzheimer disease and systemic amyloidosis. Proc Natl Acad Sci USA. 1995;92(10):4299–303. https://doi.org/10.1073/pnas.92.10.4299.
19. Jarrett JT, Lansbury PT Jr. Seeding "one-dimensional crystallization" of amyloid: a pathogenic mechanism in Alzheimer's disease and scrapie? Cell. 1993;73(6):1055–9. https://doi.org/10.1016/0092-8674(93)90635-4.
20. Arosio P, Knowles TPJ, Linse S. On the lag phase in amyloid fibril formation. Phys Chem Chem Phys. 2015;17(12):7606–18. https://doi.org/10.1039/c4cp05563b.
21. Mishra T, Pahuja M, Abidov A. Increasingly recognized role of right ventricle assessment in cardiac amyloidosis. JACC Heart Fail. 2019;7(3):277–8. https://doi.org/10.1016/j.jchf.2018.11.014.
22. Takemura G, Takatsu Y, Doyama K, Itoh H, Saito Y, Koshiji M, et al. Expression of atrial and brain natriuretic peptides and their genes in hearts of patients with cardiac amyloidosis. J Am Coll Cardiol. 1998;31(1):254–65. https://doi.org/10.1016/S0735-1097(98)00045-X.
23. Bandera F, Martone R, Chacko L, Ganesananthan S, Gilbertson JA, Ponticos M, et al. Clinical importance of left atrial infiltration in cardiac transthyretin amyloidosis. JACC Cardiovasc Imaging. 2022;15(1):17–29. https://doi.org/10.1016/j.jcmg.2021.06.022.
24. Vergaro G, Aimo A, Rapezzi C, Castiglione V, Fabiani I, Pucci A, et al. Atrial amyloidosis: mechanisms and clinical manifestations. Eur J Heart Fail. 2022;24(12):2019–28. https://doi.org/10.1002/ejhf.2650.

25. Hartnett J, Jaber W, Maurer M, Sperry B, Hanna M, Collier P, Patel DR, Wazni OM, Donnellan E. Electrophysiological manifestations of cardiac amyloidosis. JACC CardioOncology. 2021;3(4):506–15. https://doi.org/10.1016/j.jaccao.2021.07.010.
26. Khanna S, Lo P, Cho K, Subbiah R. Ventricular arrhythmias in cardiac amyloidosis: a review of current literature. Clin Med Insights Cardiol. 2020;14:1–7. https://doi.org/10.1177/117954 6820963055.
27. Eriksson A, Olofsson BO, Eriksson P. Heart valve involvement in familial amyloidosis with polyneuropathy. Pathol Res Pract. 1986;181(5):563–656.
28. Mohty D, Pradel S, Magne J, Fadel B, Boulogne C, Petitalot V, et al. Prevalence and prognostic impact of left-sided valve thickening in systemic light-chain amyloidosis. Clin Res Cardiol. 2017;106(4):331–40. https://doi.org/10.1007/s10741-023-10350-1.
29. Aimo A, Camerini L, Fabiani I, Morfino P, Panichella G, Barison A, et al. Valvular heart disease in patients with cardiac amyloidosis. Heart Fail Rev. 2024;29(1):65–77. https://doi.org/10.1007/s10741-023-10350-1.
30. Badwan O, Berglund F, Rosenzveig A, Persits I, Gharaibeh A, Kumar A, et al. Pericardial disease in cardiac amyloidosis: a comprehensive review. Am J Cardiol. 2024;223:100–8. https://doi.org/10.1016/j.amjcard.2024.05.007.
31. Sucker C, Hetzel GR, Grabensee B, Stockschlaeder M, Scharf RE. Amyloidosis and bleeding: pathophysiology, diagnosis, and therapy. Am J Kidney Dis. 2006;47(6):947–55. https://doi.org/10.1053/j.ajkd.2006.03.036.
32. Morris AD, Smith RN, Stone JR. The pathology and changing epidemiology of dialysis-related cardiac beta-2 microglobulin amyloidosis. Cardiovasc Pathol. 2019;42:30–5. https://doi.org/10.1016/j.carpath.2019.05.002.
33. Wang AK, Fealey RD, Gehrking TL, Low PA. Patterns of neuropathy and autonomic failure in patients with amyloidosis. Mayo Clin Proc. 2008;83(11):1226–30. https://doi.org/10.4065/83.11.1226.
34. Stamatelopoulos K, Georgiopoulos G, Athanasouli F, Nikolaou PE, Lykka M, Roussou M, et al. Reactive vasodilation predicts mortality in primary systemic light-chain amyloidosis. Circ Res. 2019;125(8):744–58. https://doi.org/10.1161/CIRCRESAHA.119.314862.
35. Maleszewski JJ. Cardiac amyloidosis: pathology, nomenclature, and typing. Cardiovasc Pathol. 2015;24(5):343–50. https://doi.org/10.1016/j.carpath.2015.07.008.
36. Rathore R, Coward RA, Woywodt A. What's in a name? Bence Jones protein Clin Kidney J. 2012;5(5):478–83. https://doi.org/10.1093/ckj/sfs127.
37. Bence JH. On the new substance occurring in the urine of a patient with mollities ossium. Philos Trans R Soc Lond B Biol Sci. 1848;138:55–62.
38. Lee RE, Young RH, Castleman B. James Homer Wright: a biography of the enigmatic creator of the Wright stain on the occasion of its centennial. Am J Surg Pathol. 2002;26(1):88–96.
39. Edelman GM, Gally JA. The nature of Bence-Jones proteins: chemical similarities to polypeptide chains of myeloma globulins and normal γ-globulins. J Exp Med. 1962;116(2):207–27. https://doi.org/10.1084/jem.116.2.207.
40. Glenner GG, Ein D, Eanes ED, Bladen HA, Terry W, Page DL. Creation of "amyloid" fibrils from Bence Jones proteins in vitro. Science. 1971;174(4010):712–4. https://doi.org/10.1126/science.174.4010.712.
41. Ikura H, Endo J, Kitakata H, Moriyama H, Sano M, Fukuda K. Molecular mechanism of pathogenesis and treatment strategies for AL amyloidosis. Int J Mol Sci. 2022;23(11):6336. https://doi.org/10.3390/ijms23116336.
42. Sidiqi MH, Al Saleh AS, Leung N, Jevremovic D, Aljama MA, Gonsalves WI, et al. Venetoclax for the treatment of translocation (11;14) AL amyloidosis. Blood Cancer J. 2020;10(55):1–4. https://doi.org/10.1038/s41408-020-0321-6.
43. Liao R, Jain M, Teller P, Connors LH, Ngoy S, Skinner M, Falk RH, Apstein CS. Infusion of light chains from patients with cardiac amyloidosis causes diastolic dysfunction in isolated mouse hearts. Circulation. 2001;104(14):1594–7.
44. Shi J, Guan J, Jiang B, Brenner DA, del Monte F, Ward JE, Connors LH, Sawyer DB, Semigran MJ, Macgillivray TE, Seldin DC, Falk RH, Liao R. Amyloidogenic light chains induce

cardiomyocyte contractile dysfunction and apoptosis via a non-canonical p38α MAPK pathway. Proc Natl Acad Sci USA. 2010;107(9):4188–93. https://doi.org/10.1073/pnas.0912263107.
45. Ruberg FL, Berk JL. Transthyretin (TTR) cardiac amyloidosis: contemporary reviews in cardiovascular medicine. Circulation. 2012;126(10):1286–300. https://doi.org/10.1161/CIRCULATIONAHA.111.078915.
46. Andrade C. A peculiar form of peripheral neuropathy: familial atypical generalized amyloidosis with special involvement of the peripheral nerves. Brain. 1952;75(3):408–27. https://doi.org/10.1093/brain/75.3.408.
47. Block WD, Carey JG, Curtis AC, Falls HF, Jackson CE, Rukavina JG. Primary systemic amyloidosis: a review and an experimental, genetic, and clinical study of 29 cases with particular emphasis on the familial form. Medicine (Baltimore). 1956;35(3):239–334.
48. Frederiksen T, Gotzsche H, Harboe N, Kjaer W, Mellemgaard K. Familial primary amyloidosis with severe amyloid heart disease. Am J Med. 1962;33(3):328–44.
49. Costa PP, Figueira AS, Bravo FR. Amyloid fibril protein related to prealbumin in familial amyloidotic polyneuropathy. Proc Natl Acad Sci U S A. 1978;75(9):4499–503. https://doi.org/10.1073/pnas.75.9.4499.
50. Benson MD. Partial amino acid sequence homology between an heredofamilial amyloid protein and human plasma prealbumin. J Clin Invest. 1981;67(4):1035–41. https://doi.org/10.1172/JCI110114.
51. Pomerance A. Senile cardiac amyloidosis. Br Heart J. 1965;27(5):711–8.
52. Cassidy JT. Cardiac amyloidosis: two cases with digitalis sensitivity. Ann Intern Med. 1961;55(6):989–94. https://doi.org/10.7326/0003-4819-55-6-989.
53. Rubinow A, Skinner M, Cohen AS. Digoxin sensitivity in amyloid cardiomyopathy. Circulation. 1981;63(6):1285–8. https://doi.org/10.1161/01.CIR.63.6.1285.
54. Muchtar E, Gertz MA, Kumar SK, Lin G, Boilson B, Clavell A, et al. Digoxin use in systemic light-chain (AL) amyloidosis: contraindicated or cautious use? Amyloid. 2018;25(2):86–92.
55. Cornwell GG III, Westermark P, Natvig JB, Murdoch W. Senile cardiac amyloid: evidence that fibrils contain a protein immunologically related to prealbumin. Immunology. 1981;44(4):447–52.
56. Westermark P, Sletten K, Johansson B, Cornwell GG III. Fibril in senile systemic amyloidosis is derived from normal transthyretin. Proc Natl Acad Sci U S A. 1990;87(7):2843–5. https://doi.org/10.1073/pnas.87.7.2843.
57. Robbins J. Transthyretin from discovery to now. Clin Chem Lab Med. 2002;40(12):1183–90. https://doi.org/10.1515/CCLM.2002.206.
58. Ingbar SH. Prealbumin: a thyroxine-binding protein of human plasma. Endocrinology. 1958;63:256–9.
59. Sanguinetti C, Minniti M, Susini V, Caponi L, Panichella G, Castiglione V, Aimo A, Emdin M, Vergaro G, Franzini M. The journey of human transthyretin: synthesis, structure stability, and catabolism. Biomedicines. 2022;10(8):1906. https://doi.org/10.3390/biomedicines10081906.
60. Ruberg FL, Grogan M, Hanna M, Kelly JW, Maurer MS. Transthyretin amyloid cardiomyopathy. J Am Coll Cardiol. 2019;73(22):2872–91. https://doi.org/10.1016/j.jacc.2019.04.003.
61. Sousa MM, Cardoso I, Fernandes R, Guimarães A, Saraiva MJ. Deposition of transthyretin in early stages of familial amyloidotic polyneuropathy: evidence for toxicity of nonfibrillar aggregates. Am J Pathol. 2001;159(6):1993–2000. https://doi.org/10.1016/s0002-9440(10)63050-7.
62. Goyal P, Maurer MS, Roh J. Aging in heart failure: embracing biology over chronology. JACC Heart Fail. 2024;12(5):795–809. https://doi.org/10.1016/j.jchf.2024.02.021.
63. Buxbaum JN, Tagoe C, Gallo G, Walker JR, Kurian S, Salomon DR. Why are some amyloidoses systemic? Does hepatic "chaperoning at a distance" prevent cardiac deposition in a transgenic model of human senile systemic (transthyretin) amyloidosis? FASEB J. 2012;26(6):2283–93. https://doi.org/10.1096/fj.11-189571.
64. Pedretti R, Wang L, Yakubovska A, Zhang QS, Nguyen B, Grodin JL, Masri A, Saelices L. Structure-based probe reveals the presence of large transthyretin aggregates in plasma of ATTR amyloidosis patients. JACC Basic Transl Sci. 2024;9(9):1088–100. https://doi.org/10.1016/j.jacbts.2024.05.013.

65. Fontana M, Gillmore JD, Verona G. Large transthyretin aggregates in plasma of ATTR amyloidosis patients: future clinical implications. JACC Basic Transl Sci. 2024;9(9):1101–3. https://doi.org/10.1016/j.jacbts.2024.07.005.
66. Jacobson DR, Alexander AA, Tagoe C, Garvey WT, Williams SM, Tishkoff S, et al. The prevalence and distribution of the amyloidogenic transthyretin (TTR) V122I allele in Africa. Mol Genet Genomic Med. 2016;4(5):548–56. https://doi.org/10.1002/mgg3.231.
67. Buxbaum JN, Jacobson DR, Tagoe C, Alexander A, Kitzman DW, Greenberg B, et al. Transthyretin V122I in African Americans with congestive heart failure. J Am Coll Cardiol. 2006;47(8):1724–5. https://doi.org/10.1016/j.jacc.2006.01.042.
68. Cornwell GG 3rd, Murdoch WL, Kyle RA, Westermark P, Pitkänen P. Frequency and distribution of senile cardiovascular amyloid: a clinicopathologic correlation. Am J Med. 1983;75(4):618–23. https://doi.org/10.1016/0002-9343(83)90443-6.
69. Tanskanen M, Peuralinna T, Polvikoski T, Notkola I-L, Sulkava R, Hardy J, et al. Senile systemic amyloidosis affects 25% of the very aged and associates with genetic variation in alpha2-macroglobulin and tau: a population-based autopsy study. Ann Med. 2008;40(3):232–9. https://doi.org/10.1080/07853890701842988.
70. Aimo A, Merlo M, Porcari A, Georgiopoulos G, Pagura L, Vergaro G, et al. Redefining the epidemiology of cardiac amyloidosis: a systematic review and meta-analysis of screening studies. Eur J Heart Fail. 2022;24(12):2342–51. https://doi.org/10.1002/ejhf.2532.
71. Mohammed SF, Mirzoyev SA, Edwards WD, Dogan A, Grogan DR, Dunlay SM, et al. Left ventricular amyloid deposition in patients with heart failure and preserved ejection fraction. JACC Heart Fail. 2014;2(2):113–22. https://doi.org/10.1016/j.jchf.2013.11.004.
72. Hahn VS, Yanek LR, Vaishnav J, Ying W, Vaidya D, Lee YZJ, et al. Endomyocardial biopsy characterization of heart failure with preserved ejection fraction and prevalence of cardiac amyloidosis. JACC Heart Fail. 2020;8(9):712–24. https://doi.org/10.1016/j.jchf.2020.04.007.
73. Bradwell AR, Carr-Smith HD, Mead GP, Tang LX, Showell PJ, Drayson MT, Drew R. Highly sensitive, automated immunoassay for immunoglobulin free light chains in serum and urine. Clin Chem. 2001;47(4):673–80.
74. Ali A, Turner DA, Rosenbush SW, Fordham EW. Bone scintigram in cardiac amyloidosis: a case report. Clin Nucl Med. 1981;6(3):105–8. https://doi.org/10.1097/00003072-198103000-00003.
75. Bokhari S, Castaño A, Pozniakoff T, Deslisle S, Latif F, Maurer MS. 99mTc-pyrophosphate scintigraphy for differentiating light-chain cardiac amyloidosis from the transthyretin-related familial and senile cardiac amyloidoses. Circ Cardiovasc Imaging. 2013;6(2):195–201. https://doi.org/10.1161/CIRCIMAGING.112.000132.
76. Gillmore JD, Maurer MS, Falk RH, Merlini G, Damy T, Dispenzieri A, et al. Nonbiopsy diagnosis of cardiac transthyretin amyloidosis. Circulation. 2016;133(24):2404–12. https://doi.org/10.1161/CIRCULATIONAHA.116.021612.
77. Longhi S, Guidalotti PL, Quarta CC, Gagliardi C, Milandri A, Lorenzini M, et al. Identification of TTR-related subclinical amyloidosis with 99mTc-DPD scintigraphy. J Am Coll Cardiol Cardiovasc Imaging. 2014;7(5):531–3. https://doi.org/10.1016/j.jcmg.2014.03.004.
78. Achten A, Muller SA, Sanders-van Wijk S, van der Meer MG, van der Harst P, van Tintelen P, et al. Diversity of heart failure phenotypes in transthyretin amyloid cardiomyopathy: more than just heart failure with preserved ejection fraction. Ann Med. 2024;56(1):2418965. https://doi.org/10.1080/07853890.2024.2418965.
79. Zegri-Reiriz I, de Haro-Del Moral FJ, Dominguez F, Salas C, de la Cuadra P, Plaza A, et al. Prevalence of cardiac amyloidosis in patients with carpal tunnel syndrome. J Cardiovasc Transl Res. 2019;12(6):507–13. https://doi.org/10.1007/s12265-019-09895-0.
80. Ladefoged B, Clemmensen T, Dybro A, Hartig-Andreasen C, Kirkeby L, Gormsen LC, et al. Identification of wild-type transthyretin cardiac amyloidosis in patients with carpal tunnel syndrome surgery (CACTuS). ESC Heart Fail. 2023;10(1):234–44. https://doi.org/10.1002/ehf2.14173.
81. Sperry BW, Reyes BA, Ikram A, Donnelly JP, Phelan D, Jaber WA, et al. Tenosynovial and cardiac amyloidosis in patients undergoing carpal tunnel release. J Am Coll Cardiol. 2018;72(17):2040–50. https://doi.org/10.1016/j.jacc.2018.07.092.

82. Nitsche C, Scully PR, Patel KP, Kammerlander AA, Koschutnik M, Dona C, et al. Prevalence and outcomes of concomitant aortic stenosis and cardiac amyloidosis. J Am Coll Cardiol. 2021;77(2):128–39. https://doi.org/10.1016/j.jacc.2020.11.006.
83. Sack GH Jr. Serum amyloid A—a review. Mol Med. 2018;24:46. https://doi.org/10.1186/s10020-018-0047-0.
84. Mirioglu S, Uludag O, Hurdogan O, Kumru G, Berke I, Doumas SA, et al. AA amyloidosis: a contemporary view. Curr Rheumatol Rep. 2024;26(3):248–59. https://doi.org/10.1007/s11926-024-01147-8.
85. Bunker D, Gorevic P. AA amyloidosis: Mount Sinai experience, 1997–2012. Mt Sinai J Med. 2012;79(6):749–56. https://doi.org/10.1002/msj.21342.
86. Lachmann HJ, Goodman HJB, Gilbertson JA, Gallimore JR, Sabin CA, Gillmore JD, Hawkins PN. Natural history and outcome in systemic AA amyloidosis. N Engl J Med. 2007;356(23):2361–71. https://doi.org/10.1056/NEJMoa070265.
87. Dubrey SW, Cha K, Simms RW, Skinner M, Falk RH. Electrocardiography and Doppler echocardiography in secondary (AA) amyloidosis. Am J Cardiol. 1996;77(4):313–5. https://doi.org/10.1016/s0002-9149(97)89403-9.
88. Morris AD, Smith RN, Stone JR. The pathology and changing epidemiology of dialysis-related cardiac beta-2 microglobulin amyloidosis. Cardiovasc Pathol. 2019;42:30–5.
89. Takayama F, Miyazaki S, Morita T, Hirasawa Y, Niwa T. Dialysis-related amyloidosis of the heart in long-term hemodialysis patients. Kidney Int Suppl. 2001;78:S172–6.
90. Kawano M, Muramoto H, Yamada M, Minamoto M, Araki H, Koni I, et al. Fatal cardiac beta2-microglobulin amyloidosis in patients on long-term hemodialysis. Am J Kidney Dis. 1998;31(3):E4. https://doi.org/10.1053/ajkd.1998.v31.pgE4.
91. Ioannou A, Porcari A, Patel RK, Razvi Y, Sinigiani G, Martinez-Naharro A, et al. Rare forms of cardiac amyloidosis: diagnostic clues and phenotype in Apo AI and AIV amyloidosis. Circ Cardiovasc Imaging. 2023;16: e015259. https://doi.org/10.1161/CIRCIMAGING.123.015259.
92. Saleem M, Balla S, Amin MS, Farid S, Caccamo M, Sokos G, Bianco CM. Hereditary apolipoprotein A-I–associated cardiac amyloidosis: importance of endomyocardial biopsy when suspicion remains high. JACC Case Rep. 2021;3(7):1032–7. https://doi.org/10.1016/j.jaccas.2021.02.016.

The ECG in Cardiac Amyloidosis

Bernard Belhassen

Abstract Cardiac amyloidosis (CA) is a restrictive cardiomyopathy resulting from the deposition of amyloid fibrils in the myocardial interstitium. Most cases of CA result from fibrils composed of either monoclonal immunoglobulin light chains, or transthyretin protein transthyretin (wild-type or hereditary variants). Although the diagnosis of CA is based on invasive pathology demonstration of amyloid deposits, or non-invasive criteria using advanced cardiovascular imaging techniques, the 12-lead ECG plays a crucial importance in the suspicion of the diagnosis of CA when showing (a) low QRS voltages in limb leads contrasting with marked left ventricular hypertrophy on echocardiogram, (b) marked interatrial, atrioventricular and intraventricular conduction disturbances, (c) pseudo-infarct patterns contrasting with preserved left ventricular function, and finally (d) various types of atrial and ventricular arrhythmias. The treatment of CA has dramatically improved in the last few years with the increased usage of novel therapies. An early suspicion of the diagnosis has dramatically improved the result of treatment. The ECG is playing a crucial role in establishing this early diagnosis.

Keywords ECG · Cardiac amyloidosis · Immunoglobulin light-chain · Transthyretin protein transthyretin · Bundle branch block · Atrial fibrillation

Introduction

Cardiac amyloidosis (CA) is a restrictive cardiomyopathy resulting from the deposition of amyloid fibrils in the myocardial interstitium [1]. While only nine amyloidogenic proteins accumulate in the myocardium to cause significant cardiac disease, > 98% of currently diagnosed CA results from fibrils composed of monoclonal immunoglobulin light chains (AL), the commonest cause of CA, or when they

B. Belhassen (✉)
Heart Institute, Hadassah Medical Center, Jerusalem, Israel
e-mail: bblhass@gmail.com

Tel-Aviv University, Tel-Aviv, Israel

E. Herzog (ed.), *Cardiac Amyloidosis*, https://doi.org/10.1007/978-3-031-88342-2_3

are composed of the transthyretin protein transthyretin (ATTR) [2]. In the latter instance, this can occur in the context of variant (v) or wild-type (wt) genetics as the heteritary-variant (ATTRv) or the acquired (ATTRwt) form [2].

The diagnosis of CA includes two critical phases: (a) a suspicious phase and (b) a definite diagnosis phase during which appropriate typing of the amyloid is performed allowing to guide specific treatment [2].

ECG has been used as a first-line diagnostic tool in the evaluation of both asymptomatic and symptomatic individuals [3]. ECG is abnormal in most of patients with cardiac involvement. Newly acquired knowledge on genotype–phenotype correlations has now made the ECG a useful tool to guide the etiological diagnosis ("red flags") and provide prognostic stratification [3].

Baseline Atrial Rhythm

Amyloid infiltration of atrial myocardium is associated with diastolic dysfunction, and progressive increase in atrial pressure and atrial size. This explains the high prevalence of atrial fibrillation (AF) which is the most common rhythm disturbance in CA. Evidence from prospective and retrospective studies have shown that the prevalence of AF in CA is between 10 and 69% [4] (Figs. 1, 2 and 3).

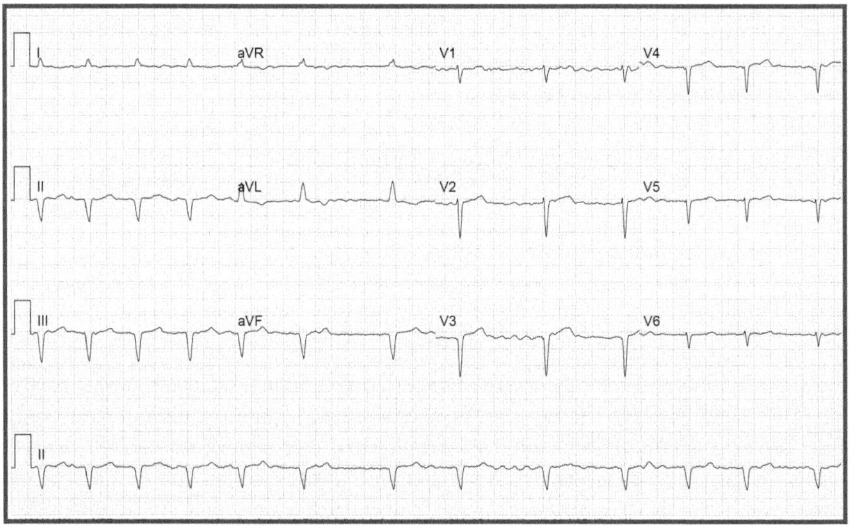

Fig. 1 A 48-year-old man with AL cardiac amyloidosis. Atrial fibrillation is present (mean heart rate of 75 bpm). There is a mild decrease of QRS voltage in limb leads (only 2 leads showing voltage of less than 0.5 mV). There is a poor R-wave progression in precordial leads with a pseudo-infarct pattern. Also note similar pseudo-infarct pattern in inferior leads. In contrast, echocardiogram showed a concentric left ventricular hypertrophy with a mild decrease of the ejection fraction. Global longitudinal strain was abnormal at − 9.7%

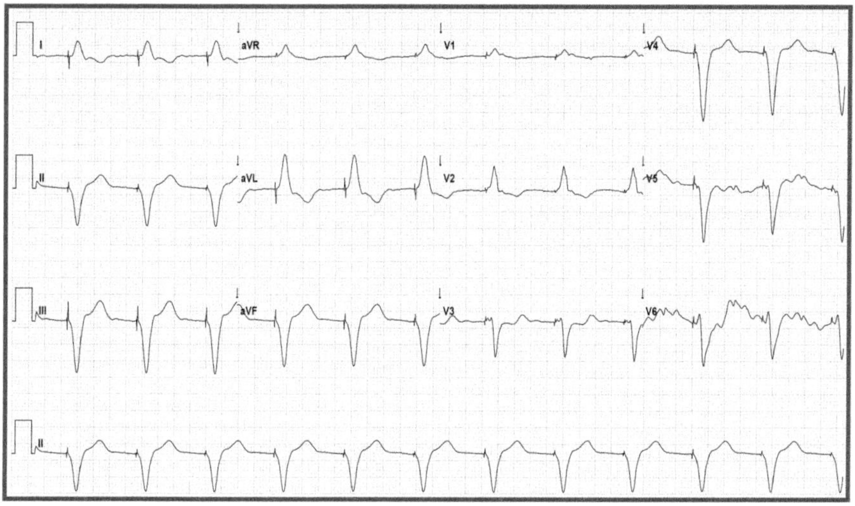

Fig. 2 An 82-year-old man with ATTRwt cardiac amyloidosis treated with Tafamidis for 2 years. The patient has a long history of chronic atrial fibrillation and received a ventricular pacemaker 8 years earlier because of complete atrioventricular infranodal block. Echocardiogram shows moderate to severe concentric left ventricular hypertrophy associated with a moderately reduced left ventricular function (45%). The global longitudinal strain is − 6.4%. Patient presentation at time of cardiac amyloidosis diagnosis frequently associates chronic atrial fibrillation and pacemaker implantation

Rapezzi and coworkers compared 3 groups of patients with CA and found that AF was more prevalent in patients with ATTRwt (27%) than in patients with AL (12%) or those with ATTRv (5%) ($p = 0.046$) [5]. Capelli et al. found that one-third of their 108 ATTRwt patients presented with AF compared with 20% of their 30 ATTRv and only 6% of those with 106 AL-CA [6].

The higher AF prevalence in the ATTRwt group when compared with AL-CA or ATTRv, has been attributed to the fact that ATTRwt patients are more likely to be elderly, male, with a longer duration of heart failure, increasing their risk [7, 8].

Approximately half of patients with ATTR-CA had AF/AFL prior to the diagnosis, another quarter were incidentally diagnosed with AF/AFL based on ambulatory monitoring while the remaining quarter were diagnosed following occurrence of symptoms [9].

When sinus rhythm is present, inter-atrial blocks, either partial or advanced, are frequent in patients with CA, being detected in 29% and 7%, respectively in a cohort of 96 CA patients (AL, $n = 40$; ATTR, $n = 56$) [10] (Fig. 4). During a median 1.5-year follow up, new-onset AF occurred in almost one third of sinus rhythm patients with CA [10]. Patients with partial or advanced inter-atrial blocks were more likely to develop atrial fibrillation during follow-up than those with no inter-atrial block.

Unexpectedly, CA rarely presents as sick sinus syndrome, and only a few cases have been reported in the literature [4, 11]. A higher index of suspicion is needed to diagnose CA in patients presenting with sick sinus syndrome.

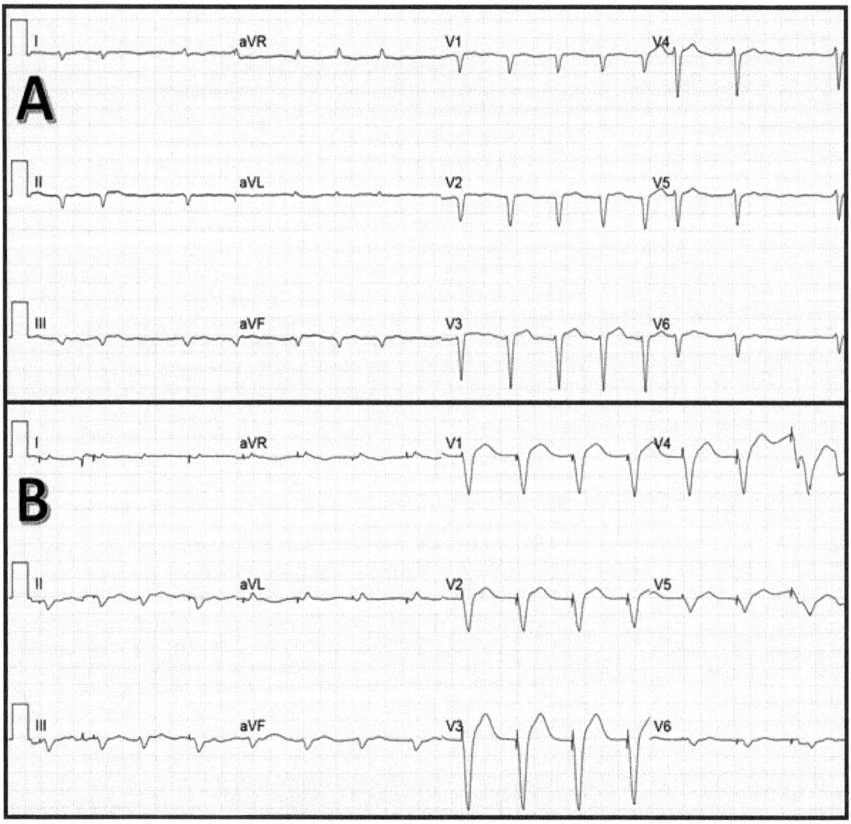

Fig. 3 A 66-year-old man with AL cardiac amyloidosis undiagnosed for several years who presented with advanced congestive heart failure and severe left ventricular dysfunction. **a** Atrial fibrillation with wide QRS complexes suggesting a left intraventricular conduction delay and a northwest QRS axis deviation. Note the poor R wave progression in precordial leads with normal QRS voltage contrasting with a markedly reduced QRS voltage (less than 0.5 mV) in all limb leads. **b** Effects of right ventricular pacing. Note the persistence of the marked discrepancy between the normal QRS voltage in precordial leads and the low QRS voltage in limb leads

Atrioventricular and Intraventricular Conduction

Conduction disease is highly prevalent in CA, and mainly affects the His-Purkinje system and the intraventricular conduction [12]. The pathophysiology to explain this remains incompletely understood. A review of autopsies of 23 patients with CA and clinical arrhythmias [13] demonstrated that only 3 of 23 patients had histologic evidence of amyloid involvement of the conduction system tissue.

In a study of 233 patients, Rapezzi et al. [5] found that first-degree AV block was present in 18% of those with AL, in 25% of those with ATTRv but in up to 33% of those with ATTRwt (P = 0.34) (Figs. 5 and 6). Right bundle branch block (19%,

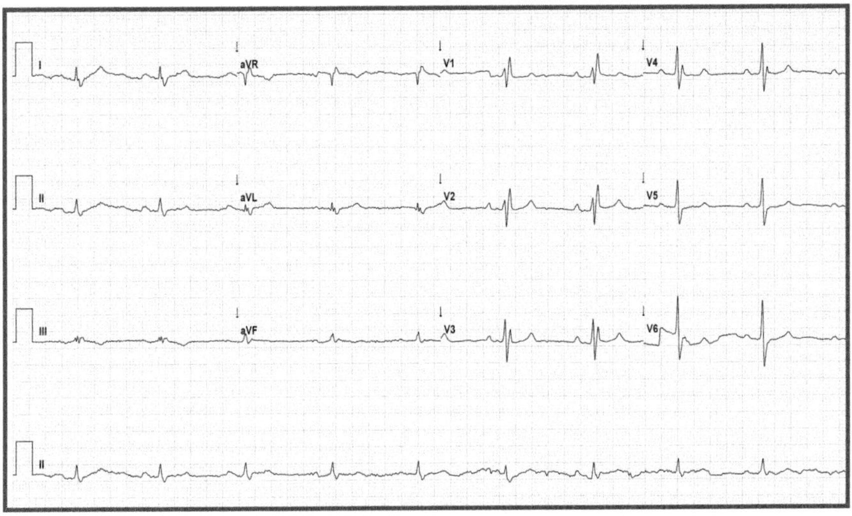

Fig. 4 An 84-year-old man with AL cardiac amyloidosis and hypertrophic cardiomyopathy (MYBC3). The ECG shows: 1) First degree intra-atrial conduction block as attested by a wide P wave duration (#160 ms); 2) Borderline PR interval (200 ms); 3) Low QRS voltage (less than 0.5 mV) in 3 of 6 limb leads (III, aVL and aVF) while the QRS voltage is between 0.5 to 0.6 mV in the remaining 3 limb leads; 4) Right bundle branch block with normal QRS voltage in precordial leads

12% and 13%) and left anterior hemiblock (29%, 30% and 20%) were present in similar proportions of patients in the Al, ATTRv and ATTRwt types, respectively (Figs. 4 and 7). However, left bundle branch block was more frequent in ATTRwt (40%) than in AL (4%) and ATTRv (7%) AC types ($P < 0.0001$) (Figs. 5 and 8).

There have been few reports dealing with the cardiac electrophysiologic findings in CA patients. In a series of 25 patients with AL-CA, Reisinger et al. [14] found that AV node conduction was borderline or within normal limits, whereas disturbances in the His-Purkinje system were common including marked prolongation of the HV interval, even in the presence of a narrow QRS complex suggesting an involvement of the distal His conduction in the latter group. Moreover, a significant association between HV interval prolongation and the occurrence of sudden death was found among those patients who died during follow-up [13].

In another study involving 18 CA patients with supraventricular tachyarrhythmias, Barbhaiya et al. [15] noted that the HV interval was prolonged (> 55 ms) in all CA patients, including 6 with normal QRS duration (≤ 100 ms), this involvement of the cardiac conduction system may lead to the need of pacemaker (PM) implantation. Rappezi et al. [5] were first to report that 13% of patients with ATTRwt-CA had pacemakers implanted prior to diagnosis compared with 3% of those with AL-CA or ATTRv-CA (Fig. 2).

In a single center retrospective study including 369 patients with ATTR-CA, Donnellan et al. showed that 9.5% had pacemakers implanted for high-grade AV

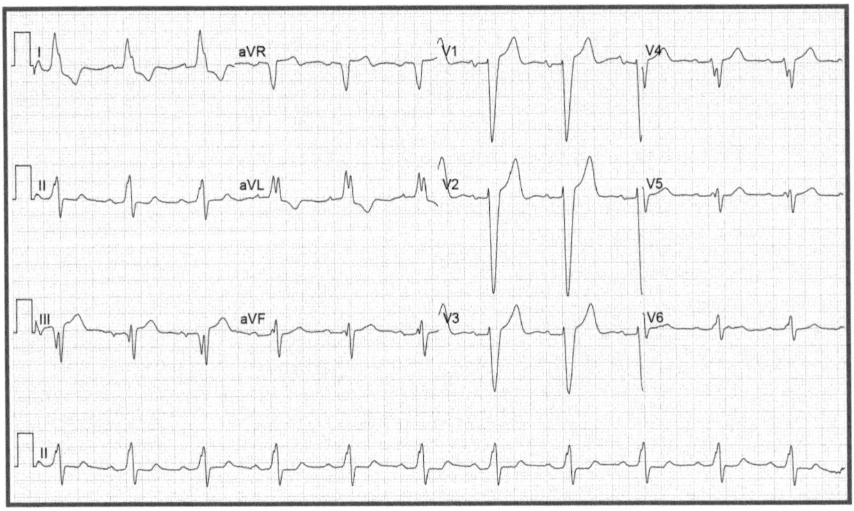

Fig. 5 An 88-year-old woman who presented with syncope with an ECG showing complete left bundle branch block. PR interval was prolonged (228 ms). Echocardiogram showed severe concentric left ventricular hypertrophy with an abnormal global longitudinal strain of – 10%. A diagnosis of cardiac amyloidosis was suspected and she was referred for complementary examinations (see Fig. 8)

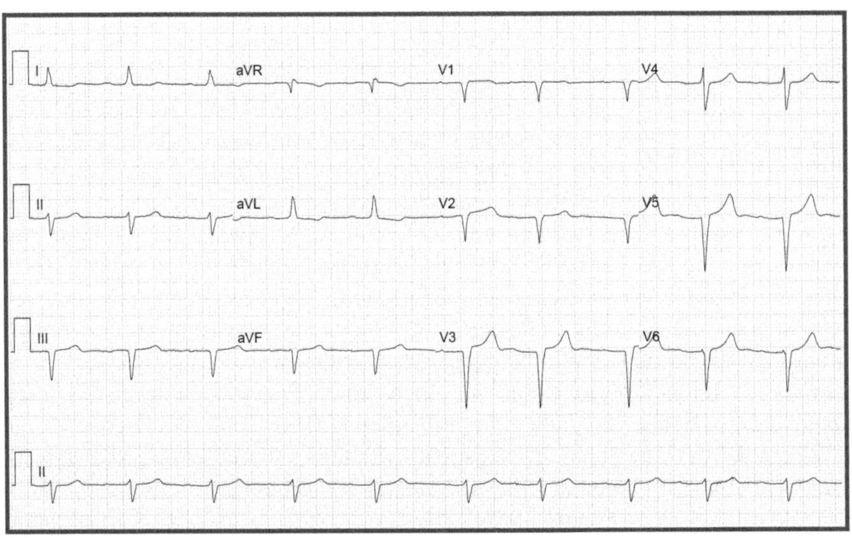

Fig. 6 A 91-year-old man with ATTRwt cardiac amyloidosis. This patient has left ventricular hypertrophy with preserved left ventricular systolic function and diastolic dysfunction. There is baseline sinus rhythm (59 bpm) with slow amplitude P waves associated with prolonged PR (240 ms). A pseudo-pattern of infarct is observed in the anterior leads

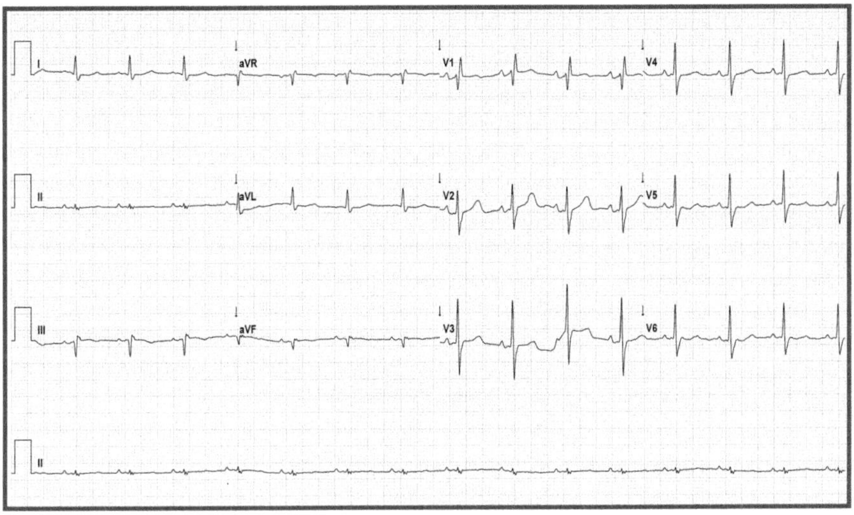

Fig. 7 An 84-year-old man with AL cardiac amyloidosis. A markedly reduced QRS voltage (less than 0.5 mV) is present in 3 limb leads (II, aVR and aVF). This contrasts with the normal QRS amplitude in precordial leads. There are Q waves in leads III and aVF which suggest a prior myocardial infarction. An incomplete right bundle branch block (QRS duration 98 ms) is also observed

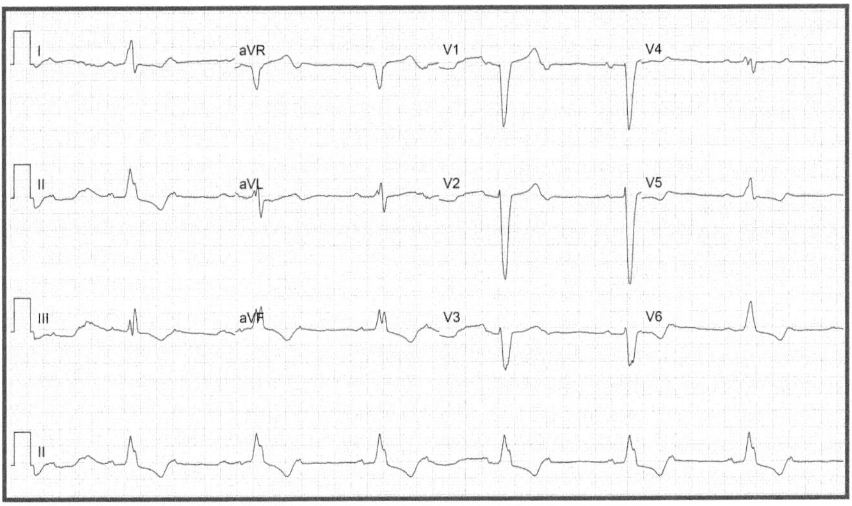

Fig. 8 Same patient as in Fig. 5. One year after the first episode of syncope, she was hospitalized due to pulmonary edema. A 2:1 atrioventricular block was now documented. Note the different QRS axis (rightward shift) as compared with previous ECG. ATTRwt cardiac amyloidosis was diagnosed in this patient

block before their diagnosis with CA [16]. During a follow-up period of 28 months, a further 11% developed a pacemaker requirement for high-degree AV block (Fig. 8). No significant differences in the development of AV block were observed across disease stages, and only a QRS duration ≥ 120 ms was associated with an elevated risk of high-grade AV block suggesting an infranodal location of the block [16].

Finally, according to the largest study to date on the prevalence and incidence of PM implantation on 459 CA patients (27.7% AL, 14.4% ATTRv and 58% ATTRwt), Porcari et al. [17] showed that the rate of PM implantation for AV conduction disorders was similar in AL-CA and ATTR-CA (8.4% and 9.1%, respectively).

Low QRS Voltage (LQRSV) in Limb Leads.

LQRSV is usually defined as a QRS voltage < 0.5 mV in each limb lead. This sign has been observed in 27% to 56% of 3 series of biopsy-proven CA [18–20] and in 54.5% of patients in a large CA group mainly diagnosed from typical echocardiographic features and pathological evidence of extra-cardiac tissue or organ [21]. An increased amyloid burden has been associated with lower voltages in CA patients [22] (Figs. 3, 4 and 7). More recent studies according to CA subtypes have shown a higher prevalence of LQRSV in AL (45–60%) than in ATTR (27.7–35.4%) [5, 6, 23, 24]. Such results suggest that amyloid infiltration is not the only determinant for LQRSV [24]. Importantly, one of the most classical landmarks of CA is the marked disproportion between QRS voltage in limb leads and left ventricular thickness or mass on cardiac imaging [5, 18, 23–26]. However, it is noteworthy that although LVQRS is more common in AL-CA than in ATTR-CA, the latter usually present greater LV thickness and mass than in AL-CA [5, 23].

Pseudo-Infarct Pattern

A pseudo-infarct pattern, defined as the presence of Q waves in ≥ 2 consecutive leads in the absence of a previously known myocardial infarction, has been frequently observed in CA patients (Figs. 1, 3, 6 and 9). It is generally explained by a phenomenon of myocardial ischemia due to obstructive intramural coronary amyloidosis [27, 28].

In the first largest series which analyzed the prevalence of pseudo-infarct pattern, Dubrey et al. [29] reported a prevalence of 74.7% in 229 patients with AL-CA. In two subsequent studies of biopsy-proven CA [18, 19] and in a large CA group mainly diagnosed from typical echocardiographic features and pathological evidence of extra-cardiac tissue or organ [21], the prevalences were 47%, 60% and 40.2%, respectively. In a series of 110 AL-CA patients, Zhao et al. [30] found a pseudo-infarct pattern in 36.4% patients. Finally, markedly different figures were found in two studies of CA patients. In a study of 233 patients, Rapezzi et al. [5] found that a pseudo-infarct pattern was present in 69%, 69% and 66% of those with AL-CA, ATTRv-CA and ATTRwt-CA, respectively. In another study of 244 patients, Capelli et al. [6] found a pseudo-infarct pattern in 39%, 23% and 34%, respectively, in the same categories of patients. A possible explanation for the discrepancy between the results of these two studies may be that the patient populations were studied at a decade interval while the patients reported in the Rapezzi's et al. paper [5] were likely diagnosed late in more advanced stages of the disease, thus having more ECG abnormalities (Prof. Giampaolo Merlini, Pavia, Italy, personal communication).

Importantly, Cheng and associates found that the combination of low QRS voltage on limb leads and a pseudo-infarct pattern had high specificity and positive predictive value for the diagnosis of CA [21]. Finally, Zhao et al. [30] found that a pseudo-infarct pattern was associated with a worse prognosis independently of indices of the extent of amyloid infiltration (such as left ventricular mass index), systolic and diastolic dysfunction.

Cardiac Amyloidosis and Bundle Branch Block

The ECG or mass/voltage criteria established for patients with a narrow QRS in the diagnosis of CA may not be applicable in patients with a bundle branch block. Sharma and coworkers found that a total QRS score/left ventricular wall thickness ratio < 92.5 mV/cm (total QRS score defined as the sum of QRS amplitude in all 12 ECG leads) was 100% sensitive and 83% specific in the diagnosis of CA [31].

Ventricular Arrhythmias

Ventricular arrhythmias, such as ventricular premature beats (VPB's), frequently multifocal, and nonsustained ventricular tachycardia (NSVT), are frequently observed on standard ECG and Holter monitoring, regardless of the amyloidosis subtype. In a systematic review and meta-analysis of data from 194 CA patients who received an ICD (67% for primary prevention and 33% for secondary prevention), Halawa et al. found that the frequency of appropriate implanted cardioverter-defibrillator treatment in CA is low and not predicted by NSVT [32]. Cappelli and coworkers reached similar conclusions after comparing CA patients with (n = 53) and without (n = 128) NSVT [33]. The presence of NSVT on 24-h ECG monitoring did not confer a worse survival, suggesting that these arrhythmias may be considered a marker of disease severity rather than a predictor of arrhythmic mortality.

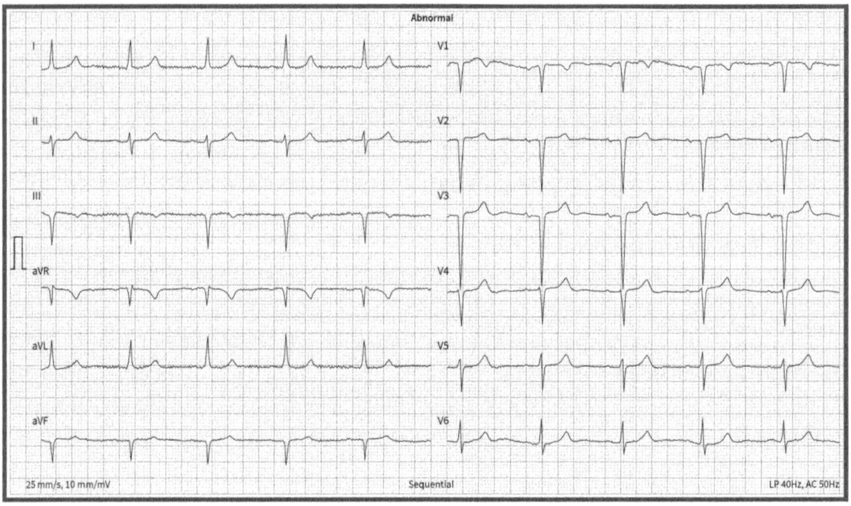

Fig. 9 ECG obtained in a 93-year-old man with AL cardiac amyloidoisis associated with severe aortic stenosis and coronary artery disease. Sinus rhythm at a rate of 59 bpm is present with normal PR and QRS durations. Note the flatted P waves in limb leads. There is a pseudo-infarct pattern in V1–V4. This patient has a preserved left ventricular ejection fraction with concentric left ventricular hypertrophy and a borderline global longitudinal strain of − 17%

Differentiation of Cardiac Amyloidosis and Nonobstructive Hypertrophic Cardiomyopathy

Clinically, some CA patients may be misdiagnosed as hypertrophic heart disease, mostly nonobstructive hypertrophic cardiomyopathy (NOHCM) by echocardiography and contrast enhanced computed tomography. Huang and coworkers [34] compared 46 CA patients with 64 patients with NOHCM and found that the ECG may be very useful in differentiating between these two diseases. Compared with NOHCM patients, CA patients showed more ECG characteristics of low voltage in limb leads (50% vs. 1.6%), pseudo-infarct pattern (84.8% vs. 39.1%), AV block (21.7% vs. 4.7%), and longer QRS duration (104 ms vs. 98 ms) (all $P < 0.05$). The combination of the R wave voltage of I and avR reached a sensitivity of 95% and a specificity of 87% for the diagnosis of CA (Fig. 9).

QRS Fragmentation

In AL-CA, the 12-lead ECG reflects myocardial amyloid infiltration with low limb voltages, pseudo-infarct patterns, and conduction abnormalities. In addition, it is not unusual to see other QRS complex abnormalities, such as notches and RsR' pattern in the absence of QRS prolongation, i.e. a fragmentation of QRS complexes (fQRS). Perlini and coworkers [35] compared the 12-lead ECG of 375 patients with AL amyloidosis (264 with and 111 without heart involvement). They found that the prevalence of QRS fragmentation (fQRS) was significantly higher in patients with cardiac AL amyloidosis (28.5% vs. 11.7%; $P = 0.0008$). In addition, they found that the presence of fQRS at diagnosis has an independent prognostic value with a significantly higher mortality in the fQRS group when compared with the no-fQRS group ($P = 0.0008$).

These results were confirmed by Guo and coworkers [36] who also found that fQRS could be used as an alternative marker when cardiac magnetic resonance is not available.

Frontal QRS-T Angle

The electrocardiographic spatial QRS-T angle reflects changes in the direction of the repolarization sequence and is a powerful predictor of outcome in patients with heart failure. In a study of 43 patients with AL-CA, Medvedovsky and associates [37] found that a frontal QRS-T angle > 102° is associated with indices of advanced amyloid disease and is an independent predictor of survival.

Early Diagnosis and Artificial Intelligence

Although likely underdiagnosed, cardiac amyloidosis is a rare disease. Since it is associated with high rates of morbidity and mortality, there is a pressing clinical need for an easy-to-deploy, scalable test for early detection, especially given the emergence of effective therapies that dramatically improve its prognosis [1]. Considering that the 12-lead ECG is almost always abnormal in CA patients, the application of artificial intelligence (AI) may be of great value for detecting minimal ECG changes years before the diagnosis is made. Grogan and coworkers from the Mayo Clinic [38] developed an AI based tool to detect CA from a standard 12-lead ECG. They found that (1) The AI 12-lead ECG alone can accurately predict CA; (2) The model performed well across amyloid subtypes; (3) Their model was able to predict CA in advance of the clinical diagnosis in almost 60% of cases; (4) The tool may be adapted to 6-lead and single-lead ECG acquisitions, allowing point-of-care screening by smartphone-enabled electrodes.

References

1. Kittleson MM, Ruberg FL, Ambardekar AV, et al. 2023 ACC expert consensus decision pathway on comprehensive multidisciplinary care for the patient with cardiac amyloidosis: a report of the American college of cardiology solution set oversight committee. J Am Coll Cardiol. 2023;81:1076–126.
2. Garcia-Pavia P, Rapezzi C, Adler Y, et al. Diagnosis and treatment of cardiac amyloidosis: a position statement of the ESC working group on myocardial and pericardial diseases. Eur Heart J. 2021;42:1554–68.
3. Silvetti E, Lanza O, Romeo F, et al. The pivotal role of ECG in cardiomyopathies. Front Cardiovasc Med. 2023;10:1178163.
4. Hartnett J, Jaber W, Maurer M, et al. Electrophysiological manifestations of cardiac amyloidosis. JACC CardioOncol. 2021;3:506–15.
5. Rapezzi C, Merlini G, Quarta CC. Systemic cardiac amyloidoses: disease profiles and clinical courses of the 3 main types. Circulation. 2009;120:1203–12.
6. Cappelli F, Vignini E, Martone R, et al. Baseline ECG features and arrhythmic profile in transthyretin versus light chain cardiac amyloidosis. Circ Heart Fail. 2020;13: e006619.
7. Longhi S, Quarta CC, Milandri A, et al. Atrial fibrillation in amyloidotic cardiomyopathy: prevalence, incidence, risk factors and prognostic role. Amyloid. 2015;22:147–55.
8. Sanchis K, Cariou E, Colombat M, et al. Atrial fibrillation and subtype of atrial fibrillation in cardiac amyloidosis: clinical and echocardiographic features, impact on mortality. Amyloid. 2019;26:128–38.
9. Dale Z, Chandrashekar P, Al-Rashdan L, et al. Routine ambulatory heart rhythm monitoring for detection of atrial arrhythmias in transthyretin cardiac amyloidosis. Int J Cardiol. 2022;358:65–71.
10. Sinigiani G, De Michieli L, Porcari A, et al. Atrial electrofunctional predictors of incident atrial fibrillation in cardiac amyloidosis. Heart Rhythm. 2024;21:725–32. https://doi.org/10.1016/j.hrthm.2024.01.056. Online ahead of print.
11. Abdelazeem B, Malik B, Baral N, Gjeka R, Kunadi A. A case report of sick sinus syndrome as an initial presentation of primary amyloidosis. Cureus. 2021;13: e13922.
12. Alreshq R, Tugal D, Siddiqi O, Ruberg F. Conduction abnormalities and role of cardiac pacing in cardiac amyloidosis: a systematic review. Pacing Clin Electrophysiol. 2021;44:2092–9.
13. Ridolfi RL, Bulkley BH, Hutchins GM. The conduction system in cardiac amyloidosis. Clinical and pathologic features of 23 patients. Am J Med. 1977;62:677–678.
14. Reisinger J, Dubrey SW, Lavalley M, Skinner M, Falk RH. Electrophysiologic abnormalities in AL (primary) amyloidosis with cardiac involvement. J Am Coll Cardiol. 1997;30:1046–51.
15. Barbhaiya CR, Kumar S, Baldinger SH, et al. Electrophysiologic assessment of conduction abnormalities and atrial arrhythmias associated with amyloid cardiomyopathy. Heart Rhythm. 2016;13:383–90.
16. Donnellan E, Wazni OM, Hanna M, et al. Atrial fibrillation in transthyretin cardiac amyloidosis: predictors, prevalence, and efficacy of rhythm control strategies. J Am Coll Cardiol EP. 2020;6:1118–27.
17. Porcari A, Rossi M, Cappelli F, Canepa M, Musumeci B, Cipriani A, et al. Incidence and risk factors for pacemaker implantation in light-chain and transthyretin cardiac amyloidosis. Eur J Heart Fail. 2022;24:1227–36.
18. Murtagh B, Hammill SC, Gertz MA, et al. Electrocardiographic findings in primary systemic amyloidosis and biopsy-proven cardiac involvement. Am J Cardiol. 2005;95:535–7.
19. Rahman JE, Helou EF, Gelzer-Bell R, et al. Noninvasive diagnosis of biopsy-proven cardiac amyloidosis. J Am Coll Cardiol. 2004;43:410–5.
20. Austin BA, Duffy B, Tan C, et al. Comparison of functional status, electrocardiographic, and echocardiographic parameters to mortality in endomyocardial-biopsy proven cardiac amyloidosis. Am J Cardiol. 2009;103:1429–33.
21. Cheng Z, Zhu K, Tian Z, Zhao D, Cui Q, Fang Q. The findings of electrocardiography in patients with cardiac amyloidosis. Ann Noninvasive Electrocardiol. 2013;18:157–62.

22. Duca F, Rettl R, Kronberger C, et al. Amyloid burden correlates with electrocardiographic findings in patients with cardiac amyloidosis-insights from histology and cardiac magnetic resonance imaging. J Clin Med. 2024;13:368–81.
23. Quarta CC, Solomon SD, Uraizee I, et al. Left ventricular structure and function in transthyretin-related versus light-chain cardiac amyloidosis. Circulation. 2014;129:1840–9.
24. Cipriani A, De Michieli L, Porcari A, Licchelli L, Sinigiani G, Tini G, et al. Low QRS voltages in cardiac amyloidosis: clinical correlates and prognostic value. JACC CardioOncol. 2022;4:458–70.
25. Carroll JD, Gaasch WH, McAdam KPWJ. Amyloid cardiomyopathy: characterization by a distinctive voltage/mass relation. Am J Cardiol. 1982;49:9–13.
26. Quarta CC, Borghi C, Perlini S, Musca F, Salinaro F. A simple voltage/mass index improves diagnosis of cardiac amyloidosis in patients with unexplained left ventricular "hypertrophy": an electrocardiographic and echocardiographic study of more than 500 patients. Circulation 2010;122:A16852 (abstract)
27. Neben-Wittich MA, Wittich CM, Mueller PS, Larson DR, Gertz MA, Edwards WD. Obstructive intramural coronary amyloidosis and myocardial ischemia are common in primary amyloidosis. Am J Med. 2005;118:1281–7.
28. Wittich CM, Neben-Wittich MA, Mueller PS, Gertz MA, Edwards WD. Deposition of amyloid proteins in the epicardial coronary arteries of 58 patients with primary systemic amyloidosis. Cardiovasc Pathol. 2007;16:75–8.
29. Dubrey SW, Cha K, Anderson J, Chamarthi B, Reisinger J, Skinner M, Falk RH. The clinical features of immunoglobulin light-chain (AL) amyloidosis with heart involvement. Quart J Med. 1998;91:141–57.
30. Zhao L, Li J, Tian Z, Fang Q. Clinical correlates and prognostic values of pseudoinfarction in cardiac light-chain amyloidosis. J Cardiol. 2016;68:426–30.
31. Sharma S, Labib SB, Shah SP. Electrocardiogram criteria to diagnose cardiac amyloidosis in men with a bundle branch block. Am J Cardiol. 2021;146:89–94.
32. Halawa A, Woldu HG, Kacey KG, Alpert MA. Effect of ICD implantation on cardiovascular outcomes in patients with cardiac amyloidosis: a systematic review and meta-analysis. J Cardiovasc Electrophysiol. 2020;31:1749–58.
33. Cappelli F, Cipriani A, Russo D, et al. Prevalence and prognostic role of nonsustained ventricular tachycardia in cardiac amyloidosis. Amyloid. 2022;29:211–2.
34. Huang J, Zhao S, Chen Z, Zhang S, Lu M. Contribution of electrocardiogram in the differentiation of cardiac amyloidosis and nonobstructive hypertrophic cardiomyopathy. Int Heart J. 2015;56:522–6.
35. Perlini S, Salinaro F, Cappelli F, et al. Prognostic value of fragmented QRS in cardiac AL amyloidosis. Int J Cardiol. 2013;167:2156–61.
36. Guo X, Chen Z, Wan K, et al. Electrocardiogram characteristics and prognostic value in light-chain amyloidosis: a comparison with cardiac magnetic resonance imaging. Front Cardiovasc Med. 2021;8: 751422.
37. Medvedovsky AT, Pollak A, Shuvy M, Gotsman I. Prognostic significance of the frontal QRS-T angle in patients with AL cardiac amyloidosis. J Electrocardiol. 2020;59:122–5.
38. Grogan M, Lopez-Jimenez F, Cohen-Shelly M, et al. Artificial intelligence–enhanced electrocardiogram for the early detection of cardiac amyloidosis. Mayo Clin Proc. 2021;96:2768–78.

Echocardiography in Cardiac Amyloidosis

David Leibowitz and Eyal Herzog

Abstract Echocardiographic imaging is crucial for the diagnostic, prognostic and therapeutic assessment of unexplained heart failure or clinically suspected cardiac amyloidosis (CA) patients. Echocardiographic imaging in CA should include cardiac morphology as well as a comprehensive assessment of systolic and diastolic function including strain imaging and hemodynamic assessment of filling pressures. Important echocardiographic findings in CA include thickening of the left ventricular walls as well as thickening of other cardiac structures. Reduced systolic function is frequently noted in CA even in the presence of normal ejection function and more advanced techniques such as global longitudinal strain are necessary to accurately assess systolic function in these patients. CA causes a broad spectrum of diastolic dysfunction (DD) with more severe DD manifesting later in the disease course. Tissue Doppler diastolic annular velocities are reduced and an elevated high E:e′ reflecting increased LV filling pressures is commonly seen in CA.

Keywords Echocardiography · Cardiac amyloidosis · Wall thickness · Strain imaging · Diastolic dysfunction · Atrial dysfunction

Introduction

Echocardiography is usually the initial imaging test performed in patients presenting with unexplained heart failure or with clinically suspected cardiac amyloidosis (CA) and is crucial for the diagnostic, prognostic and therapeutic assessment of these patients. It is important to note that many of the typical echocardiographic findings in CA are most prominent in advanced cases of the disease, and accurate echocardiographic diagnosis earlier in the disease course requires a high level of suspicion. Echocardiographic imaging in CA should include cardiac morphology as well as a

D. Leibowitz (✉) · E. Herzog
Department of Cardiology, Hadassah Medical Center, Hebrew University of Jerusalem, Jerusalem, Israel
e-mail: oleiboeve@gmail.com

E. Herzog (ed.), *Cardiac Amyloidosis*, https://doi.org/10.1007/978-3-031-88342-2_4

comprehensive assessment of systolic and diastolic function including strain imaging and hemodynamic assessment of filling pressures.

Morphologic Changes

Left Ventricle

The hallmark morphological finding on echocardiography in CA is thickening of the left ventricular (LV) walls frequently leading to decreased LV chamber size. Previously described increased myocardial echogenicity or "speckling" has a high interobserver variability and does not appear to be sensitive or specific for the diagnosis of CA [1]. LV wall thickening is generally, although not always, symmetrical as seen in Fig. 1 and must be distinguished from other causes of wall thickening such as pressure-overload hypertrophy or hypertrophic cardiomyopathy (HCM) [2–4].

Assessment of voltage on ECG may be helpful in this differential diagnosis as in pressure overload hypertrophy, wall thickening is due to cardiomyocyte hypertrophy while in CA it is due to infiltration of amyloid deposits in the myocardium [5]. Due to this difference the ECG of patients with true left ventricular hypertrophy (LVH) demonstrate high QRS amplitudes on ECG whereas patients with cardiac amyloidosis may demonstrate low QRS amplitudes as noted in Fig. 2.

Even if QRS voltage in amyloidosis is preserved, it may be inappropriate for the degree of left ventricular mass and the ratio between the LV mass index (LVMi) (obtained by echocardiogram) to QRS amplitude may be a valuable diagnostic tool in CA. It is important to note that up to one-third of patients with CA will have

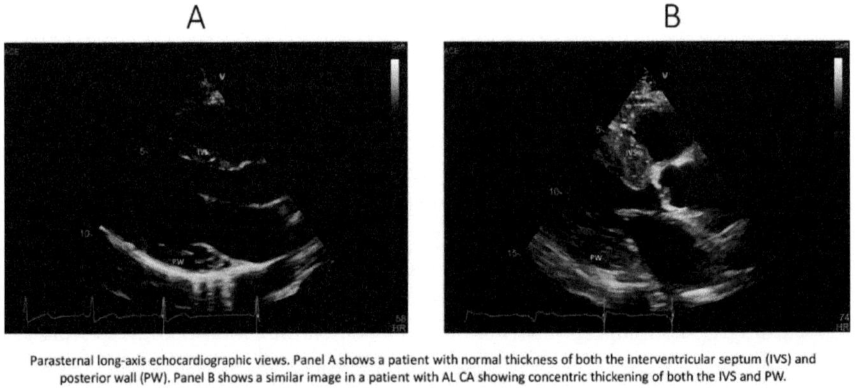

Fig. 1 Parasternal long-axis echocardiographic views. Panel A shows a patient with normal thickness of both the interventricular septum (IVS) and posterior wall (PW). Panel B shows a similar image in a patient with AL CA showing concentric thickening of both the IVS and PW

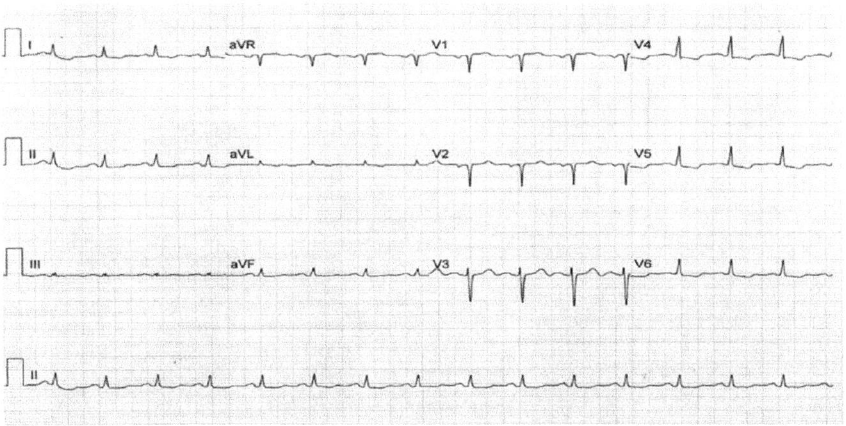

ECG of the patient depicted in Figure 1 panel B showing low QRS voltage in the presence of significant wall thickening. Low ECG voltage in this echocardiographic setting is highly suggestive of cardiac amyloidosis as explained in the text

Fig. 2 ECG of a patient depicted in Fig. 1 Panel B showing loss QRS voltage in the presence of significant wall thickening. Low ECG voltage in this echocardiographic setting is highly suggestive of cardiac amyloidosis as explained in the text

normal wall thickness and the absence of increased wall thickness does not rule out the diagnosis.

Other Cardiac Chambers

Another important echocardiographic clue to the diagnosis of CA is unexplained thickening of the other cardiac chambers which is rare in other diseases causing increased LV wall thickening such as HCM. Right ventricular (RV) wall thickness greater than 5 mm is suggestive of amyloid infiltration of these structures as seen in Fig. 3 [6]. Measurement of RV thickness should be obtained at end-diastole preferably from the subcostal view at 1 cm below the level of the tricuspid annulus [7].

Thickening of the interatrial septum of at least 6 mm is specific although not sensitive for the diagnosis of CA [6]. Biatrial enlargement due to chronically elevated ventricular filling pressures is common although not specific for CA [8]. Thickening of the atrial free walls due to amyloid deposition may be noted as well. Figure 4 demonstrates thickening of both the interatrial septum and right atrial free wall.

Patients with CA are predisposed to intracardiac thrombosis due to the hypercoagulability and vascular stasis seen in the disease and patients with concomitant atrial fibrillation are at particularly high risk as seen in Fig. 5 [9, 10].

Amyloid fibril deposition in the cardiac valves is most commonly associated with the aortic valve, however involvement of the mitral and tricuspid valves may

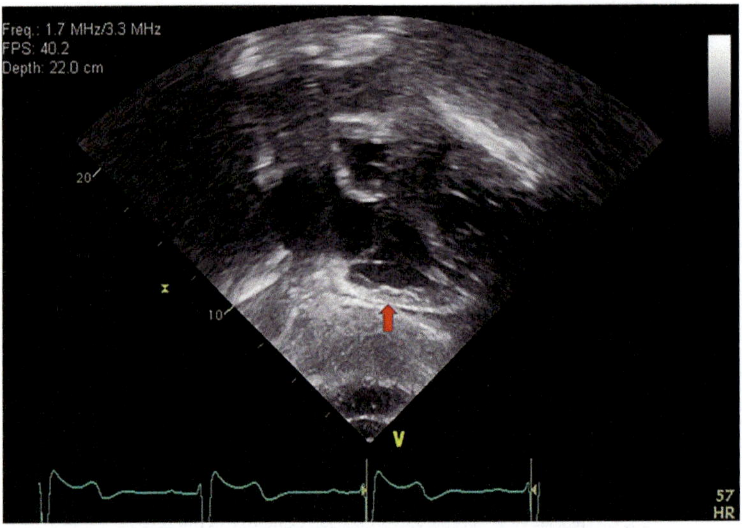

Fig. 3 Image from inverted subcostal view showing increased right ventricular wall thickness

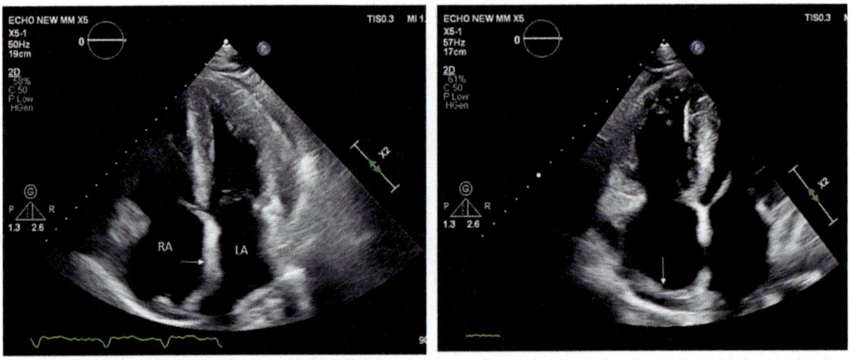

Fig. 4 Apical chamber views demonstrating a thickened interatrial septum (arrow, left image) and a thickened right atrial wall (arrow, right image) in patients with CA

be present [6]. As both degenerative aortic stenosis (AS) and CA (particularly due to wild type ATTR) are common in elderly patients, overlap of these diseases is common with up to 16% of patients undergoing TAVI having evidence of CA as well [11, 12]. Whether the overlap between AS and CA is causal or just associative remains unclear. Coexisting CA seems to be particularly common in paradoxical

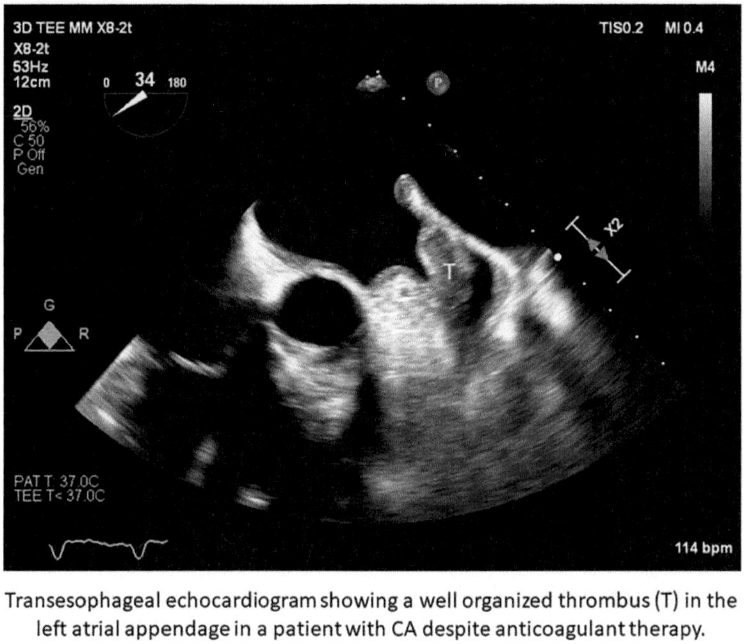

Fig. 5 Transesophageal echocardiogram showing a well organized thrombus (T) in the left atrial appendage in a patient with CA despite anticoagulant therapy

low flow low gradient AS patients due to the low stroke volume index as a result of concomitant amyloid infiltration in the myocardium.

Other Morphologic Changes

Finally, CA patients frequently present with pericardial effusions which are generally modest in size but are associated with reduced prognosis [13]. Effusions may be caused by both accumulation of amyloid fibrils in the pericardial space as well as right heart failure due to myocardial involvement. Another common morphologic finding in CA is a dilated inferior vena cava with reduced inspiratory collapse demonstrated in Fig. 6. This is due to elevated right atrial pressures frequently seen in CA.

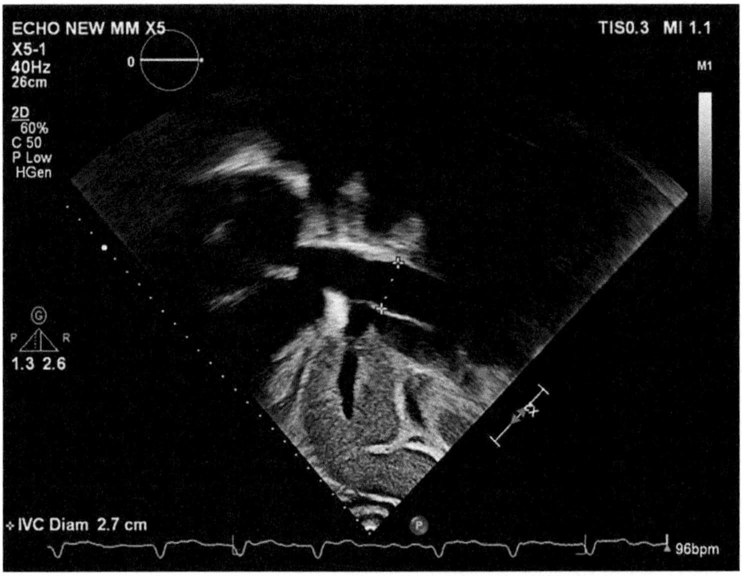

Image from inverted subcostal view a dilated inferior vena cava consistent with elevated right sided filling pressures in a patient with CA

Fig. 6 Image from inverted subcostal view a dilated inferior vena cava consistent with elevated right sided filling pressures in a patient with CA

Systolic Function

A. **Standard measurements**

Deposition and infiltration of amyloid fibrils into the myocardium impairs both systolic and diastolic function. Echocardiographic assessment of systolic function generally relies on measurement of LV ejection fraction (LVEF). LVEF relates stroke volume to end diastolic volume and does not directly include myocardial characteristics in the assessment of myocardial function. Therefore, in cardiovascular disorders with normal chamber sizes such as hypertrophic cardiomyopathy or amyloidosis, EF will not accurately reflect actual myocardial systolic function [14]. While LVEF decreases in advanced CA, systolic function may be impaired in patients with CA even in the presence of a normal LV ejection fraction [15]. Amyloid infiltration begins in the subendocardium which is primarily composed by longitudinal fibers. Techniques which assess longitudinal function may therefore be more sensitive for early systolic dysfunction than LVEF. It is therefore critical to perform additional assessment of myocardial longitudinal deformation using tissue Doppler and strain imaging [1]. Tissue Doppler imaging (TDI) measures longitudinal myocardial function by measuring annular displacement towards the ventricular apex. Systolic motion toward the annulus causes a systolic waveform (s wave) which is significantly reduced

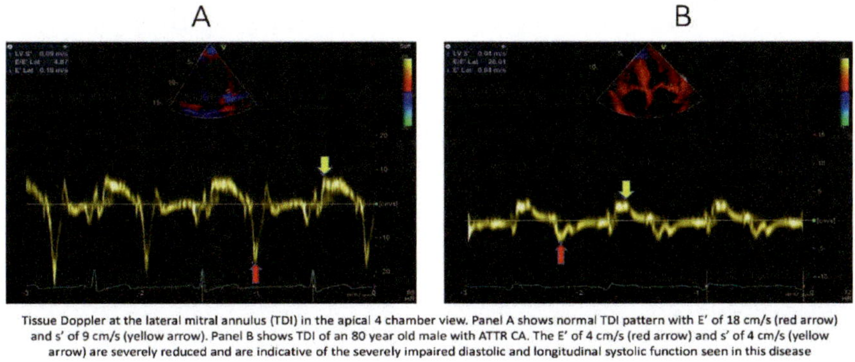

Fig. 7 Tissue Doppler at the lateral mitral annulus (TDI) in the apical 4 chamber view. Panel A shows normal TDI pattern with E′ of 18 cm/s (red arrow) and s′ of 9 cm/s (yellow arrow). Panel B shows TDI of an 80 year old male with ATTR CA. The E′ of 4 cm/s (red arrow) and 4 cm/s (yellow arrow) are severely reduced and are indicative of the severely impaired diastolic and longitudinal systolic function seen in this database

in CA due to amyloid fibrils interfering with longitudinal motion [16]. Figure 7 demonstrates reduced s wave TDI velocities in a patient with CA.

In CA, mitral annular s wave velocities are generally $\leq$ 6 cm/s. This measurement is simple to perform and does not require additional software. However, TDI cannot assess regional/segmental longitudinal motion, is angle-dependent, and velocities are influenced by translational and tethering movements.

B. **Strain imaging**

Global longitudinal strain (GLS) is a unitless measure of longitudinal deformation with more negative values indicating greater deformation/enhanced myocardial shortening. It has a high spatial and temporal resolution without many of the limitations of TDI. Generally, normal values are more negative than $-$ 18% however this measurement is vendor dependent and it is important to perform sequential studies using software from the same vendor. Reduced values of GLS may be noted in CA even if LVEF is preserved and are indicative of contractile dysfunction [17]. GLS of individual myocardial segments can also be calculated. In healthy subjects there is a base to apical gradient with increasing (i.e. more negative) GLS values in the apex, however this pattern is much more pronounced in CA with reduced longitudinal strain primarily in the basal and mid ventricular segments with apical sparing [18]. When plotted on a bull's eye map (standard for all strain software) this generates a characteristic "cherry on top" pattern as seen in Fig. 8.

This pattern appears to be caused by greater amyloid deposition in the basal segments. It is important to note that, contrary to previous reports, this pattern is not specific for CA and has been reported in patients with aortic stenosis and chronic renal failure [19, 20]. Calculating the ratio of ejection fraction to GLS is an alternative with a cutoff of > 4.1 having the highest diagnostic accuracy for a diagnosis of CA [21].

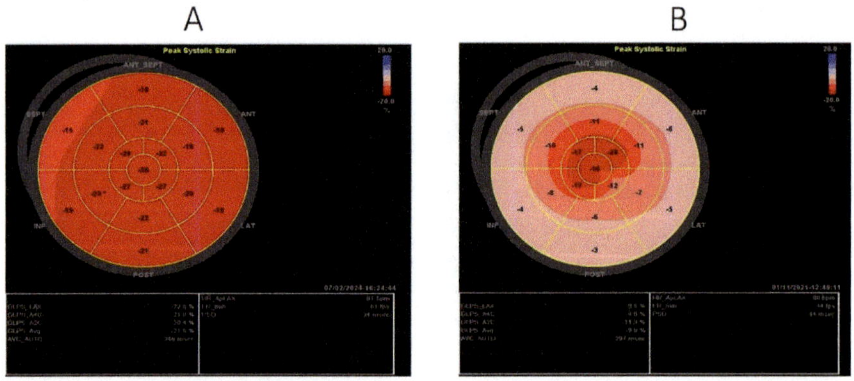

Left ventricular strain maps. Panel A shows normal strain pattern with a minimal gradient from the apical (central segments) to the base. Panel B shows a strain map in a patient with ATTR CA showing a large apical to base gradient resulting in a typical "cherry on top" pattern. Strain in the apical segments is relatively preserved while strain of the basal segments is severely reduced.

Fig. 8 Left ventricular strain maps. Panel A shows normal strain pattern with a minimal gradient from the apical (central segments) to the base. Panel B shows a strain map in a patient with ATTR CA showing a large apical to base gradient resulting in a typical "cherry on top" pattern. Strain in the apical segments is relatively preserved while strain of the basal segments is severely reduced

C. **Myocardial contraction fraction**

Systolic function in CA is also assessed utilizing the myocardial contraction fraction (MCF) [22]. The MCF is a dimensionless measure of LV function defined as the ratio of stroke volume to myocardial volume which measures the degree by which the myocardium contracts in relation to its ability to contract. It is relatively independent of chamber size and geometry and can be easily assessed using conventional 2D echo measurements. As MCF indexes stroke volume to myocardial volume it is superior to EF in the assessment of systolic function particularly in non dilated ventricles. MCF correlates with global longitudinal strain and is conceptually similar although it is a composite assessment and not a vector based assessment of myocardial shortening. Similar to strain, it can detect systolic dysfunction in patients with normal EF. Unlike strain, it does not require specialized software, is vendor independent and can be assessed even when imaging is less than optimal. In addition, unlike strain, MCF cannot assess regional abnormalities in contractile function.

Diastolic Function

Infiltration of amyloid fibrils initially results in impaired LV relaxation which causes progressive diastolic dysfunction. Any echo exam in suspected CA needs to include a comprehensive assessment of diastolic function including pulsed-wave Doppler of mitral inflow, TDI analysis of diastolic Doppler filling and pulsed-wave Doppler of pulmonary vein flow (PVF). CA causes a spectrum of diastolic dysfunction (DD)

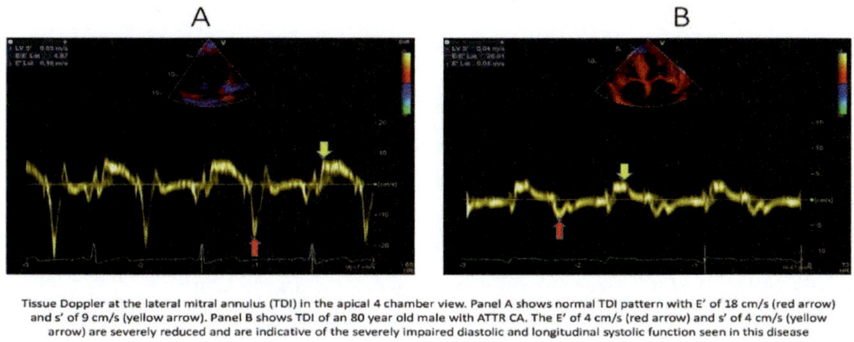

Fig. 9 Tissue Doppler at the lateral mitral annulus (TDI) in the apical 4 chamber view. Panel A shows normal TDI pattern with E′ of 18 cm/s (red arrow) and s′ of 9 cm/s (yellow arrow). Panel B shows TDI of an 80 year old male with STTR CA. The E′ of 4 cm/s (red arrow) and s′ of 4 cm/s (yellow arrow) are severely reduced and are indicative of the severely impaired diastolic and longitudinal systolic function seen in this disease

with more severe DD manifesting later in the disease course. Generally by the time the disease is diagnosed significant DD is present and Doppler shows an increased ratio of early to late diastolic filling with an E:A of > 1.5 and a shortened E wave deceleration time (150 ms) [23]. Frequently the A wave diastolic velocity is reduced due to impaired atrial function seen in this disease [24]. TDI diastolic e′ and a′ velocities are both reduced. Typical TDI findings in a patient with CA are shown in Fig. 9.

The elevated E wave along with the reduced e′ wave leads to a high E:e′ reflecting the increased LV filling pressures seen in CA. With increasing diastolic dysfunction, PVF will demonstrate a progressive decline in pulmonary systolic wave velocity with an increase in diastolic wave velocity [7]. In advanced DD, an increased PV atrial reversal velocity may be noted.

Atrial Function

Given the importance of normal atrial function in maintaining cardiac output, in recent years increasing attention has been paid to echocardiographic assessment of atrial function in CA. While the LA may be dilated in CA secondary to increased LV filling pressure, amyloid infiltration into the LA also directly impairs atrial function independently of filling pressures. Reduced atrial contraction is associated with worse prognosis in CA and should be assessed systematically [24]. As noted and as demonstrated in Fig. 10, the A wave diastolic velocity on mitral inflow Doppler is reduced due to impaired atrial function even in CA patients in sinus rhythm.

Atrial mechanical dysfunction may lead to the presence of intratrial thrombi even in sinus rhythm. The use of LA strain imaging is also useful in the assessment of

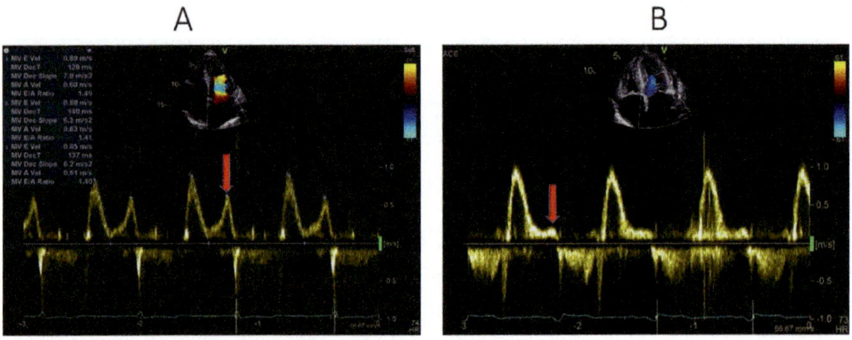

Pulse-wave Doppler of the mitral valve showing e and a waves. Panel A shows a normal a wave velocity of 60 cm/s (red arrow). Panel B in a patient with CA demonstrates a very low a wave velocity (red arrow) despite sinus rhythm, indicative of significantly impaired left atrial function.

Fig. 10 Pulse-wave Doppler of the mitral valve showing e and a waves. Panel A shows a normal a wave velocity of 60 cm/s (red arrow). Panel B in a patient with CA demonstrates a very low a wave velocity (red arrow) despite sinus rhythm, indicative of significantly impaired left atrial function

suspected CA. LA function consists of three distinct components, reservoir, conduit and pump all of which can be assessed using strain imaging. While all three components are decreased in CA, reduced reservoir and pump strains seems to be most predictive of CA [25].

Conclusion

Echocardiography is essential in the evaluation of patients with CA. It is important to emphasize that individual echocardiographic parameters in isolation may have limited diagnostic usefulness. Attempts have been made to combine the various parameters to generate risk scores and increase diagnostic accuracy. These scores combine echocardiographic findings common in CA such as elevated E;e′, increased wall thickness and reduced strain with clinical findings such as age and biomarkers such as troponin or BNP. In the future, models based on artificial intelligence which can perform more sophisticated analyses of myocardial function will presumably be useful in the echocardiographic assessment of CA.

References

1. Agrawal T, Nagueh SF. Echocardiographic assessment of cardiac amyloidosis. Heart Fail Rev. 2022;27:1505–13.
2. Ferkh A, Tjahjadi C, Stefani L, Geenty P, Byth K, De Silva K, et al. Cardiac "hypertrophy" phenotyping: 35 differentiating aetiologies with increased left ventricular wall thickness on echocardiography. Front Cardiovasc Med. 2023;10:1183485.

3. Dinwoodey DL, Skinner M, Maron MS, Davidoff R, Ruberg F. Light-chain amyloidosis with echocardiographic features of hypertrophic cardiomyopathy. Am J Cardiol. 2008;101(5):674–6.
4. Sedlis SP, Saffitz JE, Schwob VS, Jaffe AS. Cardiac amyloidosis simulating hypertrophic cardiomyopathy. Am J Cardiol. 1984;53(7):969–70.
5. Carroll JD, Gaasch WH, McAdam KP. Amyloid cardiomyopathy: characterization by a distinctive voltage/mass relation. Am J Cardiol. 1982;49(1):9–13.
6. Dorbala S, Ando Y, Bokhari S, et al. ASNC/AHA/ASE/EANM/HFSA/ISA/SCMR/SNMMI expert consensus recommendations for multimodality imaging in cardiac amyloidosis: Part 1 of 2-evidence base and standardized methods of imaging. J Nucl Cardiol 2016;2065–123.
7. Cuddy SAM, Chetrit M, Jankowski M, et al. Practical points for echocardiography in cardiac amyloidosis. J Am Soc Echocardiogr. 2022;35:31A-40A.
8. Fitzgerald BT, Scalia GM, Cain PA, Garcia MJ. Thomas JD Left atrial size–another differentiator for cardiac amyloidosis. Heart Lung Circ. 2011;20(9):574–8.
9. Feng D, Edwards WD, Oh JK, et al. Intracardiac thrombosis and embolism in patients with cardiac amyloidosis. Circulation 2007;116(21):2420–6.
10. Martinez-Naharro A, Gonzalez-Lopez E, Corovic A, Mirelis JG, Baksi AJ, Moon JC, Garcia-Pavia P, Gillmore JD, Hawkins PN, Fontana M. High prevalence of intracardiac thrombi in cardiac amyloidosis. J Am Coll Cardiol. 2019;73:1733–4.
11. Castaño A, Narotsky DL, Hamid N, et al. Unveiling transthyretin cardiac amyloidosis and its predictors among elderly patients with severe aortic stenosis undergoing transcatheter aortic valve replacement. Eur Heart J. 2017;38(38):2879–87.
12. Scully PR, Patel KP, Treibel TA, et al. Prevalence and outcome of dual aortic stenosis and cardiac amyloid pathology in patients referred for transcatheter aortic valve implantation. Eur Heart J. 2020;41(29):2759–67.
13. Binder C, Duca F, Binder T, et al. Prognostic implications of pericardial and pleural effusion in patients with cardiac amyloidosis. Clin Res Cardiol. 2021;110(4):532–43.
14. Stokke TM, Hasselberg NE, Smedsrud MK, et al. Geometry as a confounder when assessing ventricular systolic function: comparison between ejection fraction and strain. J Am Coll Cardiol. 2017;70:942–54.
15. Quarta CC, Solomon SD, Uraizee I, et al. Left ventricular structure and function in transthyretin-related versus light-chain cardiac amyloidosis. Circulation. 2014;129(18):1840–9.
16. Koyama J, Ray-Sequin PA, Davidoff R, Falk RH. Usefulness of pulsed tissue Doppler imaging for evaluating systolic and diastolic left ventricular function in patients with AL (primary) amyloidosis. Am J Cardiol. 2002;89(9):1067–71.
17. Koyama J, Ray-Sequin PA, Falk RH. Longitudinal myocardial function assessed by tissue velocity, strain, and strain rate tissue Doppler echocardiography in patients with AL (primary) cardiac amyloidosis. Circulation. 2003;107(19):2446–52.
18. Phelan D, Collier P, Thavendiranathan P, et al. Relative apical sparing of longitudinal strain using two-dimensional speckle-tracking echocardiography is both sensitive and specific for the diagnosis of cardiac amyloidosis. Heart. 2012;98(19):1442–8.
19. Singh V, Soman P, Malhotra S. Reduced diagnostic accuracy of apical-sparing strain abnormality for cardiac amyloidosis in patients with chronic kidney disease. J Am Soc Echocardiogr. 2020;33:913–16.
20. Ferreira VV, Rosa SA, Pereira-da-Silva T, Rodrigues I, Goncalves AV, Mendonca TC, et al. Prevalence 27 and prognostic impact of apical sparing contractility pattern in patients with aortic stenosis referred 28 for transcatheter aortic valve implantation. Am J Cardiovasc Dis. 2021;11:283–94.
21. Pagourelias ED, Duchenne J, Mirea O, et al. The relation of ejection fraction and global longitudinal strain in amyloidosis: implications for differential diagnosis. JACC Cardiovasc Imaging. 2016;19(11):1358–9.
22. Rubin J, Steidley DE, Carlsson M, Ong ML, Maurer MS. Myocardial contraction fraction by M-1 mode echocardiography is superior to ejection fraction in predicting mortality in transthyretin amyloidosis. J Card Fail. 2018;24:504–11.

23. Klein AL, Hatle LK, Burstow DJ, et al. Doppler characterization of left ventricular diastolic function in cardiac amyloidosis. J Am Coll Cardiol. 1989;13(5):1017–26.
24. Nochioka K, Quarta CC, Claggett B, Roca GQ, Rapezzi C, Falk RH, Solomon SD. Left atrial structure and function in cardiac amyloidosis. Eur Heart J Cardiovasc Imag. 2017;18:1128–37.
25. Rausch K, Scalia GM, Sato K, Edwards N, Lam AK, Platts DG, Chan J. Left atrial strain imaging differentiates cardiac amyloidosis and hypertensive heart disease. Int J Cardiovasc Imaging. 2021;37:81–90.

Echocardiography in Cardiac Amyloidosis for the Sonographer

Mali Mor and David Leibowitz

Abstract Echocardiography is an invaluable tool for the early detection and diagnosis of cardiac amyloidosis, a challenging and often underdiagnosed condition. Its advantages include accessibility, cost-effectiveness, ease of use, and the absence of radiation or radioactive tracers, making it superior to other imaging modalities. This chapter will demonstrate the crucial role of sonographers in identifying early signs of amyloidosis during routine echocardiographic examinations. By utilizing advanced technologies, particularly global longitudinal strain (GLS), sonographers can significantly enhance diagnostic accuracy by remaining vigilant for well-known echocardiographic markers that indicate amyloidosis. In recent years, artificial intelligence (AI)-based technologies have been introduced in echocardiography, significantly improving diagnostic capabilities. Recently, these AI technologies have advanced further with the introduction of new tools that enable automatic strain imaging within seconds after acquiring standard cardiac views. These advancements provide immediate automatic measurements of GLS, along with regional strain patterns characteristic of amyloidosis, such as apical sparing. Additionally, automatic measurements of left ventricular ejection fraction (EF) are obtained, and the recent development of regional assessments providing the Segmental Score Index further enhances diagnostic capabilities. The integration of these AI-based technologies in the echocardiographic assessment of cardiac function helps differentiate between cardiomyopathies, and aids in diagnosing amyloidosis. This chapter will demonstrate how simple, recognizable signs—further elucidated through case studies involving AL and ATTR amyloidosis—can guide sonographers to continue evaluating additional features, including the characteristic Bull's Eye pattern on GLS imaging. This pattern, known for its apical sparing contrasted with reduced strain in the basal segments, presents a hallmark appearance reminiscent of a "cherry on top" and is suggestive of amyloid infiltration. By recognizing these patterns, sonographers can effectively alert

M. Mor (✉)
Department of Cardiology, Rabin Medical Center, Sackler Faculty of Medicine, Tel Aviv University, Petah Tikva, Israel
e-mail: malima2@clalit.org.il

D. Leibowitz
Department of Cardiology, Hadassah Medical Center, Hebrew University of Jerusalem, Jerusalem, Israel

E. Herzog (ed.), *Cardiac Amyloidosis*, https://doi.org/10.1007/978-3-031-88342-2_5

the interpreting physician, prompting a more thorough assessment of the patient's clinical history and potential recommendation for further testing to confirm or rule out cardiac amyloidosis, a diagnosis that may otherwise be missed. Early diagnosis is critical for patients, as cardiac amyloidosis is a fatal disease with a significantly shortened lifespan if not treated promptly. Sonographers are often the first to encounter these patients, and through careful echocardiographic evaluation, can raise suspicion of the disease. By increasing awareness of the dangers associated with this condition and recognizing our profound ability to contribute to its diagnosis, sonographers can play a pivotal role in improving diagnosis and treatment of this illness.

Keywords Cardiac amyloidosis · Echocardiography · Global longitudinal strain (GLS) · Artificial intelligence (AI)

Introduction

Amyloidosis is a fatal, progressive disease characterized by the abnormal deposition of misfolded proteins in various tissues and organs, including the heart [1]. This accumulation impairs cardiac function, leading to heart failure, dyspnea, and arrhythmias, and is often misdiagnosed or underdiagnosed [2]. The disease primarily affects men over the age of 60 and presents with amyloid deposits that lead to heart failure and arrhythmic complications [3]. The median survival rate following the diagnosis of cardiac amyloidosis is approximately 3.5 years. Amyloidosis is a heterogeneous condition that involves multiple organs, including the heart, and presents with a range of cardiac and non-cardiac symptoms, which are often atypical of other cardiovascular diseases [4].

Echocardiography remains a key diagnostic tool in recognizing the hallmark signs of amyloidosis, which can be lifesaving [5]. Typical echocardiographic findings include thickened ventricular walls, often with diastolic dysfunction and restrictive filling patterns, as well as a characteristic "apical sparing" pattern on strain imaging [6]. The presence of these features, especially in patients with heart failure and preserved ejection fraction (HFpEF) or low-flow, low-gradient aortic stenosis, should heighten the suspicion of amyloidosis [7].

Echocardiographic Signs Consistent with Amyloidosis

Ventricles

Echocardiography may reveal several critical signs within the ventricles that raise suspicion for the disease. One of the primary findings is increased wall thickness in both the left ventricle (LV) and right ventricle (RV), which can manifest as either concentric or asymmetric thickening [2]. This thickening is frequently associated with a mismatch between the echocardiographic findings and the ECG results, where the ECG shows normal or low voltage despite the significantly increased thickness of the LV wall [3].

Another notable sign is the presence of a small or normal LV cavity, which appears disproportionate to the degree of wall thickening observed [2].

Figure 1 Panel A and B: Show parasternal long-axis views from patients with AL (A) and ATTR (B) amyloidosis. Both images demonstrate thickening of the interventricular septum (IVS) and posterior wall (PW), alongside a small LV cavity size, disproportionate to the patient's body surface area

Panel C and D: Apical four-chamber (AP4) views show thickening of the left ventricular walls as well as the right ventricular (RV) walls. This additional RV thickening reflects the extent of myocardial involvement seen in amyloidosis.

The ECG trace at the bottom of the images in the Echo machine screen, highlights low-voltage QRS complexes with a mildly widened QRS, findings that may be indicative of amyloid infiltration [3].

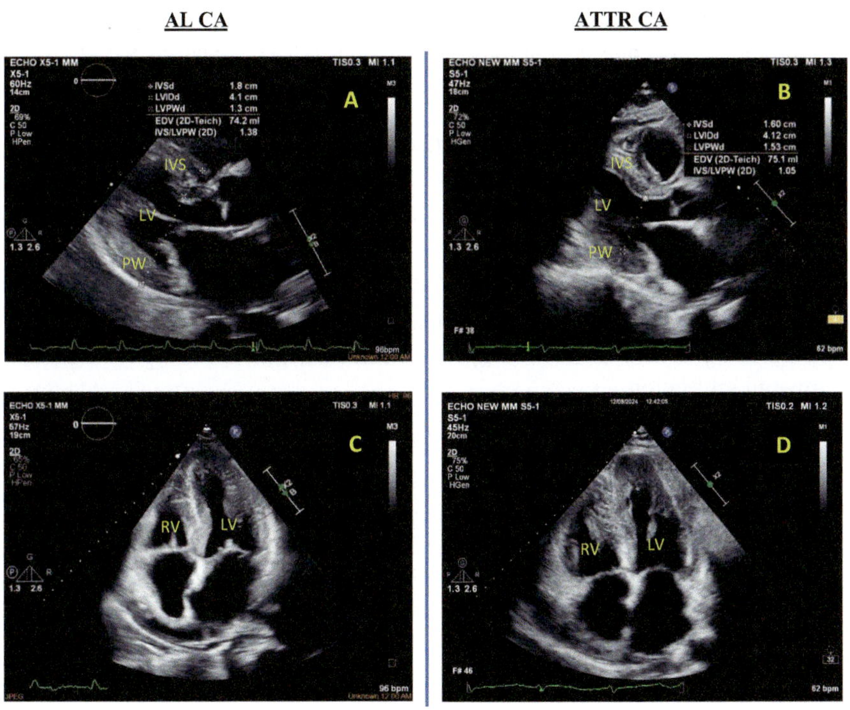

Fig. 1 Echocardiographic assessment of the ventricles in a patient with AL cardiac amyloidosis versus ATTR cardiac amyloidosis-identical signs in echo

All these findings can be observed through basic 2D echocardiography, providing early suspicion for amyloidosis before the need for more advanced imaging techniques such as strain.

In the apical views, 2D imaging may demonstrate hypokinesis of the basal segments with apical sparing. Following this, it is essential to proceed with strain imaging, which can confirm whether apical sparing is indeed present. This finding would significantly raise the echocardiographic suspicion for amyloidosis [6].

Additionally, increased myocardial echogenicity, referred to as "sparkling," can also raise suspicion of amyloidosis. However, it is important to note that advancements in echocardiographic technology, such as the introduction of Second Harmonic Imaging, have improved image clarity and reduced artifacts, making the "sparkling" appearance visible even in healthy individuals and athletes with high-quality imaging and reducing the specificity of this finding for amyloidosis [8].

Atria

In patients with amyloidosis, the atria often exhibit significant pathological changes that can be identified through echocardiography [9]. Common findings include atrial dilatation and thickening of the interatrial septum (IAS) as well as the atrial free walls. In addition, Doppler A wave velocities may be reduced even in patients in sinus rhythm. Amyloid infiltration within the atria leads to mechanical dysfunction, increasing the risk of intra-cardiac thrombus formation and systemic embolism, even in the presence of sinus rhythm [10].

These echocardiographic features are critical for recognizing atrial involvement in amyloidosis and for assessing the extent of disease progression.

Figure 2 Echocardiographic assessment of the atria in a patient with AL and ATTR Cardiac Amyloidosis. Both panels demonstrate identical echocardiographic findings, including atrial wall thickening and interatrial septal hypertrophy, suggestive of amyloid infiltration

Panel A (AL CA): The image reveals thickened left and right atrial walls and septal thickening (indicated by arrows).

Panel B (ATTR CA): Similar findings are observed, showing thickened atrial walls and septal hypertrophy, characteristic of amyloidosis.

Panel C and D: These images show the calculation of the left atrial volume (LAV) and left atrial volume index (LAVI), which is computed based on the patient's body surface area (BSA). The measurement is performed using both the apical four-chamber (AP4) and apical two-chamber (AP2) views. The LA volume is determined at end-systole by tracing the atrial borders in both views. Using the patient's height and weight, the echocardiography machine calculates the LAVI, which has become part of the routine echocardiographic assessment for detecting atrial enlargement.

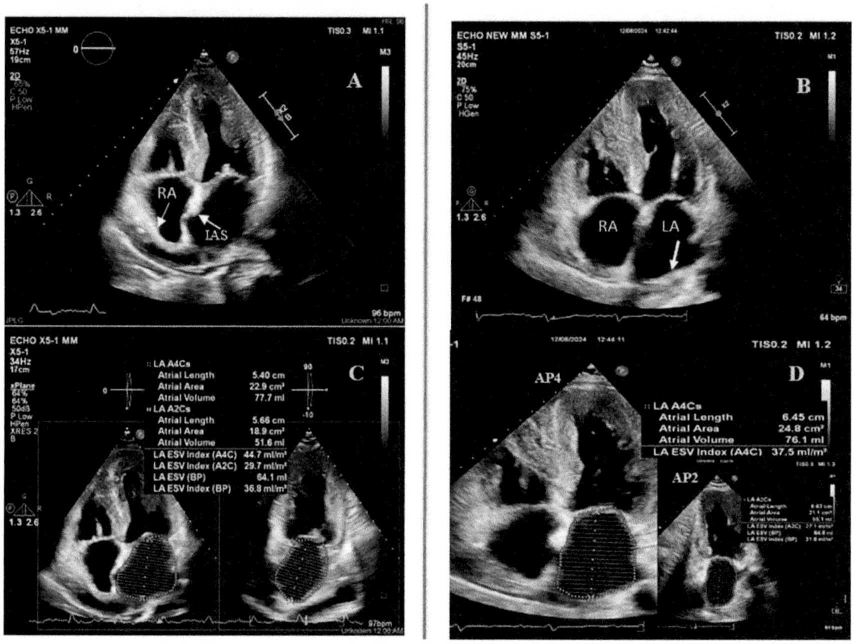

AL CA ATTR CA

Fig. 2 Echocardiographic assessment of the atria in a patient with AL cardiac amyloidosis and ATTR cardiac amyloidosis-identical signs on echo

This measurement can be performed with the 3D xPlane mode (using a 3D transducer) or with 2D imaging in the AP4 and AP2 views [11].

Valves

In patients with amyloidosis, valvular involvement is another important echocardiographic finding. This often manifests as thickening of the valve leaflets due to amyloid infiltration [9].

Additionally, patients may develop aortic stenosis, where the aortic valve narrows, leading to restricted blood flow from the heart [6, 7]. These valvular abnormalities contribute to the overall cardiac dysfunction observed in amyloidosis and are crucial to identify during echocardiographic assessments, as they play a significant role in disease progression and patient management.

Figure 3 AL CA (A, C) and ATTR CA (B, D) demonstrate valvular thickening of both the mitral and tricuspid valves. While these valves are thickened, this appearance differs from the familiar presentation in rheumatic heart disease, where significant stenosis is expected. In amyloidosis, these valves are thickened but, in most cases,

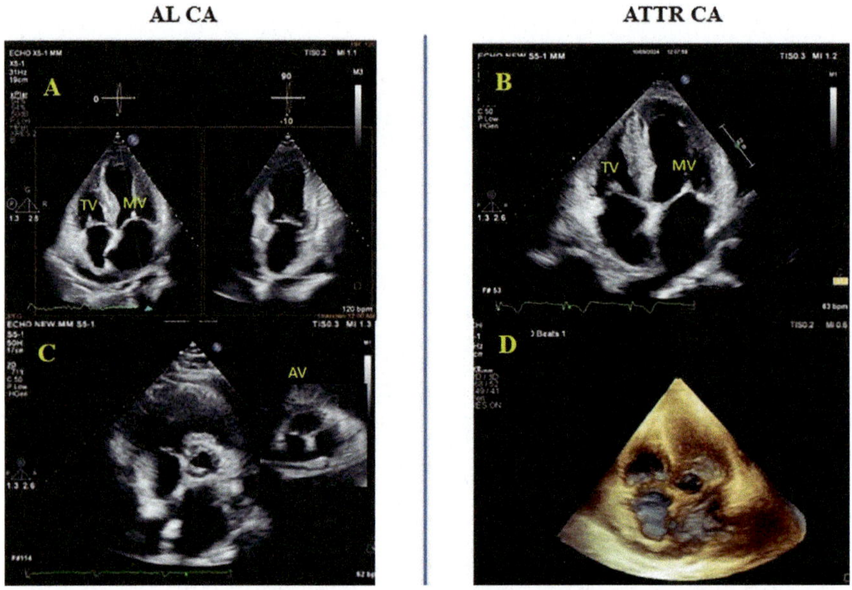

Fig. 3 Echocardiographic assessment of valvular involvement in a patient with amyloidosis

without significant stenosis, serving as an important echocardiographic indicator of the disease [2].

Additionally, in the aortic valve, although we may anticipate stenosis in cases of amyloidosis, there are instances—such as the patient in panel A with AL cardiac amyloidosis—where mild calcification occurs without significant stenosis. Panel D is a three-dimensional (3D) echocardiographic image showing the aortic valve from an apical view through the LVOT (left ventricular outflow tract) view.

This variability in valvular involvement highlights that not all valves will exhibit the same degree of thickening or stenosis. These findings demonstrate the range of red flags in amyloidosis, showing that different valves may be affected in varying degrees, and stenosis is not always present.

Additional Echocardiographic Features

In amyloidosis, several additional echocardiographic features may be observed that contribute to the overall assessment of the disease [1]. One hallmark feature is the presence of pericardial effusion, which may present as mild fluid accumulation around the heart, reflecting the severity of disease progression [5]. In addition, a common finding in advanced stages of the disease is a dilated and non-collapsing inferior vena cava indicating elevated right atrial pressure and impaired venous return [6].

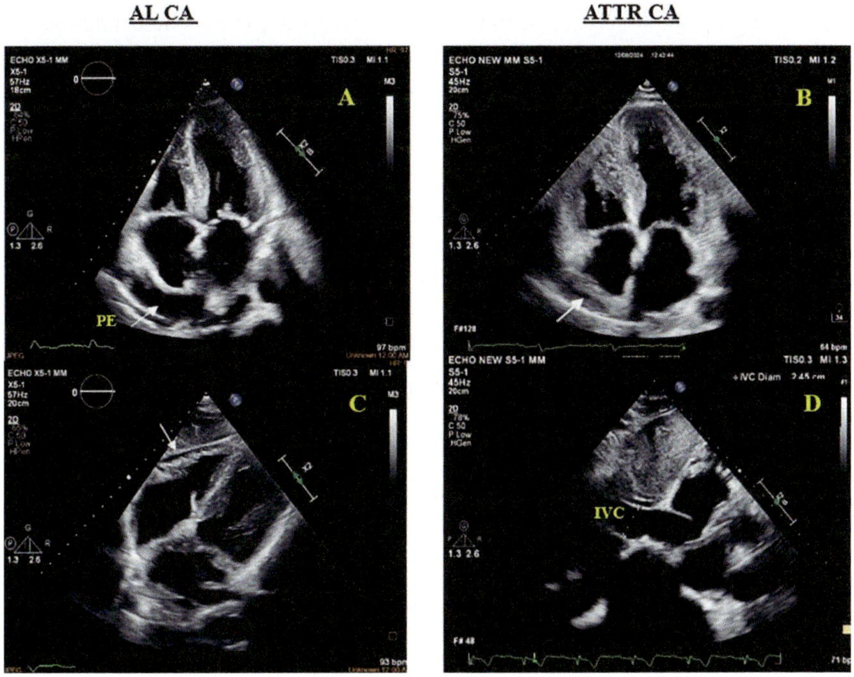

Fig. 4 Echocardiographic assessment of pericardial effusion in amyloidosis

Figure 4 Panel A and C (AL CA): These images show pericardial effusion (PE), which is small and localized near the right atrium. In some cases, pericardial effusion may be positioned or small, not necessarily visible in every patient. Panel C shows in this AL amyloidosis case, the effusion was mild, and such fluid accumulations can sometimes go undetected, especially in views other than the subcostal view, where pericardial effusion is typically best visualized.

Panel B and D (ATTR CA): In contrast, the patient with ATTR amyloidosis exhibited little to no detectable pericardial effusion. Image D demonstrates a significantly dilated inferior vena cava (IVC).

Diastolic Dysfunction

Diastolic dysfunction is also a common finding, particularly in the advanced stages of amyloidosis [1]. This typically manifests as restrictive filling patterns on Doppler echocardiography, with increased early diastolic filling (E wave) and decreased atrial contraction (A wave), often leading to an elevated E/A ratio [5]. The pulmonary veins also show characteristic flow abnormalities, with a reduced systolic wave (S wave) and a compensatory increase in the diastolic wave (D wave). These findings are essential in diagnosing restrictive cardiomyopathy secondary to amyloid infiltration.

Additionally, pulmonary hypertension may develop as a consequence of increased pulmonary pressures, further complicating the patient's clinical picture [2].

Figure 5 **A (Mitral Inflow):**

In the patient with AL CA, the mitral inflow pattern demonstrates a restrictive filling pattern, with a significantly shortened deceleration time (DT) and a high E/E′ ratio, indicating severe diastolic dysfunction (Grade 3) [1]. In contrast, the patient with ATTR CA shows a slightly higher deceleration time, but the restrictive filling pattern is still evident in both cases, indicating advanced diastolic dysfunction.

B and C (TDI on Medial and Lateral Annulus):

Both AL CA and ATTR CA show very low velocities on tissue Doppler imaging (TDI) at both the medial and lateral annuli. The S′, E′, and A′ wave velocities are all significantly reduced, approximately in the range of 5 cm/s, which is a hallmark of diastolic dysfunction [12].

Rule of 5 (5–5-5): All E′, a′, S′ Velocities < 5 cm/s. This is a Clue to the Diagnosis of CA.

In the patient with AL CA, the mitral inflow is typical of a restrictive pattern with a shorter deceleration time compared to the ATTR CA patient (though this could be incidental), but in both cases, the E/E′ ratio is elevated. This high ratio confirms significant diastolic dysfunction in both patients, suggesting Grade 2 or higher.

D (Pulmonary Veins):

In both AL CA and ATTR CA patients, the pulmonary vein flow demonstrates characteristic findings of diastolic dysfunction, with reduced systolic wave (S wave) and a compensatory increase in the diastolic wave (D wave) [5]. These findings further solidify the restrictive filling pattern observed in these patients.

Figure 6 **A: Increased Myocardial Thickness and Valve Thickening with Sparkling:**

This image is the first one typically observed in an echocardiographic exam. It demonstrates increased myocardial and valvular thickening with the characteristic "sparkling" appearance, indicative of amyloid infiltration. This is an important finding, particularly when observed diffusely with non-uniform thickening of the valves.

B: Elevated Pulmonary Pressure

Elevated pulmonary pressure is often associated with amyloidosis, but in these cases, pulmonary pressures were not significantly elevated. This finding can present in advanced cases of amyloidosis due to diastolic dysfunction and increased pulmonary pressures.

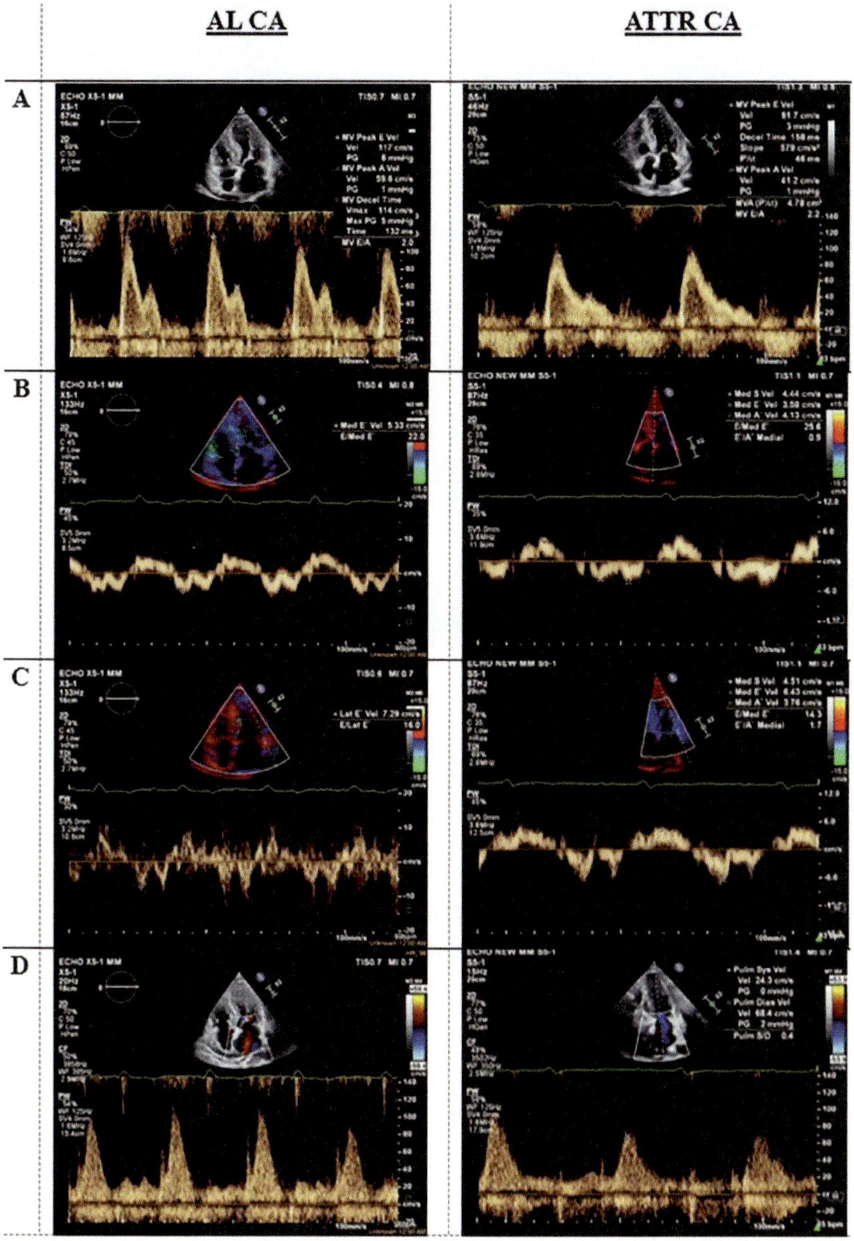

Fig. 5 Comparative echocardiographic assessment of diastolic dysfunction in patients with AL cardiac amyloidosis (AL CA) and ATTR cardiac amyloidosis (ATTR CA)

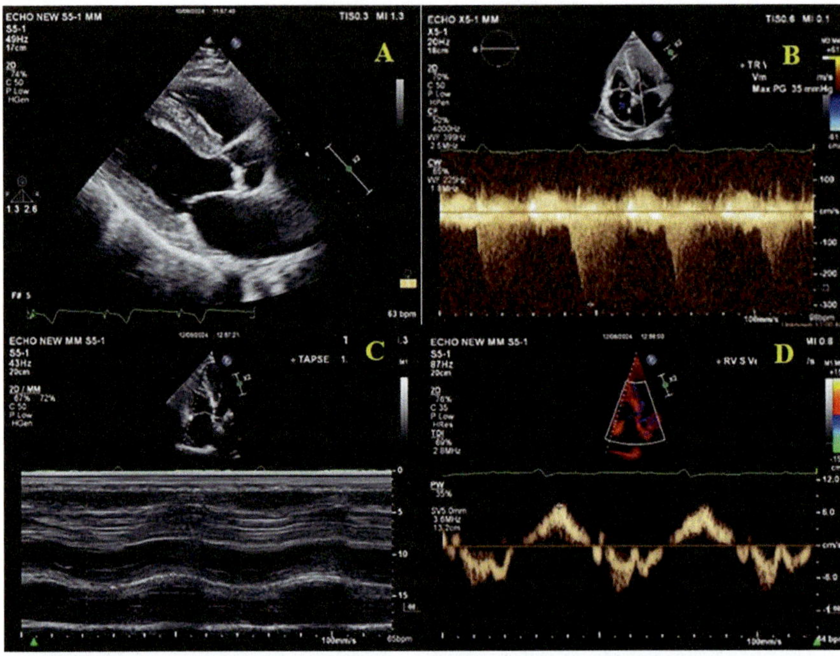

Fig. 6 Additional echocardiographic findings suggestive of cardiac amyloidosis in patients with AL and ATTR amyloidosis

C: TAPSE (Tricuspid Annular Plane Systolic Excursion)—Reduced Motion

The reduced motion of the right ventricular free wall (TAPSE) indicates impaired right ventricular systolic function. A low TAPSE value is a common finding in cardiac amyloidosis, reflecting the right ventricular dysfunction.

D: Low S′ Velocity of the Right Ventricular Free Wall

The low S′ velocity of the right ventricular free wall annulus further supports the diagnosis of impaired right ventricular systolic function, which is frequently seen in amyloidosis.

Conclusion

Each of these findings can serve as a red flag, raising suspicion for cardiac amyloidosis [1]. However, it is crucial to recognize that not all these signs need to be present in a single echocardiographic exam. Echo sonographers, should understand that even a subset of these findings could be sufficient to warrant suspicion of this severe disease which should be brought to the attention of the interpreting physician [2].

Flowchart for Diagnosing Amyloid Cardiomyopathy

Proposal for Adopting a Scoring System to Assess the Echocardiographic Suspicion of Amyloid Cardiomyopathy

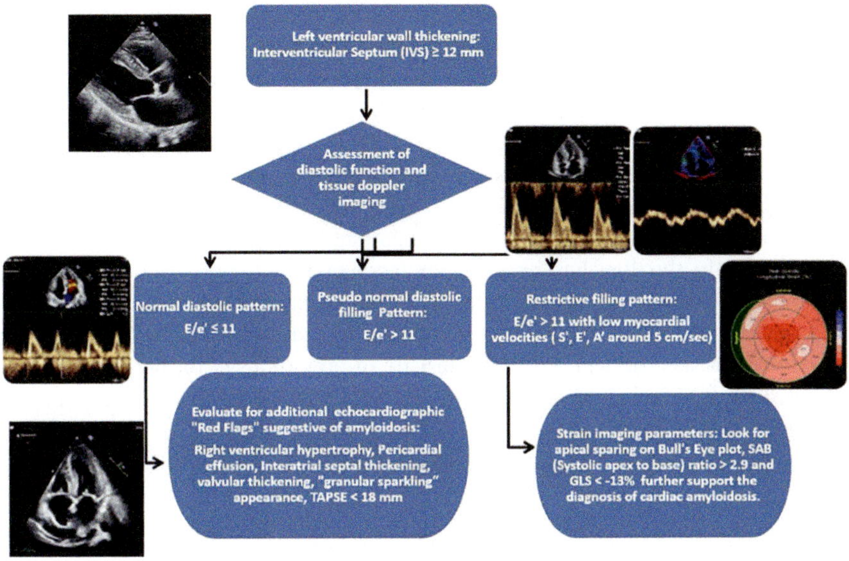

Scoring System for Suspected Amyloid Cardiomyopathy (IWT Score) [13] Table 1.

Score Summary:

- **Score 0–1**: **Low suspicion** of amyloid cardiomyopathy (no additional testing needed).
- **Score 2–7**: **Moderate suspicion** of amyloid cardiomyopathy (consider further testing).
- **Score ≥ 8**: **High suspicion** of amyloid cardiomyopathy (consider referral for advanced diagnosis or nuclear scintigraphy).

Table 1 Diagnostic flowchart for evaluating cardiac amyloidosis based on echocardiographic findings and red flag parameters

Parameter	Cut-off value	Points
RWT (relative wall thickness)	> 0.6	3
TAPSE (tricuspid annular plane systolic excursion)	≤ 19 mm	2
E/e′ (diastolic filling pressure)	> 11	1
GLS (global longitudinal strain)	≤ − 13%	1
SAB (apical to basal strain ratio)	> 2.9	3

This scoring system provides a comprehensive framework for assessing patients, helping echo sonographers flag potential cases early and improve diagnostic accuracy [5].

This flowchart provides a structured approach for evaluating patients with suspected amyloid cardiomyopathy during echocardiographic examination. The evaluation begins with identifying an increased left ventricular wall thickness (LVH) of greater than 12 mm. The flowchart suggests using a scoring system to assess the likelihood of CA [2].

The challenge lies in identifying patients who score between 2 and 7 points on the scoring table. These patients may not exhibit all the signs listed, but it is crucial to exercise clinical judgment and consider raising suspicion for amyloidosis when these intermediate scores are observed [1]. By flagging potential cases early, sonographers can facilitate timely diagnosis and improve patient outcomes.

Additionally, the flowchart provides guidance on how to proceed with the examination based on measurements from tissue Doppler imaging. The final step in the assessment involves using strain imaging, which enhances diagnostic accuracy by identifying specific patterns characteristic of amyloidosis, further aiding in the echocardiographic diagnosis of the disease.

Step 1: Left Ventricular Wall Thickness (LVH)

Begin by assessing LV wall thickness. If LV thickness $\geq$ 12 mm, proceed with further analysis.

Step 2: Diastolic Function (Mitral Inflow Doppler)

Evaluate the diastolic filling pattern:

Normal or altered release: E/A ratio is within a normal range or slightly altered. No immediate red flags but continue monitoring.

Pseudo normal or restrictive pattern: Significantly higher E/A ratio, deceleration time shortened, or a restrictive pattern suggests increased filling pressures.

Step 3: Tissue Doppler Imaging (TDI)

Measure E' and A' velocities at the septal and lateral annuli and average to calculate E/E' ratio:

If $E/E' > 11$: This suggests increased filling pressures and diastolic dysfunction. Immediately proceed to strain imaging to evaluate for apical sparing.

If $E/E' \leq 11$: Normal filling pressures, but do not stop here. If there are other echocardiographic signs like pericardial effusion, myocardial sparkling, or valve thickening, consider amyloidosis and move to the next step.

Measure S' velocities, value ≤ 5 cm/sec suggestive of amyloidosis

Step 4: Apical Sparing and Strain Imaging (Bull's Eye Map)

Perform strain imaging to check for apical sparing:

Apical Sparing Pattern: This is a hallmark of cardiac amyloidosis and provides evidence for the diagnosis.

If GLS (global longitudinal strain) $< -13\%$, this further strengthens the suspicion of cardiac amyloidosis.

Step 5: Comprehensive Clinical and Echocardiographic Review

Consider other red flags in your echocardiographic review:

Presence of pericardial effusion (even if mild or localized).

Myocardial sparkling or granular appearance.

Valve thickening (without significant stenosis, as in amyloidosis).

Check the right ventricular function: look for reduced TAPSE and diminished S′ velocity.

Step 6: Patient Clinical History

Assess shortly the patient's symptoms and background:

Ask if the patient has hypertension or any heart failure symptoms.

Discuss daily symptoms like fatigue, shortness of breath, or other unexplained discomforts that may indicate systemic involvement of amyloidosis.

Strain Imaging

In contemporary echocardiography, **Global Longitudinal Strain (GLS)** has become an essential tool for assessing myocardial deformation, particularly with the integration of AI-powered automated strain software [5, 14]. This technology, widely available in Echo systems from major manufacturers, offers real-time evaluation of myocardial strain, providing a precise analysis of cardiac function.

AI-driven software now automates the segmentation and tracking of the myocardium, allowing echocardiographers to obtain GLS and ejection fraction (EF) measurements with increased accuracy and reduced variability [15].

The automated workflow, which takes just minutes, enhances diagnostic efficiency and enables earlier detection of conditions such as diastolic heart failure and cardiac amyloidosis [13].

This chapter will focus on practical guidelines for utilizing these tools, particularly with Philips and GE machines, while outlining general principles that can be applied to other systems.

Strain measures the percentage change in the length of the myocardial fibers between two points, offering a more accurate assessment of the heart's contractile function than traditional ejection fraction measurements [8].

Strain is generally expressed as a negative value since the myocardium shortens during systole, meaning the measured distance (L) between two points is smaller than the original length (L_0). This shortening, particularly in the longitudinal direction, provides key insights into the health and function of the myocardial fibers.

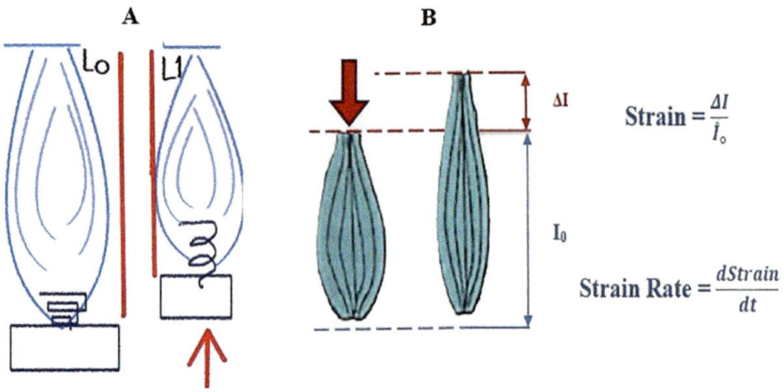

Fig. 7 Calculation of Strain and Strain rate

The formula used for calculating strain is: Strain [%] = $(L - L_0)/L_0 * 100\%$

A strain rate can also be derived, giving clinicians an idea of the rate at which the myocardial deformation occurs [1]. Strain analysis is invaluable in detecting subclinical myocardial dysfunction, particularly in conditions like amyloidosis, where ejection fraction may be normal, but strain imaging reveals significant abnormalities of myocardial systolic function [9].

This strain assessment provides valuable insights into the function of the myocardium, allowing clinicians to detect subtle dysfunction that might otherwise go unnoticed [5].

Figure 7 **Panel A** demonstrates the fundamental principle of strain, depicting a muscle fiber shortening from its initial length (L_0) to a final shortened length (L_1). The change in length is used to calculate strain, based on the formula:

Strain [%] = $(L_0 - L_1)/L_0$ * 100%, where strain is represented as a percentage to indicate the degree of myocardial deformation [8]. **Panel B** explains the strain rate, which measures how quickly this deformation occurs. The rate at which the myocardial fibers shorten gives additional insight into the heart's functionality, especially in pathological conditions such as amyloidosis or heart failure [16]. Strain rate helps clinicians assess myocardial performance over time, providing another layer of diagnostic information.

Color Scale in GLS Strain Imaging

In GLS strain imaging, the color scale is intentionally designed to reflect myocardial contractility and provide a quick visual representation of cardiac function [8]. Unlike Doppler imaging, where bright colors represent high velocities, GLS strain uses color gradients to indicate contractility: darker red shades represent areas of stronger myocardial contraction, while lighter shades to white indicate weaker contraction (low strain values). Conversely, blue tones represent myocardial lengthening or dysfunction.

The specific shade choices may vary slightly by manufacturer, depending on default settings or user adjustments.

Figure 8 In this example, taken from apical views (AP4, AP2, AP3), demonstrates a Bull's Eye (BE) strain map of a healthy myocardium. On the right side of the BE (see arrow), the color scale—from deep red to deep blue—clearly represents the strain values across myocardial segments, displayed both in color gradients and as numerical values on each segment. This figure shows the typical color distribution seen in a heart with normal GLS, offering a basis for comparison with abnormal patterns seen in various cardiac conditions.

Figure 9 **Panel A**: Strain pattern of normal myocardium. **Panel B**: Strain pattern of amyloid cardiomyopathy, showing the hallmark "Apical Sparing". **Panel C**: Strain pattern in severe asymmetric septal hypertrophic cardiomyopathy (HCM), with a septal wall thickness of 24 mm and hyperdynamic LV function. demonstrating distinct myocardial dysfunction. **Panel D**: Strain pattern of dilated cardiomyopathy, showing marked regional dysfunction in a patient with severe LV dilation and reduced global contraction, highlighting the region of damage and dysfunction

Strain imaging, specifically Global Longitudinal Strain (GLS), serves as an invaluable diagnostic tool for differentiating various cardiac conditions. Through a clear visual representation of regional and global myocardial function, GLS effectively highlights significant variations in cardiac function, which are critical in identifying diseases such as amyloidosis, hypertrophic cardiomyopathy (HCM), and dilated cardiomyopathy [5]. The characteristic "Apical Sparing" pattern observed in amyloidosis, where the apex shows preserved function while basal segments display

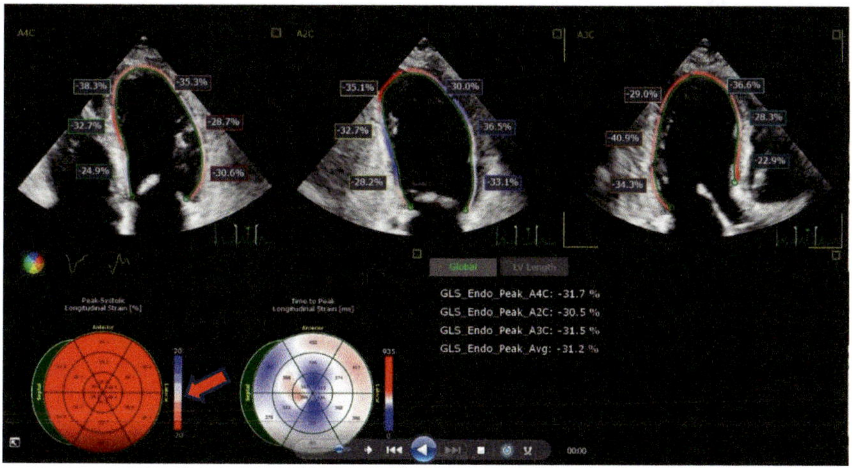

Fig. 8 Normal left ventricular GLS

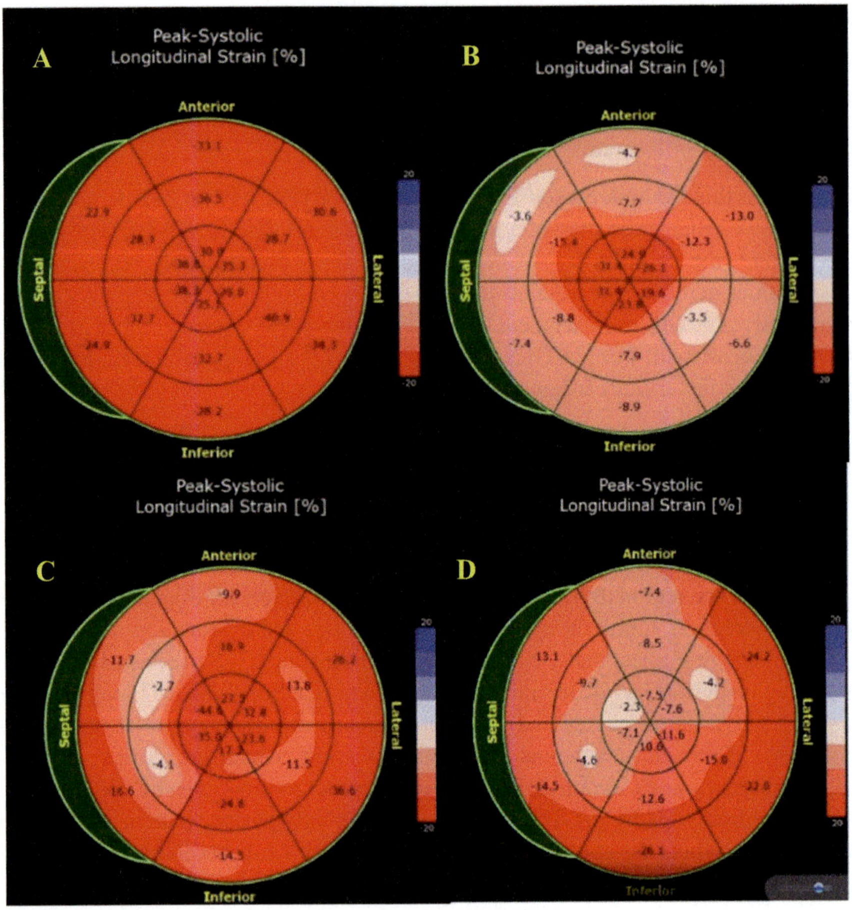

Fig. 9 Strain imaging and diagnostic differentiation

reduced strain, provides a distinct visual marker that helps differentiate it from other cardiomyopathies like HCM or myocardial infarction [13]. This level of diagnostic precision in GLS supports early detection and timely intervention, improving patient outcomes.

The examples provided in the strain maps illustrate how strain imaging visually distinguishes normal myocardial function from various pathological conditions. This technology enhances clinical decision-making by allowing echocardiographers to recognize specific strain patterns, offering insights that complement traditional imaging techniques. As strain imaging, particularly through automated systems such as Auto Strain technology, becomes more accessible, it is increasingly relied upon by clinicians for its ability to reduce variability, accelerate workflow, and deliver reliable results with consistent accuracy [8]. However, variability remains a challenge, as differences in vendor-specific algorithms, image acquisition techniques, and operator expertise can influence GLS measurements. Recent advancements, such as those detailed by Kwan et al. [15], highlight the potential of AI-driven strain imaging tools to mitigate these discrepancies, providing consistency across platforms and reducing inter- and intra-operator variability. Major manufacturers, including Philips and GE, have widely integrated these tools, simplifying myocardial deformation assessment and making it indispensable in diagnosing cardiac amyloidosis, heart failure, and other myocardial diseases.

In the following sections, we will delve into the practical applications of these strain imaging tools, focusing on systems from Philips and GE while underscoring universal principles that are adaptable across echocardiography platforms.

Auto Strain GLS in Amyloidosis

The auto Strain GLS tool, integrated into modern echocardiography machines, enhances diagnostic efficiency for amyloidosis by quickly identifying the characteristic strain patterns, such as Apical Sparing. This assists clinicians in distinguishing amyloidosis from other cardiomyopathies, aiding in timely diagnosis and treatment decisions, as recommended by Boldrini et al. [13].

For example, in Fig. 10, the auto Strain feature revealed echocardiographic signs that could be indicative of amyloidosis, helping to further refine the diagnostic process.

Panel A: Auto strain of Tomtec software from Philips in a patient with cardiac amyloidosis. The automatic analysis software autonomously recognizes, segments, and tracks the LV myocardium of the three standard apical views (four-chamber, two-chamber, and three-chamber views), and calculates the longitudinal strain of each view and GLS.

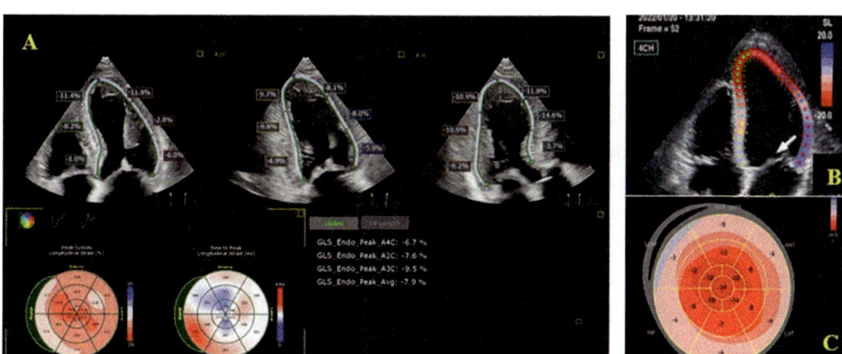

Fig. 10 Evaluation of left ventricular global longitudinal strain (LVGLS)

Panel B: Apical 4-chamber view (AP4) illustrating how to optimally track the myocardial strain using strain vectors. It demonstrates how accurate myocardial tracking is essential to obtain reliable results, ensuring the vectors follow the myocardium and not the epicardium.

Panel C: A classic strain map indicative of amyloidosis, presenting the "cherry on top" or "nipple-like" appearance (Apical Sparing), where the apical segment remains relatively unaffected compared to the basal and mid-segments. This pattern is highly suggestive of cardiac amyloidosis.

Conclusion: Strain imaging, particularly with Auto Strain technology, has become a widely adopted tool among the major echocardiography manufacturers, including Philips and GE, as well as other leading companies. This automated tool simplifies and enhances the accuracy of myocardial deformation assessments. One of the key advancements is that, instead of requiring the echocardiographer to manually select optimal images for strain analysis, the system now automatically selects the best images from the dataset collected during the study. The machine then processes these images and calculates the strain values autonomously [8, 15].

This leap forward in automation reduces variability, speeds up the workflow, and improves the reliability of the results. The technology offers greater accessibility for clinicians and sonographers who rely on precise and reproducible strain measurements for diagnosing conditions like cardiac amyloidosis, heart failure, and other myocardial diseases.

In the following sections, we will further explore the practical application of these tools, focusing on Philips and GE systems, while highlighting universal principles that can be adapted to other technologies.

Optimized GLS Imaging with Philips and GE Systems: Practical Tips

Image Acquisition and Optimization

Frame Rate: Aim for the highest frame rate possible (above 40 FPS), especially using a focused LV view. Adjust the image depth to improve frame rates and enhance the accuracy of automatic strain analysis.

Ensure **EKG** gating is accurately synchronized with the cardiac cycle to avoid errors in GLS calculation.

It is crucial to include all myocardial segments in the three standard views (AP4, AP2, and AP3) for comprehensive strain analysis.

Integration of Advanced Strain Tools in Echocardiography Systems

The integration of advanced strain tools represents a global effort to enhance the diagnostic capabilities of echocardiography. These tools, leveraging AI-driven algorithms, ensure consistent, accurate results across different echocardiographic systems and institutions. By automating critical steps and simplifying workflows, they make GLS imaging more accessible for clinicians and sonographers worldwide.

For the purposes of this chapter, the discussion on strain imaging technology is primarily based on Philips and GE echocardiography systems. These systems are commonly used in our hospitals and thus serve as representative examples for explaining the workflow and technical details. However, it is important to acknowledge that similar technologies are also available from other leading ultrasound manufacturers.

While the detailed technical explanations in this chapter focus on Philips and GE systems, it is reasonable to assume that comparable workflows and features are available in other echocardiographic platforms as well.

As outlined in Voigt et al. [8], the move toward standardization provides a robust foundation for myocardial deformation imaging, ensuring that these tools can be effectively utilized across all echocardiographic platforms. The advancements detailed in Kwan et al. [15], further emphasize the importance of reducing variability and improving diagnostic efficiency in routine clinical practice.

Tracking and ROI Adjustment

In the latest models from Philips and GE, the workflow for strain imaging has become highly similar. Both systems now allow users to acquire the three standard apical views (AP4, AP2, AP3) and, with the press of a button, instantly obtain strain, strain rate, EF, and other advanced calculations. This streamlined process, powered by AI-driven automation, has significantly enhanced efficiency and diagnostic accuracy.

Philips AutoStrain: In Philips systems, the AutoStrain feature automates the GLS (Global Longitudinal Strain) measurement, simultaneously calculating EF and the LV Segmental Score. This all-in-one step minimizes manual adjustments, saving time and ensuring consistency.

GE Systems: Similarly, in GE's newer models, the Auto GLS feature fully automates the GLS measurement, producing comparable results to Philips systems. However, in older GE models without AutoStrain, sonographers manually select and analyze each view (AP4, AP2, and AP3) individually. Despite this, even these models integrate automatic EF calculation within the strain analysis, offering significant diagnostic value.

These advancements exemplify the evolution of echocardiographic technology, making strain imaging more accessible and reliable. The importance of standardization and reducing variability across systems has been highlighted in Voigt et al. [8] while the benefits of AI-driven automation are further detailed in Kwan et al. [15] emphasizing their role in routine clinical practice (Fig. 11).

Layer Tracking: Ensure that the software accurately tracks the myocardial layer, not the epicardium, to avoid inaccurate measurements.

Image Quality: Enhance image clarity by optimizing depth and focus settings on the LV. Use Focused LV views to maximize frame rate and reduce the need for manual editing.

Quality Control: Always review the strain bull's eye map to ensure that all myocardial segments are included, especially in diagnosing conditions like amyloidosis.

Panel A: Demonstrates how to optimize the image for focused LV assessment, essential for obtaining accurate strain measurements. The software tracks the endocardium and the myocardium borders to capture precise LV deformation.

Panel B: Illustrates the segmentation points that need to be placed in each view (AP3, AP4, and AP2) on GE's Echo PAC software.

Panel C: Displays the results after strain computation for each of the three views (AP4, AP2, AP3). The Global Longitudinal Strain (GLS) for each view is visible, as well as the segmental strain values. Additionally, the Ejection Fraction (EF) is automatically calculated alongside the GLS results, offering a comprehensive analysis of the heart's function (Fig. 12).

A: Illustration of correct placement of tracking points on the myocardium in the AP4, AP2, and AP3 views. This step is essential to ensure the automated strain measurement system accurately tracks the myocardial segments for a proper strain analysis.

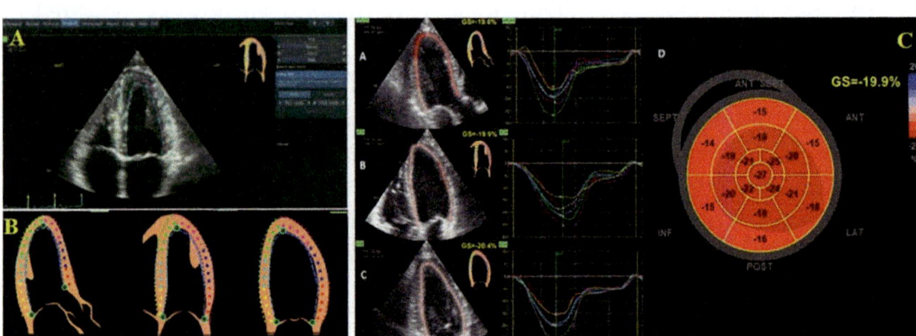

Fig. 11 Focused LV image preparation for strain analysis on GE systems

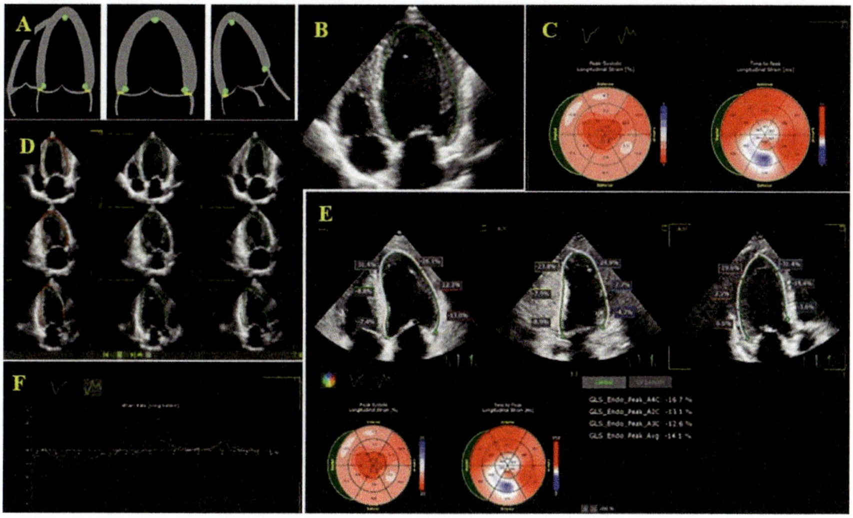

Fig. 12 Focused LV image preparation for strain analysis on PHILIPS systems

B: Focused LV view in the AP4 chamber to optimize image quality for strain analysis. The image demonstrates correct LV focus and alignment, ensuring that the tracking algorithm can evaluate all myocardial segments.

C: Bull's-eye plot showing 18-segment strain analysis, with values for each myocardial segment. In this case, a clear apical sparing pattern indicative of amyloidosis is visible, which raises suspicion for this condition.

D: Manual editing interface for adjusting segment borders in systole and diastole. This step allows for refinement of the segment tracking to improve the accuracy of the strain measurements.

E: Three views (AP4, AP2, AP3) showing longitudinal strain results for each myocardial segment. The strain values for each segment are displayed alongside the bull's-eye plot, showing global and segmental GLS results. This information provides comprehensive insight into myocardial function.

F: Strain rate curves across multiple cardiac cycles, illustrating the temporal dynamics of myocardial deformation. This data allows for detailed assessment of myocardial contraction and relaxation phases.

Left Atrium Longitudinal Strain (LA LS) and Diastolic Dysfunction

In the context of cardiac amyloidosis, assessing diastolic dysfunction is crucial, and recent advancements in echocardiography now include not only left ventricular strain but also strain analysis of the left atrium and right ventricle. These innovations provide clinicians with tools to obtain a comprehensive view of myocardial and atrial performance.

The left atrium longitudinal strain (LA LS) is a key parameter for assessing early atrial dysfunction, particularly in the context of diastolic heart failure and cardiac amyloidosis. LA LS provides detailed strain measurements, enabling the detection of subtle atrial functional changes that might otherwise go unnoticed. This parameter has now been integrated into advanced echocardiography systems from major manufacturers such as Philips, GE, and others, enhancing the automated evaluation of diastolic function.

By automating this evaluation, LA LS offers a standardized method for clinicians to identify patients at increased risk of complications such as thromboembolic events. Its ability to detect atrial dysfunction at an early stage plays a critical role in optimizing treatment plans and improving patient outcomes. As highlighted by Badano et al. [17] the standardization of left atrial deformation imaging has facilitated the broader clinical adoption of this parameter, ensuring its consistent application across echocardiographic platforms. Furthermore, Uemura et al. [18] emphasizes its significance in identifying thromboembolic risk, particularly in patients with transthyretin amyloid cardiomyopathy, underscoring its value in clinical decision-making (Fig. 13).

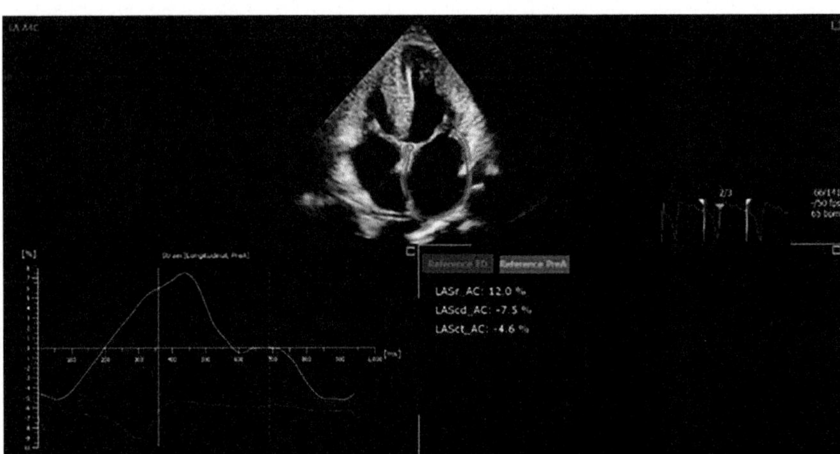

Fig. 13 Left atrium longitudinal strain (LA LS) in amyloid patient

This image illustrates the left atrium longitudinal strain (LA LS) analysis in a patient diagnosed with cardiac amyloidosis. To obtain accurate LA LS measurements, the transducer should be slightly tilted counterclockwise to maximize the size of the left atrium. After acquiring the image with the largest atrial volume, the strain values are automatically calculated with a single click.

Studies have demonstrated that LA LS provides a reliable indicator of early atrial dysfunction, particularly in patients with cardiac amyloidosis, where reduced atrial contraction function is closely linked to diastolic heart failure [17, 18]. This analysis is especially significant in detecting subtle changes in atrial performance that might otherwise go unnoticed during conventional imaging techniques.

The strain results shown here highlight reduced atrial contraction function, a key indicator of early atrial dysfunction in amyloidosis, often associated with diastolic heart failure. Automated LA LS assessment streamlines the diagnostic process, offering clinicians immediate and detailed evaluations of atrial performance, thereby aiding in both diagnosis and treatment planning [16, 19].

Auto Strain RV and Clinical Significance

Right ventricular (RV) longitudinal strain is a key parameter for evaluating RV function, particularly in diseases like pulmonary hypertension and cardiac amyloidosis. Recent technological advancements, such as the AutoStrain RV developed by TOMTEC and integrated into Philips systems, automate the assessment of RV strain. This tool provides precise and detailed evaluations of RV function, streamlining RV strain calculations and offering accurate assessments of both global and regional RV function. These advancements are critical in managing conditions that affect the right side of the heart [17, 19].

3D RV Strain: Some systems, including Philips and GE, now offer 3D RV strain, enabling a comprehensive evaluation of RV size and function. This technique provides a more complete and reproducible view, particularly valuable during follow-up studies, ensuring precise assessments of RV performance and aiding in the monitoring of disease progression more effectively [10, 20].

Additionally, GE and other major manufacturers have introduced innovations in RV strain and left atrial strain (LA LS), expanding the toolkit for diagnosing and monitoring heart conditions involving both ventricles and atria. GE's systems, for example, increasingly incorporate automated strain calculations for RV and LA, significantly improving diagnostic capabilities in complex cardiac conditions, including amyloidosis [15].

These developments underscore the importance of adopting advanced imaging techniques, such as the focused RV view, which provides a horizontal view of the heart. This view allows for more accurate and reproducible measurements of RV function, including strain, TAPSE, S′, and RV volume. Familiarity with this view is essential for echocardiographers aiming to optimize RV assessments and enhance diagnostic precision [8, 17].

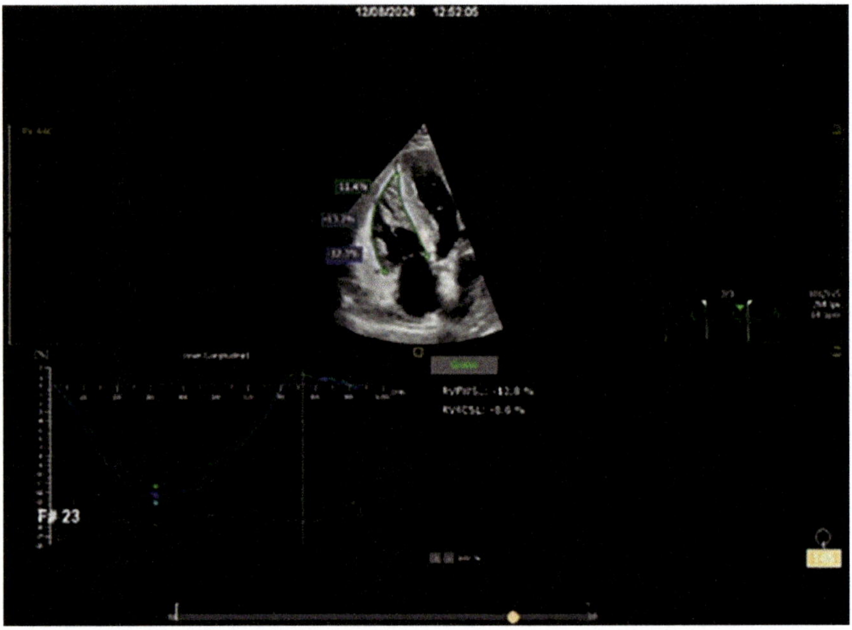

Fig. 14 Right ventricular strain in amyloidosis patient

This image demonstrates the RV longitudinal strain measured from the focused RV view in a patient with amyloidosis. The global strain values indicate reduced function, particularly in the basal and mid-segments of the right ventricle, consistent with RV involvement in amyloidosis. The strain curve highlights regional dysfunction, providing valuable insights into the severity of the disease and aiding in prognosis assessment [19].

Advanced tools like AutoStrain RV, as integrated into systems such as those from Philips and GE, enable automated and accurate analysis of RV strain from images like this. These tools simplify the workflow, ensuring precise and reproducible measurements essential for diagnosing and monitoring conditions like cardiac amyloidosis. The focused RV view, shown here in Fig. 14, plays a critical role in optimizing strain imaging and enhancing clinical decision-making [17].

Heart Model

The Heart Model by Philips represents a significant leap in echocardiographic imaging through its use of AI-based algorithms for advanced cardiac function assessment. This cutting-edge tool automates the calculation of left ventricular ejection fraction (EF) and offers a comprehensive 3D analysis of the heart's function. Its utility extends to various cardiac conditions, including cardiac amyloidosis, where precise functional evaluation is critical [15].

The Heart Model's workflow is designed for efficiency: by acquiring a single 3D volume clip, it processes data from all myocardial segments and provides real-time EF calculations. This capability minimizes variability and offers immediate, reproducible results [20]. This is particularly valuable for cardiac amyloidosis, as it enables clinicians to assess both systolic and diastolic function, streamlining the diagnostic process and facilitating timely treatment decisions.

The integration of AI-driven automation ensures that clinicians can rely on consistent and highly accurate measurements, even in challenging cases. The tool has demonstrated its ability to support advanced diagnostic workflows, making it an indispensable asset for echocardiographic imaging [17] (Fig. 15).

The image displays a 3D echocardiographic analysis using Philips' Heart Model, showing the automatic segmentation of the left ventricle and the real-time calculation of EF and other critical parameters, derived from all myocardial segments. This automated segmentation highlights the precision of the Heart Model, which provides immediate and accurate assessments, particularly valuable in conditions like cardiac amyloidosis, where comprehensive functional analysis is crucial for detecting subtle myocardial impairments and guiding treatment strategies.

Summary: Key Echocardiographic Red Flags in the Diagnosis of Cardiac Amyloidosis

Sonographers are often the first to identify subtle but significant signs that may suggest cardiac amyloidosis. The following red flags should prompt further investigation and communication with the interpreting physician [1]:

Patient Demographics: Males over the age of 60 presenting with unexplained myocardial thickening.

Echocardiographic Findings: Look for thickened ventricular walls, diastolic dysfunction, reduced tissue Doppler velocities, enlarged and thickened atria, pericardial effusion, thickened and calcified valves, (in particular aortic stenosis), a thickened, interatrial septum and apical sparing on 2D and strain imaging.

ECG Correlation: Abnormal ECG findings, such as low voltage or pseudo infarction patterns, should be cross-checked with echo findings.

Patient Symptoms: Ask about common symptoms like shortness of breath, fatigue, or swelling, and note if there is a history of hypertension.

By recognizing these red flags, sonographers can help guide physicians toward further diagnostic testing for amyloidosis, leading to timely diagnosis and treatment.

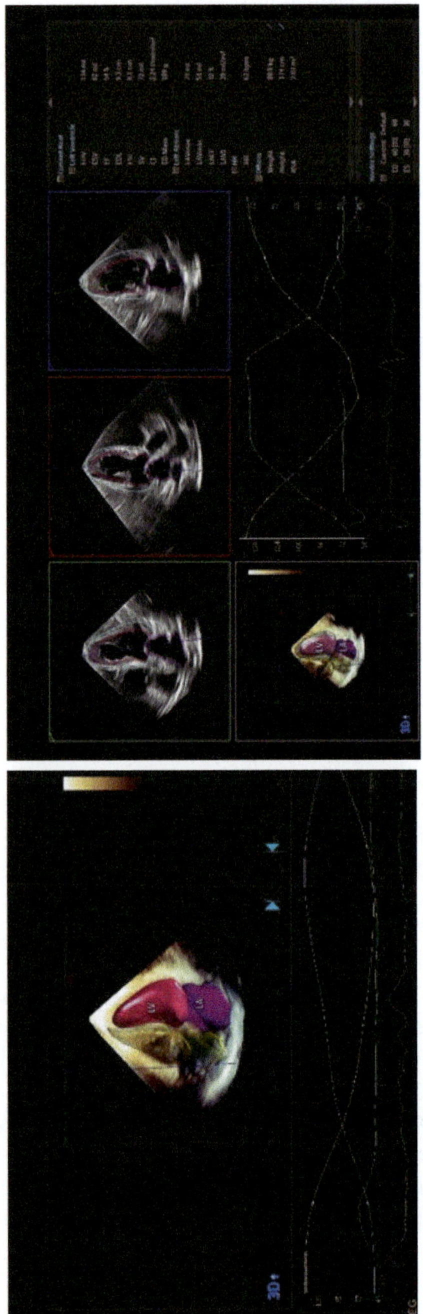

Fig. 15 3D heart model in an amyloid patient

Acknowledgements I am honored to have had the opportunity to write this chapter and contribute to the growth of our profession. To all my fellow echocardiographers and sonographers—your diligence and skill are the driving force behind these life-saving technologies. Together, we are advancing the field of echocardiography, one scan at a time.

Bibliography

1. Donnelly JP, Hanna M. Cardiac amyloidosis: an update on diagnosis and treatment. CCJM. 2017;84(12 suppl 3):12–26. https://doi.org/10.3949/ccjm.84.s3.02.
2. Brito D, Albrecht FC, De Arenaza DP, et al. World heart federation consensus on transthyretin amyloidosis cardiomyopathy (ATTR-CM). Glob Heart. 2023;18(1):59. https://doi.org/10.5334/gh.1262.
3. González-López E, Gagliardi C, Dominguez F, et al. Clinical characteristics of wild-type transthyretin cardiac amyloidosis: disproving myths. Eur Heart J. 2017;38(24):1895–904. https://doi.org/10.1093/eurheartj/ehx043.
4. Rapezzi C, Emdin M, Aimo A. Unravelling the role of sex in the pathophysiology, phenotypic expression and diagnosis of cardiac amyloidosis. Eur J Heart Fail. 2022;24(12):2364–6. https://doi.org/10.1002/ejhf.2674.
5. Garcia-Pavia P, Rapezzi C, Adler Y, et al. Diagnosis and treatment of cardiac amyloidosis: a position statement of the ESC working group on myocardial and pericardial diseases. Eur Heart J. 2021;42(16):1554–68. https://doi.org/10.1093/eurheartj/ehab072.
6. Yang C-H, Takeuchi M, Nabeshima Y, et al. Prognostic value of apical sparing of longitudinal strain in patients with symptomatic aortic stenosis. Acta Cardiol. Sin. 2022;38(3). https://doi.org/10.6515/ACS.202205_38(3).20211209A.
7. Scully PR, Patel KP, Treibel TA, et al. Prevalence and outcome of dual aortic stenosis and cardiac amyloid pathology in patients referred for transcatheter aortic valve implantation. Eur Heart J. 2020;41(29):2759–67. https://doi.org/10.1093/eurheartj/ehaa170.
8. Voigt JU, Pedrizzetti G, Lysyansky P, et al. Definitions for a common standard for 2D speckle tracking echocardiography: consensus document of the EACVI/ASE/industry task force to standardize deformation imaging. J Am Soc Echocardiogr. 2015;28(2):183–93. https://doi.org/10.1016/j.echo.2014.11.003.
9. Negishi K, Negishi T, Hare JL, Haluska BA, Plana JC, Marwick TH. Independent and incremental value of deformation indices for prediction of Trastuzumab-induced cardiotoxicity. J Am Soc Echocardiogr. 2013;26(5):493–8. https://doi.org/10.1016/j.echo.2013.02.008.
10. Eckstein J, Moghadasi N, Körperich H, et al. A machine learning challenge: detection of cardiac amyloidosis based on Bi-atrial and right ventricular strain and cardiac function. Diagnostics. 2022;12(11):2693. https://doi.org/10.3390/diagnostics12112693.
11. Lang RM, Badano LP, Mor-Avi V, et al. Recommendations for Cardiac Chamber Quantification by Echocardiography in Adults: an update from the American Society of echocardiography and the European Association of cardiovascular imaging. Eur Heart J Cardiovasc Imaging. 2015;16(3):233–71. https://doi.org/10.1093/ehjci/jev014.
12. Dorbala S, Ando Y, Bokhari S, et al. ASNC/AHA/ASE/EANM/HFSA/ISA/SCMR/SNMMI expert consensus recommendations for multimodality imaging in cardiac amyloidosis: part 1 of 2—evidence base and standardized methods of imaging. Circ: Cardiovascular Imaging. 2021;14(7). https://doi.org/10.1161/HCI.0000000000000029.
13. Boldrini M, Cappelli F, Chacko L, et al. Multiparametric echocardiography scores for the diagnosis of cardiac amyloidosis. JACC: Cardiovascular Imaging. 2020;13(4):909–920. https://doi.org/10.1016/j.jcmg.2019.10.011.
14. Biering-Sørensen T, Biering-Sørensen SR, Olsen FJ, et al. Global longitudinal strain by echocardiography predicts long-term risk of cardiovascular morbidity and mortality in a

low-risk general population: the Copenhagen city heart study. Circ: Cardiovascular Imaging. 2017;10(3):e005521. https://doi.org/10.1161/CIRCIMAGING.116.005521.
15. Kwan AC, Chang EW, Jain I, et al. Deep learning-derived myocardial strain. JACC: Cardiovascular Imaging. 2024;17(7):715–725. https://doi.org/10.1016/j.jcmg.2024.01.011.
16. Peng G, Luo S, Zhong X, et al. Feasibility and reproducibility of semi-automated longitudinal strain analysis: a comparative study with conventional manual strain analysis. Cardiovasc Ultrasound. 2023;21(1):12. https://doi.org/10.1186/s12947-023-00309-5.
17. Badano LP, Kolias TJ, Muraru D, et al. Standardization of left atrial, right ventricular, and right atrial deformation imaging using two-dimensional speckle tracking echocardiography: a consensus document of the EACVI/ASE/Industry Task Force to standardize deformation imaging. Eur Heart J—Cardiovasc Imaging. 2018;19(6):591–600. https://doi.org/10.1093/ehjci/jey042.
18. Uemura K, Ichikawa Y, Nagai S, et al. Effect of tafamidis on left atrial function of patients with transthyretin amyloid cardiomyopathy. Heart Vessels. 2024;39(9):810–7. https://doi.org/10.1007/s00380-024-02402-9.
19. Moñivas Palomero V, Durante-Lopez A, Sanabria MT, et al. Role of right ventricular strain measured by two-dimensional echocardiography in the diagnosis of cardiac amyloidosis. J. Am. Soc. Echocardiogr. 2019;32(7):845–853.e1. https://doi.org/10.1016/j.echo.2019.03.005.
20. Medvedofsky D, Mor-Avi V, Amzulescu M, et al. Three-dimensional echocardiographic quantification of the left-heart chambers using an automated adaptive analytics algorithm: multicentre validation study. Eur Heart J Cardiovasc Imaging. 2018;19(1):47–58. https://doi.org/10.1093/ehjci/jew328.

Radionuclide Imaging in Cardiac Amyloidosis

Yaniv Yechiel and Simona Ben-Haim

Abstract Cardiac amyloidosis (CA) is caused by the deposition of misfolded aggregates of light chain (AL) or transthyretin (TTR) proteins, based on the precursor proteins, in the extracellular compartment of the myocardium. It causes a restrictive cardiomyopathy and poses significant challenges in both diagnosis and management. Radionuclide imaging techniques have emerged as pivotal tools in the evaluation of cardiac amyloidosis, offering insights into the pathological processes underlying this condition. Unlike anatomical imaging modalities, radionuclide imaging allows for the detection of molecular and functional abnormalities at early stages, enabling timely intervention with novel therapies recently introduced, that may result in improved patient outcomes and prognosis. In this chapter, we explore the principles, methodologies, and clinical applications of radionuclide imaging in the context of cardiac amyloidosis with emphasis on ATTR. We delve into the specific radiotracers and imaging modalities employed, their diagnostic accuracy, and their role in guiding therapeutic strategies. Furthermore, we discuss the evolving landscape of radionuclide imaging techniques, highlighting recent advances and their potential implications for the future diagnosis and management of this complex cardiac disorder. By examining the role of radionuclide imaging through a comprehensive lens, this chapter aims to provide clinicians and researchers with a thorough understanding of its utility in the context of cardiac amyloidosis, emphasizing its contribution to personalized patient care and improved clinical outcomes.

Keywords Cardiac amyloidosis · ATTR · AL · Single-photon emission computed tomography (SPECT) · Positron emission tomography (PET)

Y. Yechiel
Department of Nuclear Medicine, Rambam Health Care Campus, Haifa, Israel

S. Ben-Haim (✉)
Department of Biophysics and Nuclear Medicine, Hadassah Medical Organization, Jerusalem, Israel
e-mail: simonabh@hadassah.org.il

Faculty of Medicine, Hebrew University of Jerusalem, Jerusalem, Israel

University College London, London, UK

E. Herzog (ed.), *Cardiac Amyloidosis*, https://doi.org/10.1007/978-3-031-88342-2_6

Introduction

Cardiac amyloidosis (CA) can present as wild type (ATTRwt), also called senile ATTR, or hereditary, also called variant ATTR (ATTRv), characterized by the deposition of transthyretin (TTR, prealbumin) protein, or as light-chain amyloidosis (AL), where light-chain amyloid deposits are produced by plasma cells. Radionuclide imaging plays a pivotal role in evaluating these conditions, as it has the capability to distinguish between the ATTR and AL variants, assess the extent of cardiac involvement, as well as involvement of other organs and monitor the effectiveness of treatment.

ATTR presents a unique diagnostic challenge due to its often subtle clinical presentation and overlap with other cardiovascular conditions. This condition results in a restrictive cardiomyopathy, most commonly presenting in men in their early 70s onwards. Patients may present with carpal tunnel syndrome or spinal stenosis (in ATTR), macroglossia, proteinuria or nephrotic syndrome (in AL), or peripheral neuropathy (both ATTR and AL). Cardiac amyloidosis should be suspected in individuals with heart failure with preserved ejection fraction (HFpEF) and thickened ventricles with grade 2 or greater diastolic dysfunction, pericardial effusion and impaired LV strain with apical sparing on echocardiography or typical findings on cardiac magnetic resonance imaging (CMR), such as diffuse late gadolinium enhancement, abnormal myocardial nulling and elevated extracellular volume [1–3]. However, these findings are not specific for CA.

In patients with clinical suspicion of CA cardiac scintigraphy with technetium-99m-labeled bone avid radiotracers (^{99m}Tc-PYP, ^{99m}Tc-DPD, ^{99m}Tc-HMDP) and screening for monoclonal light chains are the main modalities in the non-invasive diagnostic algorithm, enabling to avoid endomyocardial biopsy [1, 4]. A positive bone-avid radiotracer SPECT study and negative light chains study is highly specific for ATTR. In ATTR, gene sequencing of the transthyretin gene is recommended, to differentiate between ATTRwt and ATTRv, to define the best treatment and the need for further genetic testing of family members [4, 5]. When light chains are positive (serum and urine immunofixation, and serum free light chain assay) a biopsy is required (bone marrow, fat or myocardium) to confirm the diagnosis of AL, to avoid a false positive diagnosis in case of monoclonal gammopathy of undetermined significance (MGUS) or multiple myeloma [4–7].

This simple non-invasive diagnostic method also enables screening of at-risk populations and helps to reveal the actual prevalence of ATTR amyloidosis [8]. With recent advances in SPECT, ATTR amyloidosis has been recognized as an underdiagnosed etiology of HFpEF, with a prevalence of up to 13% of patients presenting with HFpEF and increased left ventricular wall thickness ($\geq$ 12 mm), increasing with age [9]. Furthermore, bone-avid radiotracer SPECT imaging has also contributed to increased recognition of the prevalence of ATTR in patients with severe aortic stenosis. In a screening study of 151 patients with severe aortic stenosis referred for transcatheter aortic valve replacement (TAVR), 16% had positive ^{99m}Tc-PYP cardiac scintigraphy and were diagnosed with ATTR [10]. The intensity of ^{99m}Tc-DPD uptake in ATTR is negatively correlated with the LV ejection fraction assessed by echocardiography, and shown to predict major adverse cardiac outcomes [11].

This chapter explores the pivotal role of radionuclide imaging in the assessment of cardiac amyloidosis, highlighting its impact on clinical decision-making and patient outcomes.

Mechanism/Molecular Basis

Understanding the molecular basis and mechanism underlying radionuclide imaging in cardiac ATTR amyloidosis is crucial for appreciating its diagnostic utility. Originally, radiolabeled bone-seeking SPECT agents were incidentally discovered to localize amyloid deposits. Although the exact binding mechanism of bone-seeking radiotracers to cardiac amyloid deposits remains unclear, this binding forms the basis for detecting amyloidosis using single-photon emission computed tomography (SPECT) imaging techniques. It is hypothesized that ATTR is associated with the accumulation of insoluble amyloid fibrils composed primarily of transthyretin protein variants with high calcium content, which disrupts the normal myocardial architecture and function, leading to restrictive cardiomyopathy and heart failure [12, 13]. The bone-avid radiotracers possibly bind specifically to calcium within these amyloid deposits, emitting gamma radiation that can be detected by specialized imaging equipment [14].

Currently, several radiopharmaceuticals of phosphate derivatives are used for bone scan in clinical practice. Of them ^{99m}Tc-PYP, ^{99m}Tc-HMDP and ^{99m}Tc-DPD proved effective for the evaluation of ATTR. These radiotracers have high affinity for calcium ions, likely exposed in the amyloid fibrils, resulting in selective binding to amyloid deposits. Their main advantage is avid uptake by ATTR amyloidosis. Although uptake may occur in the AL variant, it is often low grade, possibly because of lower concentration of calcium-containing deposits. Visceral uptake (i.e. liver, spleen) may also occur, more often in patients with AL.

Additional SPECT Radiopharmaceuticals

Several additional SPECT radiopharmaceuticals may have a role for the assessment of CA. ^{123}I-MIBG (Metaiodobenzylguanidine) is useful in functional cardiac evaluation, as it reveals cardiac sympathetic impairment due to amyloid deposition. Patients with familial amyloidotic polyneuropathy often exhibit myocardial adrenergic denervation while still having viable myocardium. This condition can be detected early in the course of cardiac amyloidosis, even before clinical heart disease and echocardiographic changes become apparent [15]. The main disadvantages of ^{123}I-MIBG are that it does not differentiate between amyloid subtypes and is subject to many drug interactions (e.g., opioids, labetalol, CCB, TCA).

The iodine-radiolabeled serum amyloid P component (^{123}I–SAP) is useful for the detection of extra-cardiac amyloid deposits, including those in the liver, spleen, kidneys, bones, and adrenals. However, it is not useful for the detection of cardiac amyloid deposits. In addition, ^{123}I–SAP and is also very limited in availability [16]. ^{99m}Tc-aprotinin, a protease inhibitor still under studies, with unclear mechanism of action and limited data. It is primarily used for AL and shows promise as a potential tracer for detecting CA due to the presence of anti-proteases in amyloid deposits [17].

PET Radiopharmaceuticals

Several PET radiotracers were reported for the imaging of CA. ^{11}C-PIB (Pittsburgh compound B) is one of the first PET tracers that was reported to have reliable myocardial uptake in biopsy proven cardiac amyloidosis. It was originally used for detection of β-amyloid deposits in Alzheimer's disease and is believed to bind to amyloid fibrils of any type. ^{11}C-PIB has very high accuracy in detecting cardiac involvement in the main amyloid subtypes, with 100% accuracy in AL amyloidosis [18].

Another group of PET radiotracers are primarily thioflavin T analogues that bind along the long axis of the β sheets of the amyloid protein. This group includes fluorine-18-labeled agents such as ^{18}F-Florbetapir, ^{18}F-Florbetaben and ^{18}F-flutemetamol [19]. These radiotracers offer advantages over ^{11}C-PIB, mainly the longer half-life of 110 min, which eliminates the need for an on-site cyclotron.

^{18}F-NaF is a bone-seeking PET agent. Small studies suggest that ^{18}F-NaF may have higher uptake in ATTR cardiac amyloidosis compared to AL [20].

Finally, the novel radiotracer ^{124}I-Evuzamitide, based on the pan-amyloid reactive peptide p5 + 14. ^{124}I-Evuzamitide has been developed to bind to the electronegative surface of all types of amyloid fibrils and their associated glycosaminoglycans [21].

Imaging Procedure—Bone-Avid Radiotracers

Similar principles are applicable to ^{99m}Tc-PYP, ^{99m}Tc-HMDP and ^{99m}Tc-DPD imaging. Specific patient preparation is not necessary, and scans are typically acquired at rest. The intravenously administered dose ranges between 10 and 20 mCi (370–740 MBq). Images are acquired 3 h following injection, although a 1-h acquisition is optional for ^{99m}Tc-PYP based on assessment of excess blood pool activity; if noted during 1-h images, a repeat 3-h imaging protocol is recommended [22, 23] (Fig. 1).

Planar imaging field of view (FOV) of the chest as well as SPECT images are acquired, while whole-body imaging is optional. Hybrid imaging, integrating CT

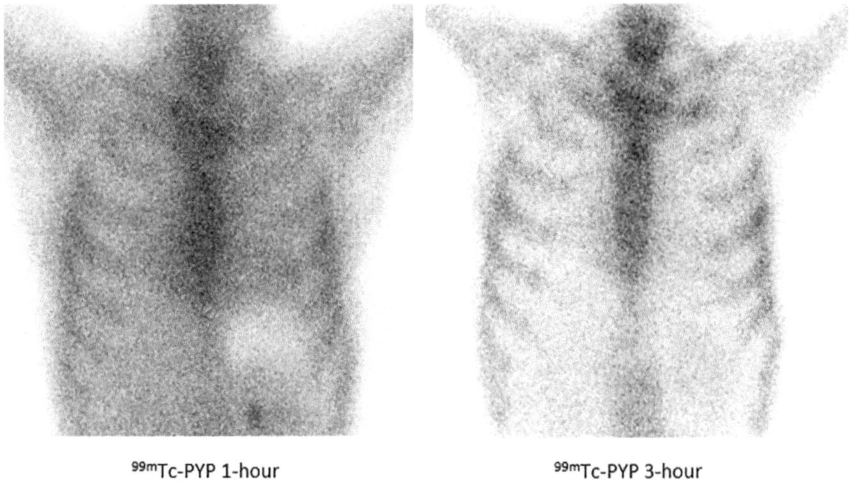

Fig. 1 ^{99m}Tc-PYP 1-h and 3-h planar images

attenuation correction of the heart is recommended. All scans are typically performed with the patient in the supine position. For optimal results, low energy, high resolution (LEHR) collimators with an energy window of 140 keV and 15–20% resolution are commonly utilized [22, 23].

Image Interpretation

The myocardial uptake patterns of ^{99m}Tc-PYP, ^{99m}Tc-DPD, and ^{99m}Tc-HMDP are categorized as absent, focal, diffuse, or focal on diffuse. Visual interpretation involves assessing planar and SPECT images to confirm diffuse radiotracer uptake in the myocardium. If excessive blood pool activity is observed on 1-h ^{99m}Tc-PYP images, it is advisable to repeat SPECT imaging at 3 h after radiotracer injection. Semi-quantitative visual analysis methods are employed to evaluate myocardial uptake relative to bone (rib) uptake. According to this grading system (Table 1 and Figs. 2 and 3), visual scores of greater than or equal to rib activity on planar or SPECT images at 3 h (grade 2, 3) are classified as ATTR positive, score 0 as ATTR negative, and score 1 as equivocal [24].

Standardized reporting should include conclusions drawn from the interpretation of overall findings, categorized into one of the following three classifications [19, 20]:

1. Not suggestive of ATTR cardiac amyloidosis (semi-quantitative visual Grade of 0).
2. Strongly suggestive of ATTR cardiac amyloidosis (semi-quantitative visual score of 2 or 3).

Table 1 Semi-quantitative visual assessment (grade) for cardiac ATTR amyloidosis

Grade	^{99m}Tc-PYP/^{99m}Tc-DPD/^{99m}Tc-HMDP myocardial uptake
0	No myocardial uptake; rib uptake is normal
1	Myocardial uptake is less than rib uptake
2	Myocardial uptake is equivalent to rib uptake
3	Myocardial uptake exceeds rib uptake; rib uptake is mild or absent

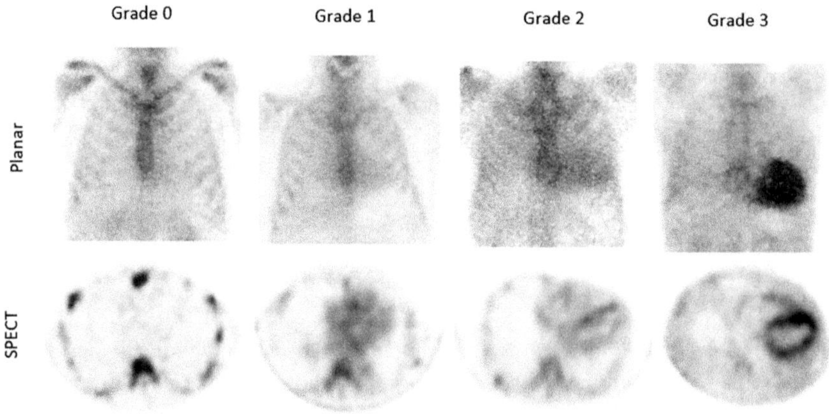

Fig. 2 Grading of myocardial ^{99m}Tc-PYP uptake

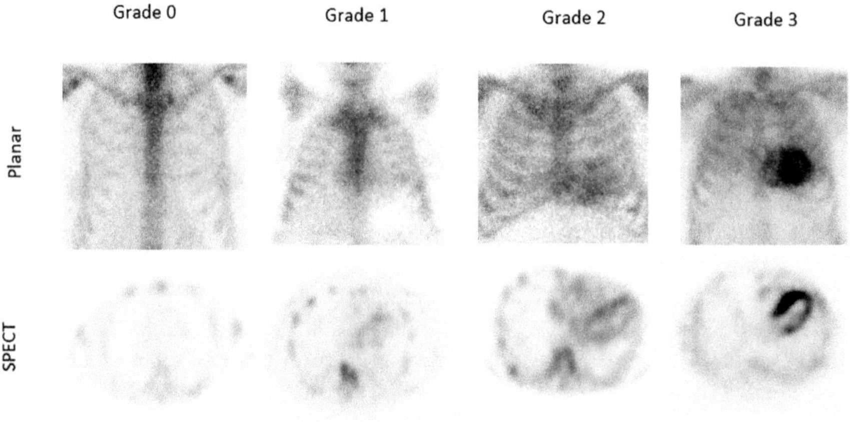

Fig. 3 Grading of myocardial ^{99m}Tc-DPD/HMDP uptake

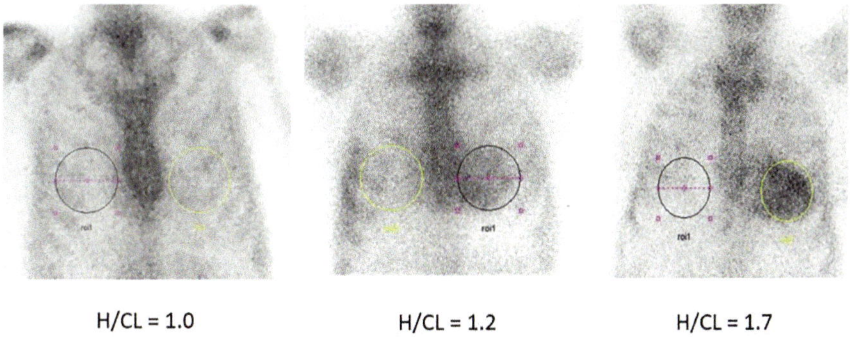

Fig. 4 Quantitation of cardiac ^{99m}Tc-PYP uptake using heart-to-contralateral lung (H/CL) ratio

3. Equivocal for ATTR cardiac amyloidosis (semi-quantitative visual score of 1).

On ^{99m}Tc-PYP scan, quantitative assessment of the Myocardial-to-Contralateral lung uptake ratio can be performed. Circular target Regions of Interest (ROI) are delineated over the heart on the anterior planar images and mirrored onto the contralateral chest to correct for background and rib interference.

Care should be taken to avoid sternal overlap and ensure the ROIs are sized appropriately to maximize coverage of the heart while excluding adjacent lung tissue. Both ROIs should be of equal size and positioned above the diaphragm (Fig. 4).

H/CL $= 1$ is negative. When myocardial uptake is seen on SPECT images, H/CL ratios of ≥ 1.5 at one hour (≥ 1.3 at 3 h) are classified as ATTR positive, while ratios of < 1.5 at 1 h (< 1.3 at 3 h) as ATTR negative [22, 25] (Fig. 4) and < 1.3 (3 h) or $<$ 1.5 (1 h) as equivocal.

Pitfalls

False-positive results are primarily caused by excessive cardiac blood pool activity within the left ventricular cavity, particularly noticeable on planar images but often resolved with SPECT imaging (Figs. 1 and 5). Other factors that can complicate scan interpretation include bone pathologies such as rib cage fractures and metastases. Care must be taken not to include such focal bone pathology in the ROI, to avoid erroneous interpretation. Aortic and mitral valves calcification may also lead to increased counts in the heart area. Additionally, myocardial pathologies/damage, such as perimyocarditis, cardiac toxicity from medications (including chemotherapy), and infarction, can contribute to false positive results due to increased nonspecific uptake. The addition of CT component as part of the scan may help to reduce these pitfalls by demonstrating morphological findings such as those described, as well as localized uptake both on blood pool and LV myocardium (Fig. 5). A positive study can also occur in AL in up to 30% of patients, although in most cases cardiac activity is low.

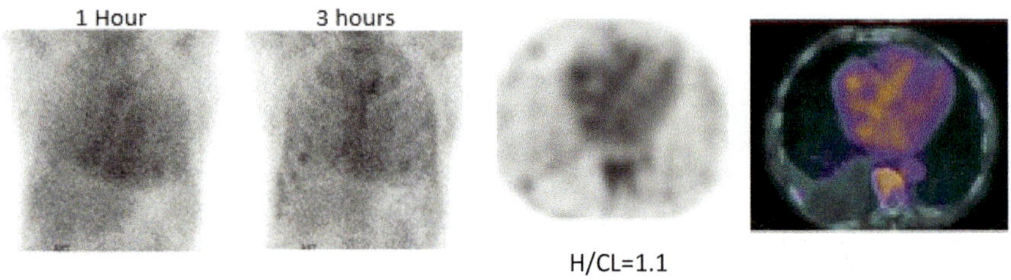

Fig. 5 ^{99m}Tc-PYP 1-h and 3-h planar and SPECT/CT images

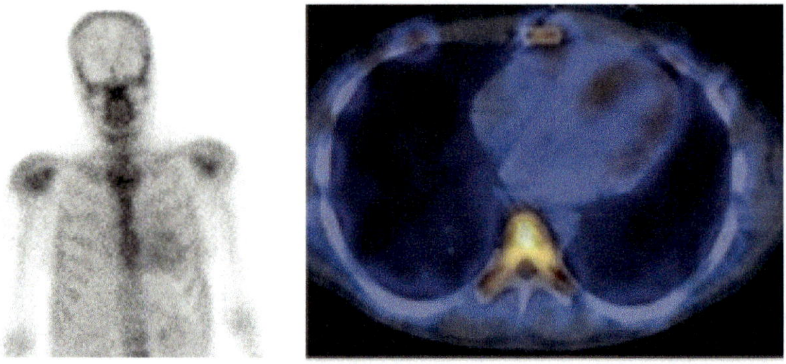

Fig. 6 Planar and SPECT/CT ^{99m}Tc-DPD in ATTRv

Therefore, the concomitant results of hematological tests have an important role in the diagnostic algorithm [23].

False-negative results can occur with certain types of CA, particularly those associated with specific genetic mutations such as Phe64Leu, Val30Met, Ser77Tyr (Fig. 6) and other variants [24, 26]. Additionally, scar tissue from a previous infarction, which does not perfuse, can also lead to false-negative results. Lastly, minimal or absent uptake may be observed in the early stages of the disease due to low levels of myocardial amyloid deposition.

PET

PET tracers, originally developed for brain beta-amyloid imaging, were also shown to accumulate in CA [20, 27]. PET may offer a solution for AL, as well as more accurate quantitation, enabling improved capabilities for the diagnosis, disease monitoring and follow up. ^{11}C-PIB was an early PET radiotracer used for this purpose but had limitations [28]. Consequently, newer radiotracers based on ^{18}F, such as ^{18}F-Florbetapir, ^{18}F-Florbetaben, ^{18}F-flutemetamol and ^{18}F-Sodium Fluoride, are

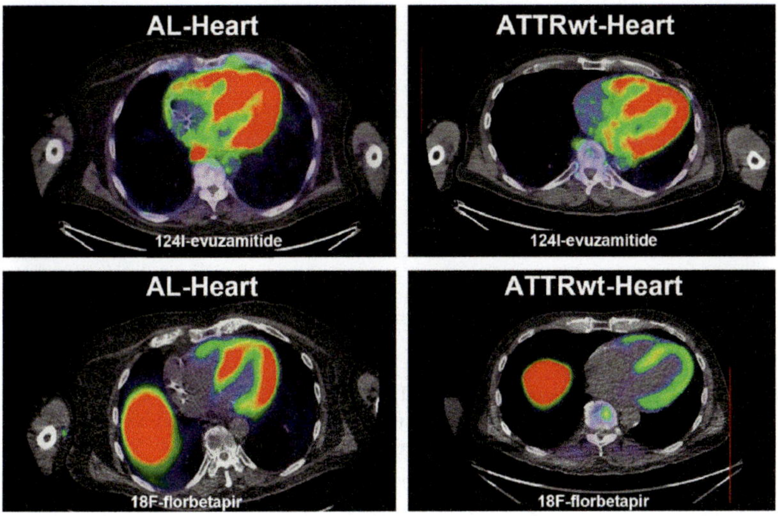

Fig. 7 PET/CT imaging of ATTR and AL (modified from Clerc et al. [8])

becoming promising alternatives for imaging CA and are under clinical investigation [20, 29–33]. Those tracers exhibit a pooled sensitivity of 95% and pooled specificity of 98% [29]. Moreover, myocardial uptake of these radiotracers is notably higher in AL amyloidosis compared to ATTR amyloidosis, highlighting their efficacy in imaging AL amyloidosis, unlike bone-avid SPECT radiotracers [29]. Some studies suggest that differences in PET radiotracer kinetics, such as delayed ^{18}F-Florbetaben cardiac uptake, could potentially differentiate cardiac amyloidosis due to AL from that caused by TTR [30].

Additional novel PET radiotracers are ^{18}F-NaF and ^{124}I-Evuzamitide mentioned above.

Studies have suggested that ^{124}I-Evuzamitide is highly accurate for a wide variety of CA and may exhibit a superior affinity for ATTRwt compared to ^{18}F-Florbetapir [8] (Fig. 7).

Quantitative Assessment

Semiquantitative metrics for ^{99m}Tc-PYP/DPD/HMDP using SPECT/CT are emerging, although less developed compared to those for PET/CT. A pilot study by Dorbala et al. found that quantitative ^{99m}Tc-PYP measures were consistent with visual grade. Using quantitative parameters such as SUV_{max}, SUV_{mean}, CAA (cardiac amyloid activity), and %ID (percentage injected dose). The study demonstrated a strong correlation between quantitative ^{99m}Tc-PYP metrics and extracellular volume (ECV) on cardiac MRI [31]. Ben-Haim et al. demonstrated that quantitative SPECT/

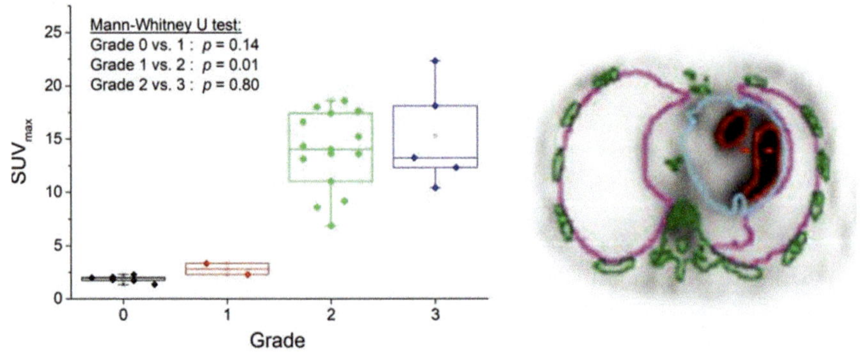

Fig. 8 SPECT/CT segmentation of cardiac and extra-cardiac activity of ^{99m}Tc-DPD in a 80-year-old male patient with suspected CA (right). Correlation between the grade of visual cardiac uptake and quantitation of myocardial activity (left). (modified from [32])

CT parameters of cardiac ^{99m}Tc-DPD uptake are effective in distinguishing between grades 2 and 3 myocardial uptake and grades 0 and 1 [32] (Fig. 8). These studies and other have demonstrated that quantitative SPECT/CT can be used to estimate amyloid burden and thus may have a role in monitoring response to targeted therapy.

CA PET scans are typically interpreted visually. Semiquantitative assessment using SUV-based metrics normalized to body weight can be calculated by SUV and myocardium–to–blood-pool activity concentration ratios on static images. Another semiquantitative measure is the percentage injected dose, which is independent of body weight [19].

Monitoring Disease Activity and Treatment Response

The primary assessment tools in the follow up of patients with CA are echocardiography and cardiac MRI. There is limited data on changing scan appearances, whether due to disease progression or treatment response in cardiac amyloidosis. Figure 9 illustrates progression of CA over a 4-year follow-up period on ^{99m}Tc-DPD scintigraphy. Current therapies targeting precursor proteins aim to enhance natural amyloid resorption, improve cardiac structure and function, and potentially reduce amyloid burden. A recent phase I study evaluated the effectiveness of an antibody-based therapy designed to remove ATTR fibrils. The study reported a reduction in myocardial uptake of bone-avid ^{99m}Tc tracer as early as four months after treatment began, along with an improvement in extracellular volume [34]. These results highlight the importance of cardiac imaging in evaluating treatment response. However, visual identification of changes on serial amyloid scans is challenging. Therefore, serial quantitative amyloid SPECT/CT or PET imaging may offer a more accurate assessment of treatment efficacy.

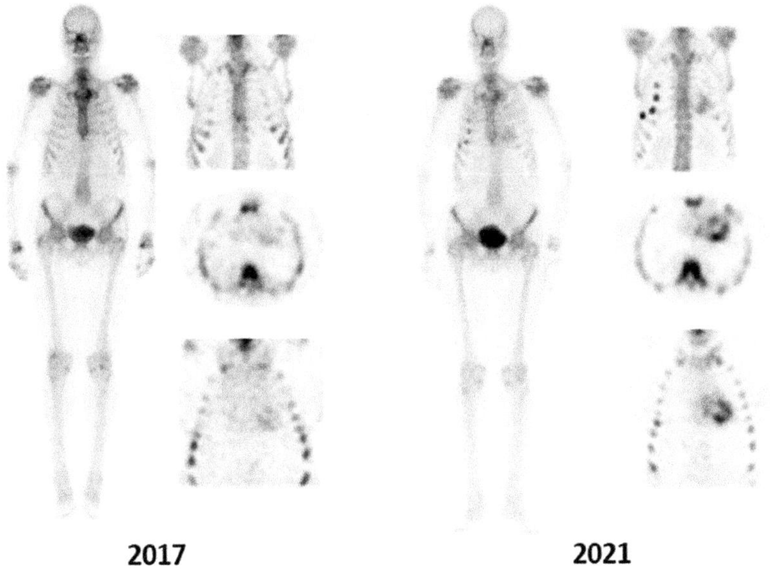

Fig. 9 ^{99m}Tc-DPD planar and SPECT: progression of ATTR over a 4-year period

Conclusions

Radionuclide imaging has emerged as a pivotal component of the diagnostic approach for cardiac amyloidosis, leveraging advancements in SPECT and PET technologies to achieve high levels of accuracy. SPECT radiotracers have revolutionized the diagnosis of ATTR cardiac amyloidosis, offering a non-invasive alternative to traditional diagnosis with endomyocardial biopsy. This shift has not only alleviated the need for invasive procedures but has also revealed a higher prevalence of ATTR cardiac amyloidosis than previously appreciated. The early detection enabled by these imaging modalities is particularly significant, as it allows for earlier therapeutic interventions with potential prognostic implications given the progressive nature of amyloidosis, where timely treatment may significantly impact patient outcomes. Moreover, PET amyloid-binding radiotracers, the most promising is ^{124}I-Evuzamitide, have demonstrated exceptional sensitivity and specificity in detecting various types of amyloidosis, including both ATTR and AL amyloidosis. This broader diagnostic scope enhances our ability to identify and differentiate between different amyloid types, thereby guiding more precise treatment strategies. Looking forward, further research is needed to accurately determine the true prevalence and incidence of cardiac amyloidosis within different populations. Additionally, ongoing studies should focus on refining diagnostic protocols and exploring the utility of follow-up imaging in assessing treatment response. These efforts are essential for advancing our understanding of cardiac amyloidosis and optimizing patient care through improved diagnostic and monitoring techniques.

References

1. Gillmore JD, Maurer MS, Falk RH, Merlini G, Damy T, Dispenzieri A, Wechalekar AD, Berk JL, Quarta CC, Grogan M, Lachmann HJ, Bokhari S, Castano A, Dorbala S, Johnson GB, Glaudemans AW, Rezk T, Fontana M, Palladini G, Milani P, Guidalotti PL, Flatman K, Lane T, Vonberg FW, Whelan CJ, Moon JC, Ruberg FL, Miller EJ, Hutt DF, Hazenberg BP, Rapezzi C, Hawkins PN. Nonbiopsy diagnosis of cardiac transthyretin amyloidosis. Circulation. 2016;133(24):2404–12. https://doi.org/10.1161/CIRCULATIONAHA.116.021612.
2. González-López E, Gallego-Delgado M, Guzzo-Merello G, de Haro-Del Moral FJ, Cobo-Marcos M, Robles C, Bornstein B, Salas C, Lara-Pezzi E, Alonso-Pulpon L, Garcia-Pavia P. Wild-type transthyretin amyloidosis as a cause of heart failure with preserved ejection fraction. Eur Heart J. 2015;36(38):2585–94. https://doi.org/10.1093/eurheartj/ehv338. Epub 2015 Jul 28.
3. Redfield MM. Heart failure with preserved ejection fraction. N Engl J Med. 2016;375(19):1868–77. https://doi.org/10.1056/NEJMcp1511175.
4. Garcia-Pavia P, Rapezzi C, Adler Y, Arad M, Basso C, Brucato A, Burazor I, Caforio ALP, Damy T, Eriksson U, Fontana M, Gillmore JD, Gonzalez-Lopez E, Grogan M, Heymans S, Imazio M, Kindermann I, Kristen AV, Maurer MS, Merlini G, Pantazis A, Pankuweit S, Rigopoulos AG, Linhart A. Diagnosis and treatment of cardiac amyloidosis: a position statement of the ESC working group on myocardial and pericardial diseases. Eur Heart J. 2021;42(16):1554–68. https://doi.org/10.1093/eurheartj/ehab072.
5. Dorbala S, Ando Y, Bokhari S, Dispenzieri A, Falk RH, Ferrari VA, Fontana M, Gheysens O, Gillmore JD, Glaudemans AWJM, Hanna MA, Hazenberg BPC, Kristen AV, Kwong RY, Maurer MS, Merlini G, Miller EJ, Moon JC, Murthy VL, Quarta CC, Rapezzi C, Ruberg FL, Shah SJ, Slart RHJA, Verberne HJ, Bourque JM. ASNC/AHA/ASE/EANM/HFSA/ISA/SCMR/SNMMI expert consensus recommendations for multimodality imaging in cardiac amyloidosis: part 1 of 2-evidence base and standardized methods of imaging. J Nucl Cardiol. 2019;26(6):2065–123. https://doi.org/10.1007/s12350-019-01760-6.Erratum.In:JNuclCardiol.2021Aug;28(4):1761-1762.doi:10.1007/s12350-021-02711-w.
6. Stats MA, Stone JR. Varying levels of small microcalcifications and macrophages in ATTR and AL cardiac amyloidosis: implications for utilizing nuclear medicine studies to subtype amyloidosis. Cardiovasc Pathol. 2016 Sep–Oct;25(5):413–7. https://doi.org/10.1016/j.carpath.2016.07.001. Epub 2016 Jul 9.
7. Ruberg FL, Grogan M, Hanna M, Kelly JW, Maurer MS. Transthyretin amyloid cardiomyopathy: JACC state-of-the-art review. J Am Coll Cardiol. 2019;73(22):2872–91. https://doi.org/10.1016/j.jacc.2019.04.003.
8. Clerc OF, Vijayakumar S, Dorbala S. Radionuclide imaging of cardiac amyloidosis: an update and future aspects. Semin Nucl Med. 2024;S0001–2998(24):00053–9. https://doi.org/10.1053/j.semnuclmed.2024.05.012.
9. AbouEzzeddine OF, Davies DR, Scott CG, Fayyaz AU, Askew JW, McKie PM, Noseworthy PA, Johnson GB, Dunlay SM, Borlaug BA, Chareonthaitawee P, Roger VL, Dispenzieri A, Grogan M, Redfield MM. Prevalence of transthyretin amyloid cardiomyopathy in heart failure with preserved ejection fraction. JAMA Cardiol. 2021;6(11):1267–74. https://doi.org/10.1001/jamacardio.2021.3070.
10. Nitsche C, Scully PR, Patel KP, Kammerlander AA, Koschutnik M, Dona C, Wollenweber T, Ahmed N, Thornton GD, Kelion AD, Sabharwal N, Newton JD, Ozkor M, Kennon S, Mullen M, Lloyd G, Fontana M, Hawkins PN, Pugliese F, Menezes LJ, Moon JC, Mascherbauer J, Treibel TA. Prevalence and outcomes of concomitant aortic stenosis and cardiac amyloidosis. J Am Coll Cardiol. 2021;77(2):128–39. https://doi.org/10.1016/j.jacc.2020.11.006.
11. Harapoz M, Evans S, Geenty P, Kwok F, Stewart G, Taylor MS, Farlow D, Thomas L. Correlation between quantitative uptake of 99mTC-DPD and echocardiographic parameters in cardiac ATTR: a novel follow-up strategy. Front Cardiovasc Med. 2021;8: 663929. https://doi.org/10.3389/fcvm.2021.663929.

12. Perugini E, Guidalotti PL, Salvi F, Cooke RM, Pettinato C, Riva L, et al. Noninvasive etiologic diagnosis of cardiac amyloidosis using 9mTc-3,3-diphosphono-1,2-propanodicarboxylic acid scintigraphy. J Am Coll Cardiol. 2005;46(6):1076–84.
13. Pilebro B, Suhr OB, Näslund U, Westermark P, Lindqvist P, Sundström T. (99m)Tc-DPD uptake reflects amyloid fibril composition in hereditary transthyretin amyloidosis. Ups J Med Sci. 2016;121(1):17–24. https://doi.org/10.3109/03009734.2015.1122687.
14. Bokhari S, Castaño A, Pozniakoff T, Deslisle S, Latif F, Maurer MS. (99m)Tc-pyrophosphate scintigraphy for differentiating light-chain cardiac amyloidosis from the transthyretin-related familial and senile cardiac amyloidoses. Circ Cardiovasc Imaging. 2013;6(2):195–201. https://doi.org/10.1161/CIRCIMAGING.112.000132.
15. Tanaka M, Hongo M, Kinoshita O, Takabayashi Y, Fujii T, Yazaki Y, Isobe M, Sekiguchi M. Iodine-123 metaiodobenzylguanidine scintigraphic assessment of myocardial sympathetic innervation in patients with familial amyloid polyneuropathy. J Am Coll Cardiol. 1997;29(1):168–74. https://doi.org/10.1016/s0735-1097(96)00438-x.
16. Hawkins PN, Lavender JP, Pepys MB. Evaluation of systemic amyloidosis by scintigraphy with 123I-labeled serum amyloid P component. N Engl J Med. 1990;323(8):508–13. https://doi.org/10.1056/NEJM199008233230803.
17. Aprile C, Marinone G, Saponaro R, Bonino C, Merlini G. Cardiac and pleuropulmonary AL amyloid imaging with technetium-99m labelled aprotinin. Eur J Nucl Med. 1995;22(12):1393–401. https://doi.org/10.1007/BF01791147.
18. Rosengren S, Skibsted Clemmensen T, Tolbod L, Granstam SO, Eiskjær H, Wikström G, Vedin O, Kero T, Lubberink M, Harms HJ, Flachskampf FA, Baron T, Carlson K, Mikkelsen F, Antoni G, Frost Andersen N, Hvitfeldt Poulsen S, Sörensen J. Diagnostic accuracy of [^{11}C]PIB positron emission tomography for detection of cardiac amyloidosis. JACC Cardiovasc Imaging. 2020;13(6):1337–47. https://doi.org/10.1016/j.jcmg.2020.02.023.
19. Dorbala S, Kijewski MF. Molecular imaging of systemic and cardiac amyloidosis: recent advances and focus on the future. J Nucl Med. 2023;64(Suppl 2):20S-28S. https://doi.org/10.2967/jnumed.
20. Abulizi M, Sifaoui I, Wuliya-Gariepy M, Kharoubi M, Israël JM, Emsen B, Bodez D, Monnet A, Didierlaurent D, Tacher V, Luciani A, Damy T, Deux JF, Itti E. ^{18}F-sodium fluoride PET/MRI myocardial imaging in patients with suspected cardiac amyloidosis. J Nucl Cardiol. 2021;28(4):1586–95. https://doi.org/10.1007/s12350-019-01885-8.
21. Clerc OF, Cuddy SAM, Robertson M, Vijayakumar S, Neri JC, Chemburkar V, Kijewski MF, Di Carli MF, Bianchi G, Falk RH, Dorbala S. Cardiac amyloid quantification using 124I-evuzamitide (124I–P5+14) versus 18F-florbetapir: a pilot PET/CT study. JACC Cardiovasc Imaging. 2023;16(11):1419–32. https://doi.org/10.1016/j.jcmg.2023.07.007.
22. Dorbala S, Bokhari S, Miller E, Bullock-Palmer R, Soman P, Thompson R. ASNC cardiac amyloidosis practice points. 99mTechnetiumPyrophosphate imaging for transthyretin cardiac amyloidosis. 2021.
23. Jerome S, Farrell MB, Warren J, Embry-Dierson M, Schockling EJ. Cardiac amyloidosis imaging, part 3: interpretation, diagnosis, and treatment. J Nucl Med Technol. 2023;51(2):102–16. https://doi.org/10.2967/jnmt.123.265492.
24. Dorbala S, Bokhari S, Glaudemans AWJM, Miller E, Bullock-Palmer R, Slart RHJA, Soman P, Thompson R, Verberne HJ. ASNC and EANM cardiac amyloidosis practice points. 99mTechnetium3,3-diphosphono1,2-propanodicarboxylic acid (DPD) and 99mTechnetiumhydroxymethylene diphosphonate (HMDP) imaging for transthyretin cardiac amyloidosis. 2019.
25. Dorbala S, Cuddy S, Falk RH. How to image cardiac amyloidosis: a practical approach. JACC Cardiovasc Imaging. 2020;13(6):1368–83. https://doi.org/10.1016/j.jcmg.2019.07.015. Epub 2019 Oct 11.
26. Musumeci MB, Cappelli F, Russo D, Tini G, Canepa M, Milandri A, Bonfiglioli R, Di Bella G, My F, Luigetti M, Grandis M, Autore C, Perlini S, Perfetto F, Rapezzi C. Low sensitivity of bone scintigraphy in detecting Phe64Leu mutation-related transthyretin cardiac amyloidosis. JACC Cardiovasc Imaging. 2020;13(6):1314–21. https://doi.org/10.1016/j.jcmg.2019.10.015.

27. Dorbala S, Vangala D, Semer J, Strader C, Bruyere JR Jr, Di Carli MF, Moore SC, Falk RH. Imaging cardiac amyloidosis: a pilot study using 1^{8}F-florbetapir positron emission tomography. Eur J Nucl Med Mol Imaging. 2014;41(9):1652–62. https://doi.org/10.1007/s00259-014-2787-6.
28. Antoni G, Lubberink M, Estrada S, Axelsson J, Carlson K, Lindsjö L, Kero T, Långström B, Granstam SO, Rosengren S, Vedin O, Wassberg C, Wikström G, Westermark P, Sörensen J. In vivo visualization of amyloid deposits in the heart with 11C-PIB and PET. J Nucl Med. 2013;54(2):213–20. https://doi.org/10.2967/jnumed.111.102053.
29. Law WP, Wang WY, Moore PT, Mollee PN, Ng AC. Cardiac amyloid imaging with 18F-florbetaben PET: a pilot study. J Nucl Med. 2016;57(11):1733–9. https://doi.org/10.2967/jnumed.115.169870. Epub 2016 Jun 15.
30. Genovesi D, Vergaro G, Giorgetti A, Marzullo P, Scipioni M, Santarelli MF, Pucci A, Buda G, Volpi E, Emdin M. [18F]-florbetaben PET/CT for differential diagnosis among cardiac immunoglobulin light chain, transthyretin amyloidosis, and mimicking conditions. JACC Cardiovasc Imaging. 2021;14(1):246–55. https://doi.org/10.1016/j.jcmg.2020.05.031.
31. Dorbala S, Park MA, Cuddy S, Singh V, Sullivan K, Kim S, Falk RH, Taqueti VR, Skali H, Blankstein R, Bay C, Kijewski MF, Di Carli MF. Absolute quantitation of cardiac ^{99m}Tc-pyrophosphate using cadmium-zinc-telluride-based SPECT/CT. J Nucl Med. 2021;62(5):716–22. https://doi.org/10.2967/jnumed.120.247312.
32. Ben-Haim S, Chicheportiche A, Goshen E, Arad M, Smekhov M, Menezes LJ, Elliott PM, O'Mahoney E, Stern E, Yuzefovich B, Bomanji JB. Quantitative SPECT/CT parameters of myocardial ^{99m}Technetium-3,3-diphosphono-1,2-propanodicarboxylic acid (DPD) uptake in suspected cardiac transthyretin amyloidosis. EJNMMI Res. 2021;11(1):86. https://doi.org/10.1186/s13550-021-00828-0.
33. Kim YJ, Ha S, Kim YI. Cardiac amyloidosis imaging with amyloid positron emission tomography: a systematic review and meta-analysis. J Nucl Cardiol. 2020;27(1):123–32. https://doi.org/10.1007/s12350-018-1365-x.
34. Garcia-Pavia P, Aus dem Siepen F, Donal E, Lairez O, van der Meer P, Kristen AV, Mercuri MF, Michalon A, Frost RJA, Grimm J, Nitsch RM, Hock C, Kahr PC, Damy T. Phase 1 trial of antibody NI006 for depletion of cardiac transthyretin amyloid. N Engl J Med. 2023 Jul 20;389(3):239–250. https://doi.org/10.1056/NEJMoa2303765.

Cardiovascular Magnetic Resonance in the Diagnosis and Prognosis of Cardiac Amyloidosis

Vladimir Kaplinskiy, Emad Albayouk, and Warren Manning

Abstract Cardiovascular magnetic resonance (CMR) has become an important clinical tool in the diagnosis of cardiac amyloidosis (CA). Its ability to provide high-resolution functional images and tissue characterization has led to its prominent role on the pathway to amyloid diagnosis or exclusion. In addition to identifying classic features of the pathology, a CMR study can provide important prognostic information. In this chapter, the authors review the utility of CMR and provide a simplified rubric for understanding the relevant features of a CMR study in the diagnosis of CA.

Keywords Cardiac magnetic resonance imaging · Late gadolinium enhancement · Extracellular volume · Native T1 mapping · Cardiac amyloidosis · Radiofrequency pulse · Relaxation time

Introduction to CMR

Cardiovascular magnetic resonance (CMR) image generation is dependent on modifying and analyzing the magnetic properties of hydrogen protons of the scanned organs. Important CMR sequences include non-contrast cine bright blood (functional) imaging, phase-contrast (flow) imaging, T1- and T2- weighted (anatomic) imaging, assessment of extracellular volume (ECV), contrast-enhanced inversion-recovery to assess for gadolinium enhancement (LGE) and native parametric mapping of the left ventricular (LV) myocardium [1].

V. Kaplinskiy (✉)
Division of Cardiology, Hadassah Medical Center, Hebrew University of Jerusalem, Jerusalem, Israel
e-mail: vkaplins@gmail.com

E. Albayouk · W. Manning
Departments of Medicine (Cardiovascular Division), Harvard Medical School, Boston, MA, USA

W. Manning
Radiology Beth Israel Deaconess Medical Center, Harvard Medical School, Boston, MA, USA

E. Herzog (ed.), *Cardiac Amyloidosis*, https://doi.org/10.1007/978-3-031-88342-2_7

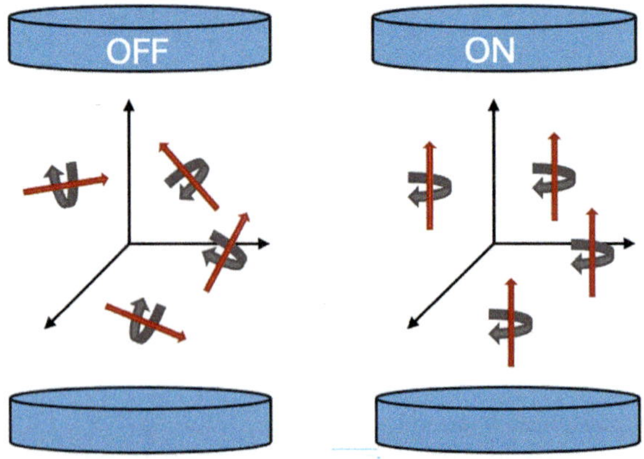

Fig. 1 Alignment of proton spins in CMR magnet. In absence of a magnetic field (off), proton spins (red arrows) orient randomly and the net/summation of spins is 0 (left side). In the presence of a magnetic field (on), proton spins align along the axis of the magnetization (along the bore of the magnet) (represented by blue disks). Proton spins align along and rotate around (precess) around the major axis of the magnetic field

CMR is feasible because hydrogen protons have orientation in space (spin) which can be influenced by a magnetic field. In the absence of a magnetic field (magnet off), protons align randomly with no net magnetic vector. In the presence of a magnetic field, the spins align along the major axis of the magnet (Fig. 1). Subsequent brief radiofrequency pulses displace (flip) the proton spins off axis. The re-orientation of these proton spins toward the baseline position is known as the relaxation time, which differs by tissue type and pathologic process.

T1 relaxation is the time that it takes for the protons to re-align along the magnetic field of the magnet. T1 is high in blood, water and muscle and therefore results in a darker signal in those tissues. T1 relaxation time is low (short) for fat hydrogen protons and this results in a bright signal (Fig. 2). Tissue with fewer protons (e.g., lungs) will also have dark signal. T2 relaxation is the time it takes for proton spins to move out of phase with each other in the transverse plane (Fig. 3). On this sequence, water protons appear bright while fibrous or calcified tissues appear dark.

Myocardial T1 and T2 mapping measures the T1 signal of each tissue pixel. Native (non-contrast) myocardial T1 before and after administration of gadolinium contrast, as well as measurement of the native T2 signal can yield important information about pathological processes. Elevated T1 is often associated with fibrosis and elevated T2 is often associated with edema (Fig. 4). Comparing the pre- and post-contrast native T1 allows an estimation of the extracellular volume (ECV). This serves as a proxy for extracellular processes such as edema and fibrosis.

Myocardial late gadolinium enhancement (LGE) is a key CMR tool for tissue characterization because it can identify evidence of fibrosis or scar. Gadolinium is an extracellular contrast agent which has a slow washout period in a collagen/scar matrix. Gadolinium shortens the T1 relaxation time and makes scar tissue appear

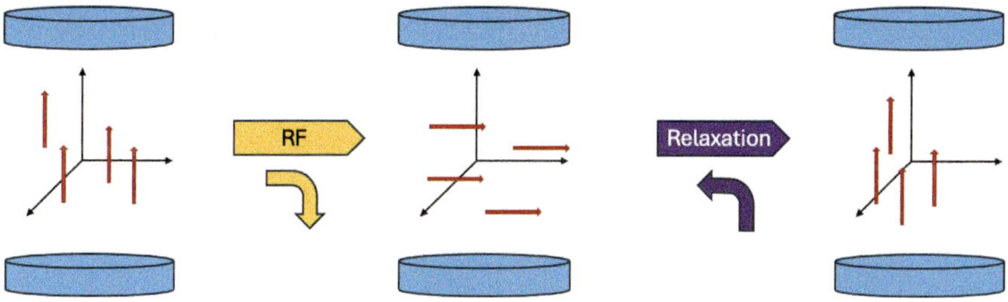

Fig. 2 Radiofrequency pulse followed by T1 relaxation. With the magnet turned on, the proton spins are aligned along the major axis of the magnet bore. A radiofrequency (RF) pulse can tip the spins by 90° (middle panel). When the pulse is turned off, the proton spins realign themselves to their original orientation along the axis of the magnet bore. The speed with which the spins re-align themselves along the major axis is known as the T1 relaxation time

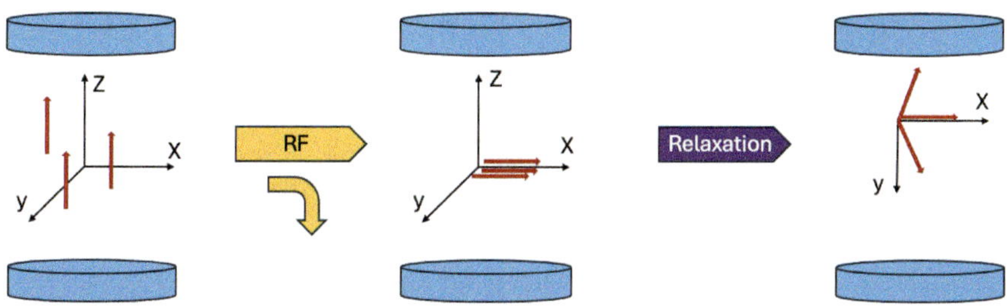

Fig. 3 Radiofrequency pulse followed by T2 relaxation. After a radiofrequency pulse displaces the spin vector into the XY plane, all spins are initially aligned in a single direction. The spins move out of phase along the XY plane with time. This is recorded as T2 relaxation

brighter on T1-weighted imaging, in contrast to normal healthy myocardium which will appear "black." To maximize the contrast, the time at which normal myocardium appears black is first identified by the technologist by an iterative process referred to as "nulling of the myocardium".

Cine imaging allows for a motion image of all cardiac chambers in 3 dimensions. Due to its high spatial resolution and high endocardial border definition, CMR cine imaging provides a detailed assessment of myocardial mass, volume and regional/global systolic function. Lastly, myocardial strain, the percentage change in myocardial length throughout the cardiac cycle, can also be measured via CMR post-processing techniques (see later). The various CMR techniques that can be applied to assessment of CA are summarized in Table 1.

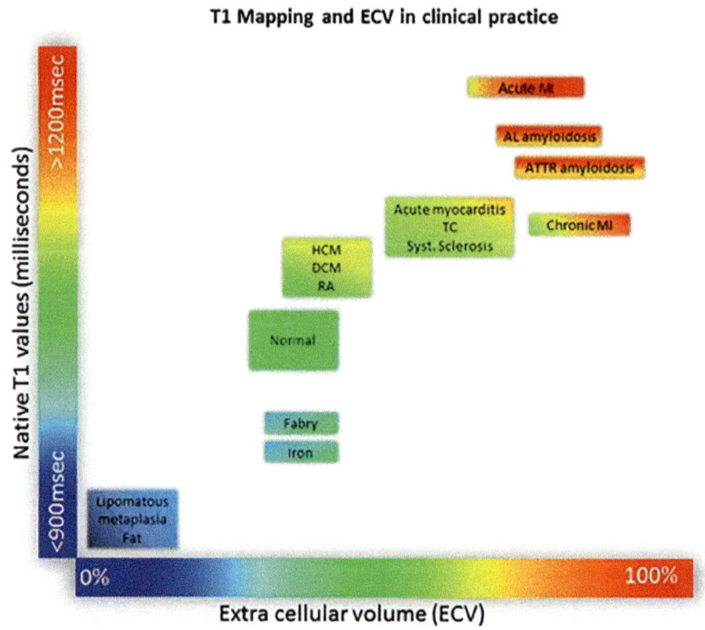

Fig. 4 T1 Mapping and ECV in clinical practice [2]. ECV and native T1 are associated with various clinical entities. Both values are highly elevated in the setting of amyloidosis. [2] Adapted from: Haaf et al.. https://doi.org/. AL = light chain; ATTR = amyloid transthyretin protein; DCM = dilated cardiomyopathy; HCM = hypertrophic cardiomyopathy

Table 1 CMR sequences in the assessment of CA

Cine imaging	T1 weighted	T2 weighted	Gadolinium enhancement	Native T1 mapping	Extracellular volume	Strain
Atrial volume Ejection fraction Wall motion Myocardial mass	Vascular anatomy Fat/fluid characterization	Inflammation/ edema	Fibrosis/scar	Scarring and fibrosis	Inflammation/ edema Fibrosis	Quantitative assessment of subtle regional anomalies

Patient Selection and Test Limitations

While CMR is a low-risk non-invasive imaging modality, careful patient selection is required to ensure safety and optimal image quality. Patients undergoing the test should be able to lay on their back for 30–60 min and, ideally, be able to follow breathing instructions, which will often require repeated 10–20 s breath-holds. As such, patients with decompensated heart failure, altered mental status or claustrophobia are potential barriers to a successful study. In certain patients, claustrophobia can be anticipated and, if appropriate, managed with anxiolytic use.

Since single CMR images are usually generated from data derived from multiple successive cardiac cycles, motion of any kind can significantly degrade image quality. In certain sequences, inability to perform a breath-hold can be managed by a longer duration "free breathing real time" sequences which have inferior spatial and temporal resolution; but this is not possible for all sequences. Similarly, arrhythmias often negatively impact image quality.

Since the exam takes place in the presence of a strong static magnetic field, a thorough evaluation is needed to ensure that there are no risks to the patient. Due to risk of movement/dislodgement of metallic objects, all implants and foreign bodies are chronicled and strict contraindications identified. Radiofrequency pulses generated by the coils can also result in focal heating of certain mechanical implants. For these reasons, many metallic objects, such as older cerebral aneurysm clips and residual metallic fragments from shrapnel injury are contraindications to CMR.

Patients with implanted cardiac devices should be evaluated on a case-by-case basis. Most modern pacemakers and defibrillators, valvular clips, annular rings, prosthetic valves and occluder devices are considered CMR conditional. This means that a CMR can be performed if certain conditions are met. For example, it is recommended to wait for 6 weeks post implantation for any conditional device that has ferromagnetic qualities, and some devices are only approved at 1.5 Tesla field strength. The presence of an intracardiac device often introduces local imaging artifacts.

A highly morbid but fortunately very rare complication of gadolinium contrast is nephrogenic systemic fibrosis, which can occur in patients with advanced renal disease who receive gadolinium-based contrast. For this reason, contrast-based CMR was previously contraindicated in patients with end stage renal disease (ESRD) and used with extreme caution in patients with advanced kidney disease or acute kidney injury. With the advent of new and safer macrocyclic gadolinium-based contrast media (e.g., Gadovist, ProHance, Dotarem), the guidelines now support the use of these macrocyclic gadolinium contrast in patients with ESRD [3]. Given nuances in contrast types, protocols vary by institution.

Finally, costs associated with CMR must be considered, as CMR is more costly than cardiac ultrasound and cardiac computed tomography; though less expensive that positron emission tomography (PET) and many radionuclide studies.

CMR Findings in Amyloid Cardiomyopathy

Although not specific, there are several findings that are commonly seen in CA patients. Myocardial infiltration by light chain (AL) or transthyretin protein (ATTR) leads to several characteristic changes, including left ventricular (LV) wall thickening and bi-atrial dilation (Fig. 5).

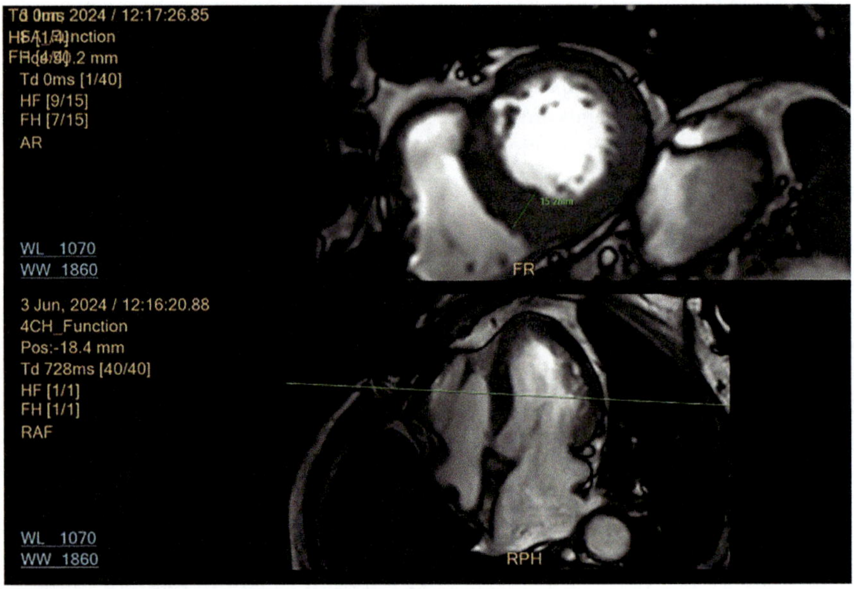

Fig. 5 Cine imaging in CA. Cine images demonstrate increased LV myocardial wall thickness (green line) and mass in a patient with amyloid cardiomyopathy

Cine imaging allows an overall assessment of the cardiac function [4]. This modality often provides high image resolution and accurate 3D-based measurements of myocardial mass, volume and biventricular regional/global systolic function.

1.5 Tesla native T1 (Fig. 6) is elevated in CA (i.e. 1140 ms vs. 958 ms in normal subjects and 979 ms in subjects with aortic stenosis). Native T1 is obtained *without* gadolinium contrast. Small studies have suggested a diagnostic accuracy (for "possible" or "definite" involvement) of up to 92% [5]. Native T1 has been shown to identify very early onset of CA in genetically predisposed patients [6]. Native T2 may also be increased in CA [7], though the association is not as well-established.

ECV is also markedly elevated in amyloidosis. In one study, patients with known CA had an average ECV of 44% compared to only 25% in healthy subjects [9]. ECV was also independently associated with a higher risk for mortality in CA patients. ECV tracks closely with LGE burden in patients with CA and also has a strong prognostic value for mortality, adjusted for other confounders such as LV ejection fraction and LV mass [10]. ECV has also been proposed as a proxy to track disease activity in response to therapy [11].

LGE is commonly seen in CA. The pattern is very heterogenous and has been described as diffuse/subendocardial (but not based on coronary distribution), patchy and even transmural (Fig. 7) [12].

As above, during the acquisition of LGE images, the technologist chooses a "null point" at which normal myocardium appears black. This is a challenge in CA because infiltration of amyloid proteins fundamentally alters the tissue characteristics. The

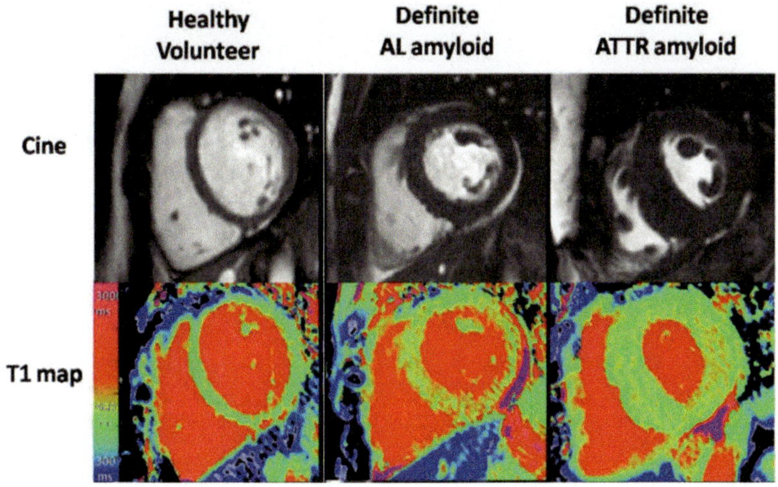

Fig. 6 Characteristic examples from CMR scans. CMR end-diastolic cine images (upper panel) and native T1 mapping (lower panel) for a healthy volunteer, AL CA and ATTR CA. Myocardial native T1 is markedly elevated in AL amyloid and ATTR amyloid (red color; higher in AL than ATTR patient), compared to the healthy volunteer. Adapted and edited for simplification: Fontana et al. [8]. https://creativecommons.org/publicdomain/zero/1.0/

inability to null the myocardium (prior to nulling of the blood pool) correlates highly with CA, yielding a sensitivity of 93% and a specificity of up to 96% [13, 14]. While in the normal condition, blood is nulled earlier than the myocardium, in some cases of CA, the nulling time of the myocardium occurs earlier than that of the blood pool.

LGE has been shown to predict mortality in all types of CA, though precise quantification is a challenge due to inability to ensure myocardial nulling [10] and findings remain controversial [15].

Beyond the diagnosis of CA, CMR parameters can aid in differentiating various forms of CA. For instance, ATTR is associated with higher ECV values compared to AL amyloidosis [16, 17]. The patterns and extent of LGE also serve as distinguishing features; transmural involvement is more frequently observed in ATTR amyloidosis, while diffuse subendocardial involvement is more commonly seen in AL amyloidosis [12, 18]. Additionally, ATTR amyloidosis typically exhibits more extensive LGE, often involving the right ventricle (RV). Dungo et al. proposed the Query Amyloid Late Enhancement (QALE) scoring system, which quantifies LGE involvement [19]. Scores greater than 13 suggest ATTR amyloidosis. At present, this scoring system requires further validation [20, 21].

Myocardial strain is another marker of subclinical myocardial dysfunction and holds significant prognostic value across a wide range of myocardial diseases [22]. Traditionally, speckle-tracking echocardiography (STE) has been the standard technique for global longitudinal strain (GLS) measurement. However, CMR feature tracking (FT) has emerged as a reliable alternative to STE, leveraging cine CMR images in the apical 2, 3, and 4-chamber orientations without tissue tagging or

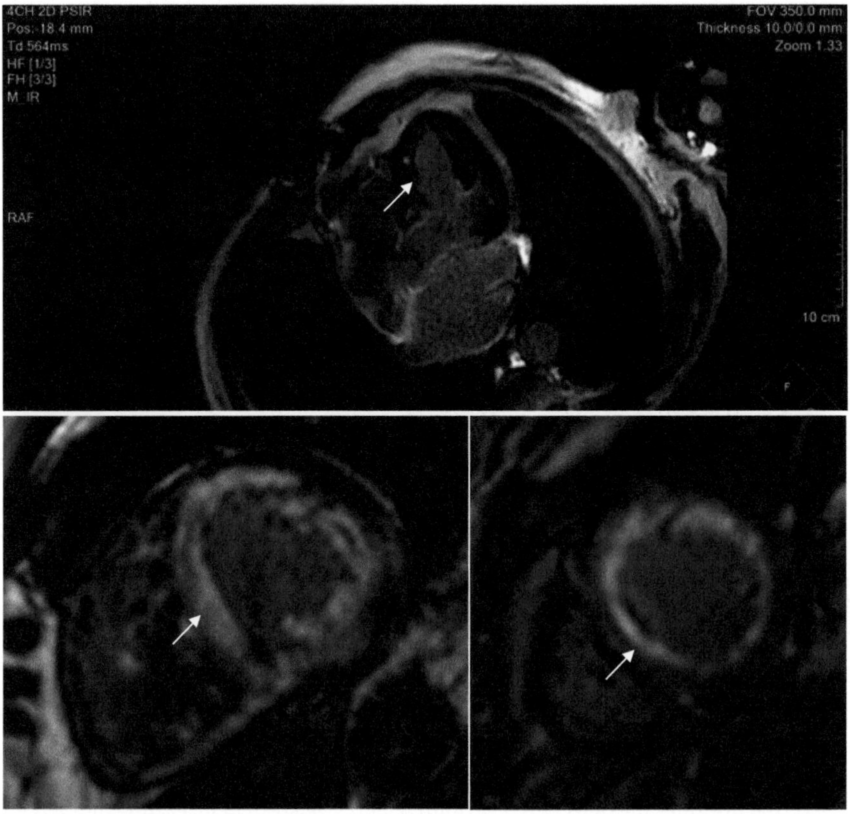

Fig. 7 Late gadolinium enhancement in CA. Diffuse, predominantly subendocardial late gadolinium enhancement (white arrow) visualized on an inversion-recovery sequence in patients with amyloid cardiomyopathy

gadolinium [23]. FT-CMR involves identifying specific patterns within images of the same myocardial regions captured at different time points during the cardiac cycle. The quantification of displacement among myocardial segments enables the calculation of deformation parameters, providing insights into myocardial mechanics. This technique is applicable in both 2-dimensional and 3-dimensional analyses [24].

The comparability of STE and FT-CMR GLS remains somewhat inconclusive [25, 26]. Nonetheless, similar to STE, CA is characterized by significantly reduced FT-CMR GLS strain values. The basal myocardial segments are typically the most affected with relative preservation of apical strain [27]. FT-CMR can facilitate early diagnosis and may assist in differentiating CA from other causes of LV hypertrophy [28]. Additionally, FT-CMR has prognostic value and is associated with all-cause mortality, particularly in patients with AL amyloidosis [29].

Additional ancillary findings in CA include increased wall thickness, increased LV mass [30], and bi-atrial enlargement in the setting of pleural and pericardial

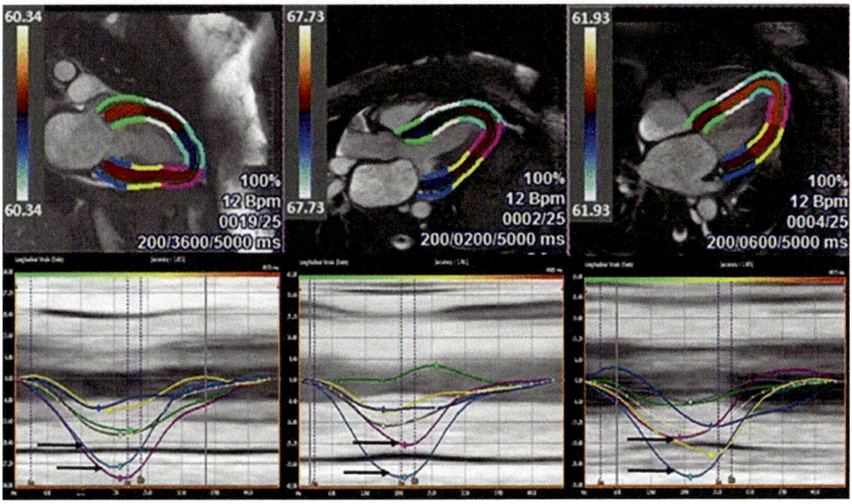

Fig. 8 Strain analysis in CA. Example of left ventricular global longitudinal strain analysis and curves in long axis views in a patient with cardiac amyloidosis. The colors of the strain curves in the lower panels correspond to segments in upper panels. The turquoise and pink curves correspond to the apical segments and have highest strain values. [33] Adapted from: Williams et al.. https://doi.org/.

effusions [31]. As above, GLS may show abnormal basal strain with relative apical sparing [32, 33] (Fig. 8). There is also a reduction in atrial strain and atrial strain rate [34]

The sequence of CMR interpretation when there is suspicion for CA can be conceptualized by a schematic below (Fig. 9).

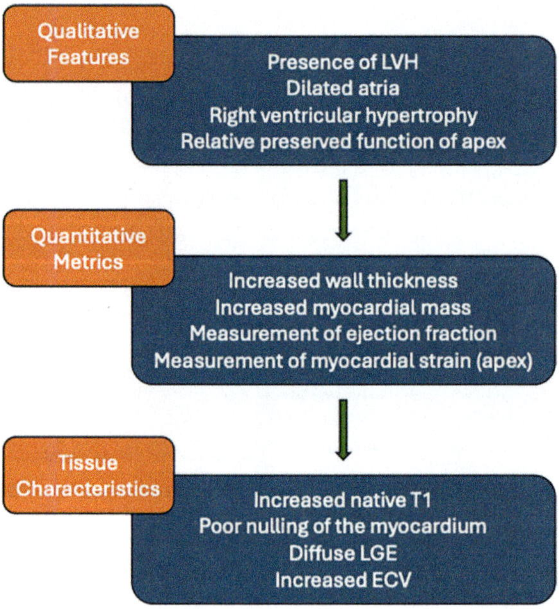

Fig. 9 Systematic analysis of CMR in patient with possible CA. Simplified schematic for review of CMR in assessment for cardiac amyloidosis. LVH: Left ventricular hypertrophy. LGE: Late gadolinium enhancement. ECV: Extracellular volume

Conclusion

CMR is an important and evolving imaging modality in the diagnosis and prognostic assessment of CA. The characteristic CMR findings of CA include increased LV thickness/mass, include high native T1, high ECV and diffuse/atypical patterns of LGE. Despite its limitations and need for careful patient selection, CMR can provide valuable insight in terms of tissue characterization, myocardial function and disease burden in patients with suspected CA.

References

1. Manning WJ, Pennell DJ. Cardiovascular magnetic resonance: a companion to Braunwald's heart disease. Elsevier Health Sciences; 2018.
2. Haaf P, Garg P, Messroghli DR, Broadbent DA, Greenwood JP, Plein S. Cardiac T1 mapping and extracellular volume (ECV) in clinical practice: a comprehensive review. J Cardiovasc Magn Reson. 2016;18:89.
3. Weinreb JC, Rodby RA, Yee J, Wang CL, Fine D, McDonald RJ, Perazella MA, Dillman JR, Davenport MS. Use of intravenous gadolinium-based contrast media in patients with kidney disease: consensus statements from the American college of radiology and the national kidney foundation. Kidney Med. 2021;3:142–50.
4. Boretto P, Patel NH, Patel K, et al. Prognosis prediction in cardiac amyloidosis by cardiac magnetic resonance imaging: a systematic review with meta-analysis. Eur Heart J Open. 2023;3:oead092.

5. Karamitsos TD, Piechnik SK, Banypersad SM, et al. Noncontrast T1 mapping for the diagnosis of cardiac amyloidosis. JACC Cardiovasc Imaging. 2013;6:488–97.
6. Fontana M, Banypersad SM, Treibel TA, et al. Native T1 mapping in transthyretin amyloidosis. JACC Cardiovasc Imaging. 2014;7:157–65.
7. Grazzini G, Pradella S, Bani R, Fornaciari C, Cappelli F, Perfetto F, Cozzi D, Giovannelli S, Sica G, Miele V. The role of T2 mapping in cardiac amyloidosis. Diagnostics (Basel). 2024. https://doi.org/10.3390/diagnostics14101048.
8. Fontana M, Banypersad SM, Treibel TA, et al. Native T1 mapping in ATTR cardiac amyloidosis—comparison with AL cardiac amyloidosis—a 200 patient study. J Cardiovasc Magn Reson. 2014;16(Suppl 1):O4. https://doi.org/10.1186/1532-429X-16-S1-O4
9. Banypersad SM, Fontana M, Maestrini V, et al. T1 mapping and survival in systemic light-chain amyloidosis. Eur Heart J. 2015;36:244–51.
10. Fontana M, Pica S, Reant P, et al. Prognostic value of late gadolinium enhancement cardiovascular magnetic resonance in cardiac amyloidosis. Circulation. 2015;132:1570–9.
11. Martinez-Naharro A, Abdel-Gadir A, Treibel TA, et al. CMR-verified regression of cardiac AL amyloid after chemotherapy. JACC Cardiovasc Imaging. 2018;11:152–4.
12. Maceira AM, Joshi J, Prasad SK, Moon JC, Perugini E, Harding I, Sheppard MN, Poole-Wilson PA, Hawkins PN, Pennell DJ. Cardiovascular magnetic resonance in cardiac amyloidosis. Circulation. 2005;111:186–93.
13. Dorbala S, Cuddy S, Falk RH. How to image cardiac amyloidosis: a practical approach. JACC Cardiovasc Imaging. 2020;13:1368–83.
14. White JA, Kim HW, Shah D, et al. CMR imaging with rapid visual T1 assessment predicts mortality in patients suspected of cardiac amyloidosis. JACC Cardiovasc Imaging. 2014;7:143–56.
15. Cuddy SAM, Jerosch-Herold M, Falk RH, et al. Myocardial composition in light-chain cardiac amyloidosis more than 1 year after successful therapy. JACC Cardiovasc Imaging. 2022;15:594–603.
16. Fontana M, Banypersad SM, Treibel TA, et al. Differential myocyte responses in patients with cardiac transthyretin amyloidosis and light-chain amyloidosis: a cardiac MR imaging study. Radiology. 2015;277:388–97.
17. Chamling B, Bietenbeck M, Drakos S, Korthals D, Vehof V, Stalling P, Meier C, Yilmaz A. A compartment-based myocardial density approach helps to solve the native T1 vs. ECV paradox in cardiac amyloidosis. Sci Rep. 2022;12:21755.
18. Caobelli F. Imaging of inflammation and infection in cardiovascular diseases. Springer Nature; 2021.
19. Dungu JN, Valencia O, Pinney JH, et al. CMR-based differentiation of AL and ATTR cardiac amyloidosis. JACC Cardiovasc Imaging. 2014;7:133–42.
20. Ridouani F, Damy T, Tacher V, Derbel H, Legou F, Sifaoui I, Audureau E, Bodez D, Rahmouni A, Deux J-F. Myocardial native T2 measurement to differentiate light-chain and transthyretin cardiac amyloidosis and assess prognosis. J Cardiovasc Magn Reson. 2018;20:58.
21. Slivnick JA, Matthew S, Tong DO, Wallner A, Raman SV, Zareba KM. Novel cardiovascular magnetic resonance model to distinguish immunoglobulin light chain from transthyretin cardiac amyloidosis. Cardiovascular Imaging. 2021.https://doi.org/10.1016/j.jcmg.2020.07.030
22. Liu B, Dardeer AM, Moody WE, Hayer MK, Baig S, Price AM, Leyva F, Edwards NC, Steeds RP. Reference ranges for three-dimensional feature tracking cardiac magnetic resonance: comparison with two-dimensional methodology and relevance of age and gender. Int J Cardiovasc Imaging. 2018;34:761–75.
23. Vo HQ, Marwick TH, Negishi K. MRI-derived myocardial strain measures in normal subjects. JACC Cardiovasc Imaging. 2018;11:196–205.
24. Claus P, Omar AMS, Pedrizzetti G, Sengupta PP, Nagel E. Tissue tracking technology for assessing cardiac mechanics: principles, normal values, and clinical applications. JACC Cardiovasc Imaging. 2015;8:1444–60.
25. Onishi T, Saha SK, Delgado-Montero A, Ludwig DR, Onishi T, Schelbert EB, Schwartzman D, Gorcsan J 3rd. Global longitudinal strain and global circumferential strain by speckle-tracking

echocardiography and feature-tracking cardiac magnetic resonance imaging: comparison with left ventricular ejection fraction. J Am Soc Echocardiogr. 2015;28:587–96.

26. Pryds K, Larsen AH, Hansen MS, et al. Myocardial strain assessed by feature tracking cardiac magnetic resonance in patients with a variety of cardiovascular diseases—a comparison with echocardiography. Sci Rep. 2019;9:11296.
27. Pandey T, Alapati S, Wadhwa V, Edupuganti MM, Gurram P, Lensing S, Jambhekar K. Evaluation of myocardial strain in patients with amyloidosis using cardiac magnetic resonance feature tracking. Curr Probl Diagn Radiol. 2017;46:288–94.
28. Pezeshki PS, Ghorashi SM, Houshmand G, Ganjparvar M, Pouraliakbar H, Rezaei-Kalantari K, Fazeli A, Omidi N. Feature tracking cardiac magnetic resonance imaging to assess cardiac manifestations of systemic diseases. Heart Fail Rev. 2023;28:1189–99.
29. Illman JE, Arunachalam SP, Arani A, Chang IC-Y, Glockner JF, Dispenzieri A, Grogan M, Araoz PA. MRI feature tracking strain is prognostic for all-cause mortality in AL amyloidosis. Amyloid. 2018;25:101–8.
30. Baggiano A, Boldrini M, Martinez-Naharro A, et al. Noncontrast magnetic resonance for the diagnosis of cardiac amyloidosis. JACC Cardiovasc Imaging. 2020;13:69–80.
31. Shah O, Choh N, Shera T, Shera F, Gojwari T, Shaheen F, Robbani I. Magnetic resonance imaging in cardiac amyloidosis: unraveling the stealth entity. Int J Angiol. 2022;31:40–7.
32. Korthals D, Chatzantonis G, Bietenbeck M, Meier C, Stalling P, Yilmaz A. CMR-based T1-mapping offers superior diagnostic value compared to longitudinal strain-based assessment of relative apical sparing in cardiac amyloidosis. Sci Rep. 2021;11:15521.
33. Williams LK, Forero JF, Popovic ZB, Phelan D, Delgado D, Rakowski H, Wintersperger BJ, Thavendiranathan P. Patterns of CMR measured longitudinal strain and its association with late gadolinium enhancement in patients with cardiac amyloidosis and its mimics. J Cardiovasc Magn Reson. 2017;19:61.
34. Sciacca V, Eckstein J, Körperich H, et al. Magnetic resonance imaging based left atrial strain and left atrial strain rate as diagnostic parameters in cardiac amyloidosis. J Clin Med Res. 2022. https://doi.org/10.3390/jcm11113150.

Hematological Manifestations and Testing in the Diagnosis of Cardiac Amyloidosis

Neta Sternbach, Iuliana Vaxman, and Morie A. Gertz

Abstract Systemic amyloidosis is a group of disorders marked by the extracellular deposition of misfolded proteins forming amyloid fibrils, which accumulate in organs and cause dysfunction. In AL amyloidosis, the amyloidogenic proteins are immunoglobulin light chains produced by clonal plasma cells. AL amyloidosis often arises in the context of plasma cell disorders, including monoclonal gammopathy of undetermined significance (MGUS) and multiple myeloma (MM), although it can occasionally emerge from other B-cell disorders. Clinical manifestations vary by organ involvement, with major impacts on the heart, kidneys, nervous system, and gastrointestinal tract. Diagnostic strategies include detecting monoclonal proteins through serum electrophoresis, immunofixation, and free light chain assays, while tissue biopsies with Congo red staining confirm amyloid deposition. In particular, amyloid fibril typing is essential to distinguish AL amyloidosis from other types, such as transthyretin amyloidosis. Recent treatment advances have improved outcomes; standard therapy now includes daratumumab with bortezomib, cyclophosphamide, and dexamethasone. This regimen has shown efficacy in reducing plasma cell burden and improving survival rates. Emerging therapies, including anti-amyloid antibodies and BCMA-targeted treatments, offer promising results. The revised Mayo Clinic Amyloid Staging system now incorporates amyloidogenic FLC levels to better predict long-term outcomes based on organ progression. With advances in early diagnosis and innovative therapies, the prognosis in AL amyloidosis has improved, but early intervention remains critical to prevent irreversible organ damage and improve patient survival.

Keywords AL amyloidosis · ATTR amyloidosis · Plasma cell disorders · Daratumumab therapy

---

N. Sternbach · I. Vaxman (✉)
Institute of Hematology, Davidoff Cancer Center, Rabin Medical Center, Petah-Tikva, Israel
e-mail: Juliava1@clalit.org.il

School of Medicine, Faculty of Medical and Health Sciences, Tel-Aviv University, Tel-Aviv, Israel

M. A. Gertz
Division of Hematology, Mayo Clinic, Rochester, MN, USA

E. Herzog (ed.), *Cardiac Amyloidosis*, https://doi.org/10.1007/978-3-031-88342-2_8

Introduction

Systemic amyloidosis encompasses a diverse group of disorders characterized by the extracellular accumulation of misfolded proteins, which form insoluble beta-pleated sheet fibrils. These fibrils deposit in various organs throughout the body, leading to organ dysfunction and potentially fatal consequences [1]. The characteristic appearance of amyloid fibrils under electron microscopy and their affinity for Congo red staining under polarized light are key diagnostic features of amyloidosis [2].

Thirty-six proteins are known to cause systemic amyloidosis, of which immunoglobulin light chain (historically referred to as primary amyloidosis) is the most common form [3]. AL amyloidosis is a type of systemic amyloidosis in which the amyloidogenic proteins are monoclonal immunoglobulin (Ig) light chains (either κ or λ) secreted by a clonal population of plasma cells in the bone marrow. These abnormal light chains can be deposited either as intact molecules or as fragments. The development of AL amyloidosis is often preceded by an increase in the level of serum free light chains, which can be detected many years before the onset of clinical symptoms, so called light chain MGUS [4]. In AL amyloidosis, the underlying pathology is associated with a clonal B-cell proliferative disorder, with most cases being related to plasma cell dyscrasias, particularly monoclonal gammopathy of undetermined significance (MGUS) and multiple myeloma (MM). However, it's important to note that AL amyloidosis can also arise from other types of B-cell disorders, albeit less commonly. These include certain subtypes of lymphoma, such as lymphoplasmacytic lymphoma (often Waldenström macroglobulinemia), CLL, or other lymphoproliferative disorders characterized by the production of monoclonal Ig light chains [5].

The clinical presentation of amyloidosis can vary significantly depending on the organs affected, and signs and symptoms can overlap between different types of amyloidosis. The major different types of systemic amyloidosis are shown in Table 1. In cardiac amyloidosis, the accumulation of amyloid fibrils in the interstitial space between cardiac myocytes can lead to restrictive cardiomyopathy. The second most common type of systemic amyloidosis involving the heart is amyloid transthyretin (formerly known as pre-albumin produced in the liver), either mutant (mATTR) or wild type (wtATTR). Differentiating between AL and TTR is often challenging.

Light chain toxicity refers to the harmful effects associated with the accumulation of free light chains. The internalization of these proteins has been linked to alterations in cellular processes, including inflammation, apoptosis, and the formation of toxic aggregates that disrupt normal cellular function. In cardiac cells, the presence of toxic light chains can lead to cardiomyocyte injury and heart failure, while in renal cells, it can result in tubular dysfunction and proteinuria [6].

Treatment of AL amyloidosis is intended to suppress light-chain production by the underlying clonal process and is anti-plasma cell-directed. The combination of daratumumab, a monoclonal antibody targeting CD38 on plasma cells, with bortezomib, cyclophosphamide, and dexamethasone (D-VCd) has shown efficacy in the treatment of AL amyloidosis and is currently the standard of care for AL amyloidosis

Table 1 The different systemic amyloidosis

Type	Precursor protein	Site of origin	Affected organs
AL amyloidosis	Immunoglobulin light chain	Bone marrow plasma cell or B cell clone	Heart, kidney, nerve, GI, liver, soft tissue, spleen, lung
wtATTR amyloidosis	Transthyretin	Liver	Heart, soft tissue, nerve
mATTR amyloidosis	Transthyretin	Liver	Heart, kidney, soft tissue, nerve
AA amyloidosis	Amyloid A protein	Liver	Kidney, liver, spleen, GI
Aβ2M amyloidosis (dialysis-related)	Beta-2 microglobulin	Component of the major histocompatibility complex class I molecules, removed by the kidneys	Joints and tendons

treatment [7, 8]. Other treatment options for AL amyloidosis may include high-dose melphalan followed by an autologous stem cell transplantation (ASCT), which is often reserved for eligible patients with preserved organ functions and good performance status [9]. New therapeutic options are emerging, and ongoing research is underway to shape clinical practice. There are several phase 3 trials using antibodies designed to dissolve amyloid fibrils by activating macrophages.

Epidemiology

Although AL amyloidosis is the most common form of systemic amyloidosis, it is considered a rare disease. The exact incidence of AL amyloidosis is challenging to determine precisely due to several factors, including underdiagnosis and varying diagnostic practices across different regions and healthcare settings. In the United States, the incidence ranges from 9.7 to 14.0 cases per million person/year [10], making it roughly one-sixth as common as MM. Conversely, a practicing hematologist should expect at least one AL amyloidosis patient for every 6 MM patients; otherwise, the likelihood of underdiagnosis is significant. AL amyloidosis incidence rates increase with age [10], with only 5% of patients being diagnosed before the age of 40, and the median age at diagnosis is commonly reported to be in the range of 60–70 years [11, 12]. There is a slight male predominance, with males accounting for 60% of patients [10]. AL amyloidosis can occur across all geographical regions and ethnicities. While the disease is generally considered to affect individuals of all races, there is emerging evidence suggesting racial disparities [13].

Plasma Cell Disorders and the Relation to AL Amyloidosis

Plasma cell (PC) disorders are clonal neoplasms of PCs resulting in a spectrum of clinical conditions—ranging from early asymptomatic states of minimal clonal expansion to symptomatic disease states with end-organ damage. The hallmark feature of plasma cell disorders is the presence of a monoclonal protein, also known as an M protein or paraprotein, in the serum and/or urine. This monoclonal protein is produced by the abnormal, clonal population of plasma cells and is composed of a heavy chain of any immunoglobulin class (IgG, IgA, IgM, IgD, or IgE) and a light chain, which can be either κ or λ.

Monoclonal gammopathy of undetermined significance represents the earliest detectable stage of PC disorders. It is characterized by the presence of an M protein in the serum at levels less than 30 g/L, clonal plasma cells in the bone marrow comprising less than 10% of all plasma cells, and the absence of end-organ damage related to the monoclonal protein.

Multiple Myeloma represents the other end of the spectrum of plasma cell disorders and is characterized by the presence of a higher burden of clonal plasma cells in the bone marrow, exceeding 10%, along with evidence of symptomatic disease: bone pain with osteolytic lesions, unexplained anemia, hypercalcemia or acute kidney failure (CRAB criteria). Additionally, the diagnosis of MM can also be established in patients with more than 60% clonal plasma cells in the bone marrow, involved/uninvolved FLC ratio of 100 or more with the involved FLC being greater than or equal to 100 mg/L or MRI with more than one focal marrow lesions, regardless of the presence of symptoms or end-organ damage (SLIM criteria).

Smoldering myeloma (SMM) represents an intermediate stage between MGUS and MM. it is characterized by a significant clonal expansion of plasma cells in the bone marrow, exceeding 10% but less than 60%, without evidence of end-organ damage or symptomatic disease.

Waldenström macroglobulinemia is a related but different condition in which a mature B cell (malignant lymphoplasmacytic cell) produces monoclonal IgM. The overproduction of monoclonal IgM antibodies in WM can lead to various clinical manifestations, including hyperviscosity syndrome (due to increased serum viscosity), neuropathy (resulting from IgM binding to peripheral nerves), cytopenias (due to bone marrow infiltration), lymphadenopathy, hepatosplenomegaly, and symptoms related to immune dysfunction.

A small percentage of patients with MGUS may progress to develop AL amyloidosis over time. The risk of progression from MGUS to AL amyloidosis is relatively low, estimated to be around 1% over 20 years [14]. However, this risk may vary among individuals and may be influenced by factors such as the size and type of the monoclonal protein, the presence of an abnormal serum-free light chain ratio, and other patient-specific characteristics.

When MM and AL amyloidosis are diagnosed in the same patient, it is more common for the MM to be diagnosed before or around the same time as the amyloidosis diagnosis. This is because MM typically presents with symptoms that prompt further evaluation and diagnosis. In some cases, however, MM may develop more than six months after the diagnosis of AL amyloidosis. This scenario, known as delayed progression or sequential development, is less common but can occur. The mechanisms underlying the delayed progression from AL amyloidosis to MM are not fully understood but may involve the continued proliferation and evolution of the underlying plasma cell clone [15, 16].

When to Suspect AL Amyloidosis

Amyloidosis lacks a single definitive diagnostic test, and its clinical manifestations can be nonspecific, often resembling those of more common disorders. Clinical suspicion plays a crucial role in identifying patients who may have amyloidosis. Early diagnosis of amyloidosis is crucial for initiating timely treatment and improving patient outcomes. Treatment strategies for amyloidosis aim to suppress the production of amyloidogenic proteins, reduce amyloid deposition, and manage organ-specific complications. Early intervention may help prevent or delay the progression of organ dysfunction and improve overall prognosis. Early mortality in AL amyloidosis is high with advanced cardiac involvement, and it remains unchanged despite advances in treatment in the past decade.

Regardless of the cell of origin or the underlying condition—all patients with *increased secretion of either light chain* should be routinely screened for AL amyloidosis by a focused history and physical examination, and routine assessment of urine albumin. Patients under observation for MGUS or SMM who become unwell and develop symptoms such as unintentional weight loss or fatigue should raise suspicion for AL amyloidosis. An asymptomatic MGUS patient with a positive Congo red stain on BM biopsy has only a 2.7% chance of developing AL amyloidosis [17]. Therefore, routine bone marrow biopsy with Congo red staining is not indicated in asymptomatic patients.

The greatest diagnostic challenge arises from the subset of cases where routine laboratory testing does not reveal a significant increase in monoclonal light chains. This scenario, which occurs in less than 2% of cases, can result from various factors, including a low burden of amyloidogenic proteins or the insufficient sensitivity of standard laboratory assays for detecting abnormal light chains [18, 19]. These cases require an even higher level of suspicion and attention to relevant clinical syndromes.

AL amyloidosis can involve almost any organ except for brain parenchyma, which is typically spared. The majority of patients manifest with multi-organ involvement. The affected organs include the heart (70%), kidney (60%), the nervous system either peripheral (15%) or autonomic (10%), the liver (20%), the gastrointestinal tract (15%), and soft tissue (10%) [20, 21]. The most common clinical scenarios that should raise suspicion include:

- preserved ejection fraction heart failure with left ventricular "hypertrophy" in the absence of hypertension or aortic stenosis

- nephrotic range proteinuria in the absence of diabetes
- peripheral or autonomic neuropathy in the absence of an apparent cause
- hepatomegaly with an elevated ALP and no liver texture abnormality on imaging studies
- specific findings on physical examination, including macroglossia and periorbital purpura (Figs. 1 and 2).

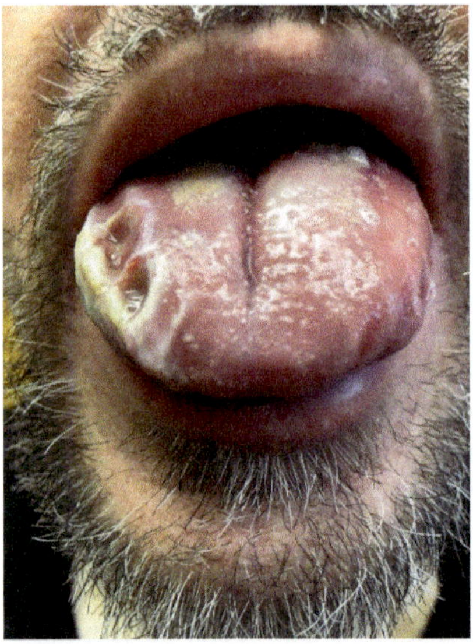

Fig. 1 Macroglossia

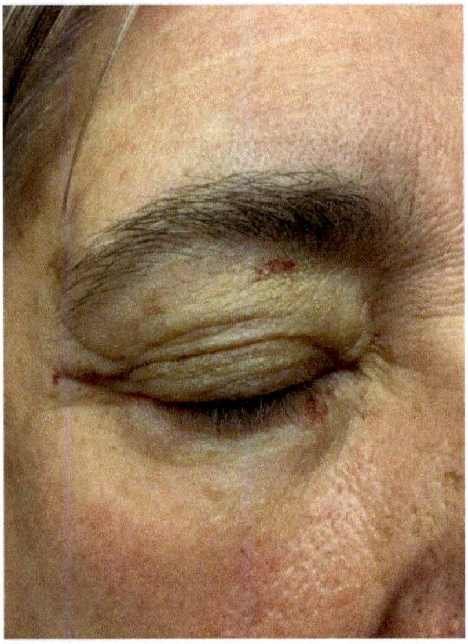

Fig. 2 Periorbital purpura

Clinical features of AL amyloidosis according to the system involved are detailed in Table 2.

Diagnosis

The diagnosis of AL amyloidosis requires histological confirmation of the presence of amyloid deposition in any body tissue and proof that this amyloid arises from clonal Ig light chains by amyloid subtyping. In addition, the identification of a monoclonal protein in the serum or urine and serum-free light chain assay results provide supportive information for the diagnosis and a measure to follow disease response.

Laboratory Features

Appropriate screening for patients with suspicious clinical scenarios should include serum protein electrophoresis (SPEP), immunofixation (IFE) of the serum, IFE of the urine, and an Ig-free light chain (FLC) assay [23]. SPEP is a quantitative test that involves separation of proteins based on their charge and mass using a gel, enabling the detection of monoclonal proteins, which appear as characteristic narrow spikes in the gamma (γ) and occasionally beta (β) regions (Fig. 3). IFE is a more sensitive technique used to characterize the type of monoclonal proteins or to detect and quantify them at lower levels than serum SPEP. IFE uses antibodies directed against each of the heavy chains and the κ and λ light chains (Fig. 4). This complimentary technique allows the identification of the type of monoclonal protein as well as the detection of small amounts of monoclonal protein otherwise undetectable on SPEP.

The serum FLC assay measures the concentrations of κ and λ light chains in the blood, along with their ratio. These FLCs are not bound to the heavy chain of immunoglobulins and can be detected due to their exposure of epitopes that are normally hidden when bound as part of the intact immunoglobulin molecule. An abnormal κ/λ ratio suggests a monoclonal plasma cell disorder, aiding in early detection and monitoring of disease progression. Aging is associated with physiological changes in immunoglobulin production, which can lead to elevated FLC levels and altered κ/λ ratios, even in the absence of plasma cell disorders. Similarly, impaired kidney function significantly affects FLC clearance, particularly for lambda chains, often resulting in increased levels and a skewed κ/λ ratio. The iStopMM study, conducted in Iceland, exemplifies the significance of light chain testing in large-scale screening and underscored the importance of accounting for these factors when interpreting FLC results. Adjusting cutoffs based on renal function and age-specific trends helps to differentiate between benign variations and true pathological findings. This approach ensures accurate identification of high-risk individuals while minimizing false positives in large-scale screening efforts. Reference Intervals for Individuals

Table 2 Clinical features of AL amyloidosis

Organ	Symptoms and signs on PE	Laboratory and imaging studies	ISA consensus definition for organ involvement [22]
Heart	Fatigue, dyspnea on exertion, orthopnea, paroxysmal nocturnal dyspnea, syncope, sudden cardiac death PE: jugular venous distention, peripheral edema, hypotension or normotension in previously hypertensive	ECG: QRS voltage to mass discordance, pseudo infract pattern (poor R wave progression), conduction abnormalities, arrhythmias ECHO: thick walled ventricles, preserved ejection fraction, atrial enlargement, restrictive pattern on Doppler studies CMR: diffuse subendocardial late gadolinium enhancement, thick walled ventricles, preserved ejection fraction, atrial enlargement BIOMARKERS: elevated BNP, NT-pro-BNP and troponin	NT-pro-BNP > = 332 ng/L in the absence of renal failure or atrial fibrillation Left ventricular wall thickness > = 12 mm on Echo
Kidney	Foamy urine PE: peripheral edema	Nephrotic range proteinuria, hyperlipidemia Enlarged kidneys on imaging (rare)	24 h protein > 500 mg/day, predominantly albumin
Nervous system	Numbness, paresthesia and pain due to peripheral nerve involvement Postural hypotension, erectile dysfunction, bladder and bowel dysfunction due to autonomic neuropathy	EMG: often not helpful when small fibers dominantly affected	
Liver	Weight loss, fatigue, abdominal distention, early satiety, bleeding disorders PE: hepatomegaly, jaundice (liver failure uncommon)	Elevated liver enzyme especially ALKP, PT, and PTT prolongation Hepatomegaly on abdominal imaging	Liver span > 15 cm in the absence of heart failure ALKP > 1.5*ULN
GI tract	Weight loss, irregular bowel habits ranging from diarrhea to constipation, GI bleeding, gastroparesis, dysphagia, bacterial overgrowth, malabsorption, intestinal pseudo-obstruction	Hypoalbuminemia, anemia	

(continued)

Table 2 (continued)

Organ	Symptoms and signs on PE	Laboratory and imaging studies	ISA consensus definition for organ involvement [22]
Soft tissue	Macroglossia, hoarseness, obstructive sleep apnea, dysarthria, enlarged salivary glands, dry mouth, paroxysmal muscle weakness, arthropathy, jaw claudication, carpel tunnel syndrome		
Spleen	Adnominal distention, early satiety. (Spontaneous spleen rupture uncommon)	Howell jolly bodies on peripheral blood smear, splenomegaly on abdominal imaging	
Coagulation system	Bleeding disorder, periorbital and other bruising	Altered coagulation profile with acquired factor X deficiency In addition—decreased synthesis of coagulation factor in patients with advanced liver disease	
Lung	Dyspnea, dry cough	Interstitial pattern on CT	Interstitial radiographic finding in the absence of pulmonary edema

PE physical examination; *ISA* the International Society of Amyloidosis; *ECG* electrocardiogram; *CMR* Cardiac magnetic resonance; *BNP* Brain natriuretic peptide; *NT-pro-BNP* N-Terminal Pro-BNP; *ALKP* alkaline phosphatase; *PT* prothrombin time; *PTT* partial thromboplastin time; *CT* computed tomography

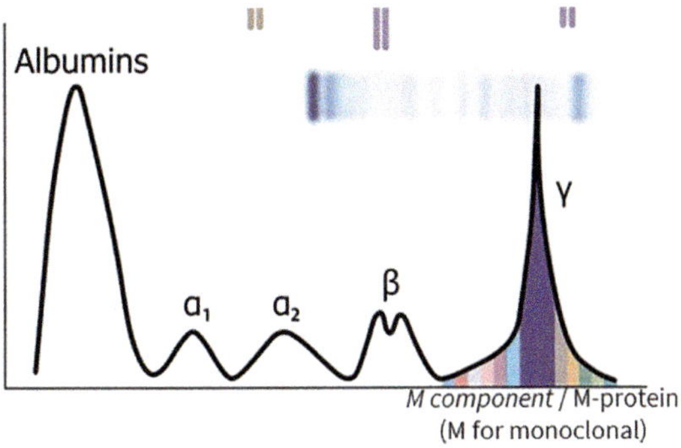

Fig. 3 Serum protein electrophoresis

Fig. 4 Immunofixation

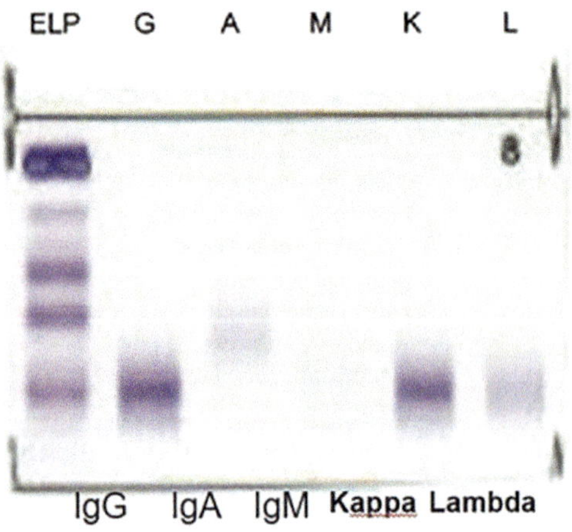

with Normal and reduced Kidney Function are shown in (Tables 3 and 4) [24]. These findings need to be further validated in additional and various patient populations.

The combination of these three tests allows for the identification of more than 98% of patients with plasma cell disorders. Most patients with AL amyloidosis have little to no intact monoclonal Ig, and they exhibit elevated evels of monoclonal FLCs in the serum. The hallmark of AL amyloidosis is the high frequency of an elevated light chain, λ type in 70% of cases [25]. If SIFE is negative and the FLC ratio is normal, AL amyloidosis is unlikely, unless the index of suspicion is very high.

Table 3 Reference intervals for individuals with normal kidney function (eGFR ≥ 60 mL/min/1.73 m^2)

Age group	Kappa FLC (mg/L)	Lambda FLC (mg/L)	FLC ratio
< 70 years	6.3–39.0	5.9–36.7	0.44–2.16
≥ 70 years	7.0–55.8	6.4–48.0	0.46–2.59

GFR glomerular filtration rate; *FLC* free light chain

Table 4 Reference intervals for individuals with reduced kidney function (eGFR < 60 mL/min/1.73 m^2)

eGFR (mL/min/1.73 m^2)	FLC ratio
45–59	0.46–2.62
30–44	0.48–3.38
< 30	0.54–3.30

GFR glomerular filtration rate; *FLC* free light chain

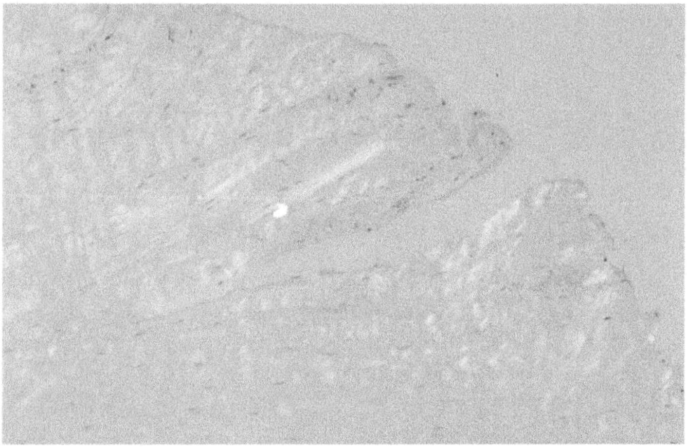

Fig. 5 Amyloid appearance in bone marrow biopsy

Pathological Features

Amyloid deposits can be demonstrated on a biopsy from either an affected organ or a surrogate site, such as the BM and abdominal subcutaneous fat. Biopsies of affected organs such as the heart, kidneys, or liver are less feasible, more invasive, and pose an increased risk of post-procedure complications, including hemorrhage. A combined biopsy with Congo red staining of BM and abdominal subcutaneous fat can identify amyloid deposits in more than 85% of cases and is often sufficient [26]. In addition, a BM examination is usually necessary since it also allows the classification of the primary PC disorder. Minor salivary gland biopsy is also sensitive in the detection of amyloid (68%), is noninvasive, and safe [27]. In case surrogate site biopsies are all negative, a biopsy from a suspected affected organ may be warranted. On the hematoxylin and eosin (H&E) stained biopsy section, amyloid appears as a pink, amorphous, waxy substance and binds strongly to Congo red (Fig. 5). The presence of amyloid can be confirmed by its characteristic appearance on electron microscopy. The PC proliferation in AL amyloidosis is typically low burden, with < 10% PCs in over half of the patients (Fig. 6).

Amyloid Typing

Amyloid typing is an important step in the diagnosis. Monoclonal gammopathies are common in older patients, and their presence in pathologically confirmed amyloidosis patients does not necessarily indicate AL amyloidosis. About 10% of patients with a pathological diagnosis of amyloidosis and positive M protein are eventually proven to have TTR amyloidosis [28]. In addition, 25% of wtATTR patients also demonstrated

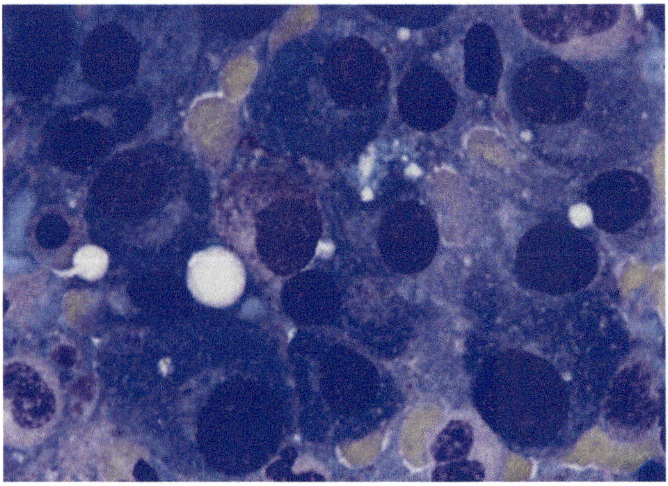

Fig. 6 Plasma cell proliferation in bone marrow biopsy

a monoclonal protein [29]. Mass spectrometry has emerged as a powerful tool in the diagnosis of amyloidosis, offering high sensitivity and specificity of more than 98% in identifying the specific type of amyloid fibrils present in tissue samples. By analyzing the amino acid sequence of the proteins within the amyloid deposits, mass spectrometry can determine the specific type of amyloid present, whether it originates from immunoglobulin light chains (AL amyloidosis), serum amyloid A protein (AA amyloidosis), transthyretin (ATTR amyloidosis), or other less common types. The technique can be applied to almost any tissue source [30].

A pathway to the diagnosis of AL amyloidosis is shown in (Fig. 7).

Clinical Evaluation and Disease Staging

In addition to a detailed history and physical examination (including the measurement of orthostatic hypotension), the following workup should be performed in all AL amyloidosis patients:

- Laboratory studies: complete blood cell count with differential, chemistry panel with liver enzymes and renal function, coagulation screening including prothrombin time and partial prothrombin time (a detailed coagulation test should be considered in patients with a bleeding disorder), serum and urine protein electrophoresis with immunofixation, serum FLC assay, 24-h urine protein, NT-pro-BNP, troponin, and thyroid stimulating hormone.
- BM aspirate and biopsy with cytogenetic studies for MM.
- Bone imaging to assess for osteolytic lesions associated with MM.
- Electrocardiogram.

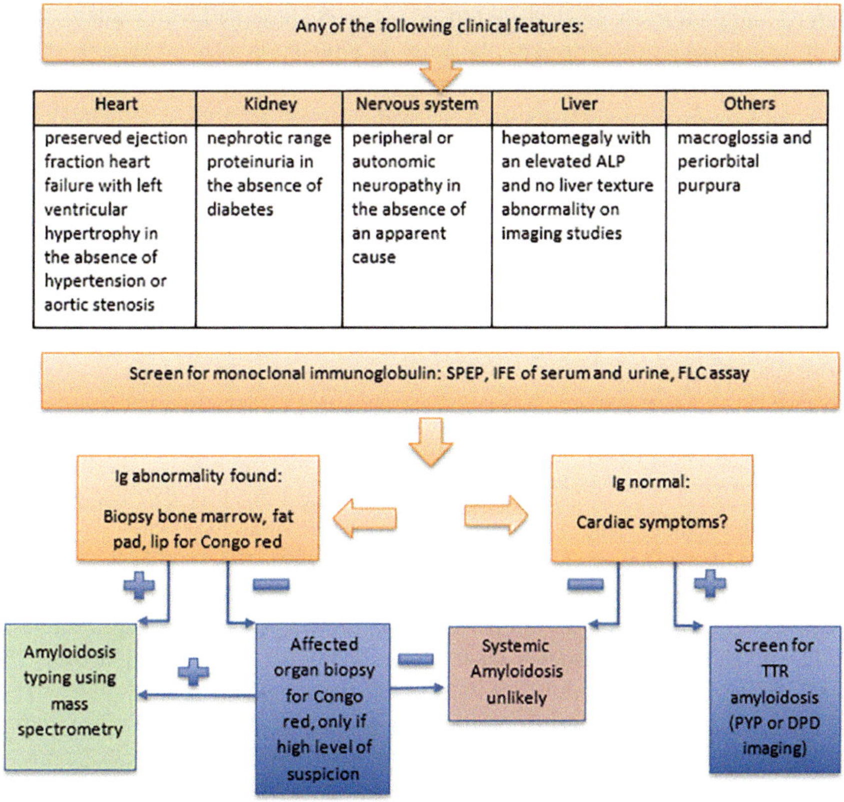

Fig. 7 A pathway to the diagnosis of AL amyloidosis

- Cardiac imaging, including transthoracic Echo. Cardiac MRI can provide helpful information if an Echo is non-diagnostic.
- Abdominal imaging to assess liver span and splenic size.
- Electromyography and nerve conduction studies in patients with neuropathy symptoms.
- Additional evaluation is based on suspected organ involvement.

The revised Mayo Clinic Amyloid Staging system classifies encompasses the following risk factors: NT-pro-BNP $\geq$ 1800 ng/L, cardiac troponin T $\geq$ 0.025 g μ/L, and a difference of involved and uninvolved serum FLCs $\geq$ 18 mg/dL. Patients are classified as having stage I, II, III, IV, based upon the identification of 0, 1, 2, or 3 of the risk factors [31]. Injury to cardiac muscle leads to the release of troponins, which are considered sensitive and specific markers of cardiac damage. Additionally, NT-pro-BNP is released from myocardial cells in response to increased wall stress, with its levels rising in both asymptomatic and symptomatic cases of left ventricular dysfunction. Previous staging systems have included only cardiac markers, which are strongly predictive of early mortality. However, the long-term prognosis for patients with AL amyloidosis is more likely influenced by the progression of organ involvement, which is, in turn, driven by the ongoing production of amyloidogenic FLC; therefore, this factor was incorporated into the staging system.

Treatment

Up until recently, the three most common treatment approaches consisted of high-dose melphalan followed by ACST, melphalan and dexamethasone, and bortezomib-based combinations. However, the introduction of daratumumab, a highly effective therapy targeting plasma cells capable of inducing deep responses, has led to a notable advancement in treatment outcomes. The combination of daratumumab, cyclophosphamide, bortezomib, and dexamethasone was studied in the ANDROMEDA trial, where it showed efficacy in inducing deep responses and improving overall survival and has become the standard of care [7]. Whether ASCT is still warranted in patients who achieve deep responses after induction therapy is a matter of ongoing debate. Immunomodulator-based regimens, including medications such as thalidomide, lenalidomide, and pomalidomide, have been extensively investigated in AL amyloidosis. Studies have shown hematological response rates ranging from 50 to 80%, with up to 50% of patients experiencing improvement in organ function [32–37]. However, immunomodulatory therapy has been associated with a higher risk for cardiac toxicity, manifesting as increasing levels of NT-pro-BNP and deteriorating cardiac function, and thus should be used cautiously [38, 39]. Future prospects include immune-directed therapy and anti-amyloid antibodies. BCMA-targeting bi-specific Antibodies are an enticing treatment option for AL amyloidosis due to their ability to induce deep and durable hematological response (As shown in MM patients) with a relatively low incidence of cytokine release syndrome as compared to other T-cell redirecting immunotherapies. Two anti-BCMA immunoconjugates have been studied and found efficacious and safe in relapsed refractory AL amyloidosis patients. Belantamab mafadotin was able to induce a rapid and durable reduction in involved FLC and improve organ function in five of six patients, achieving complete responses in three [40]. Taclistamab led to very good partial response (VGPR) or better in all seven patients (100%) [41]. BCMA-chimeric antigen receptor (CART) cells are another potential promising treatment option, with a first study providing a proof-of-concept that this therapy is safe and highly efficacious for the treatment of patients with relapsed refractory AL amyloidosis [42]. Anti-amyloid antibodies are designed to bind amyloid fibrils and lead to macrophage activation and amyloid dissolution. There are now three antibodies under clinical investigation.

Response assessment in AL amyloidosis is composed of hematological response, with FLC levels being the marker of choice and improvement in organ function. The prognosis of AL amyloidosis varies considerably depending on the extent of organ involvement, primarily the heart. Patients with advanced disease have a poor long-term prognosis, with a median survival of seven months [21]. On the other hand, patients with limited organ involvement can expect a median survival of more than five years with current therapy [43].

In the past two decades, outcomes among patients with AL amyloidosis have improved with earlier diagnosis, higher rates of hematological responses, lower early mortality, and improved survival [44].

Conclusion

The primary goal in managing AL amyloidosis is achieving an early and accurate diagnosis, given that treatment primarily focuses on decreasing Ig light chain production and is currently unable to consistently reverse organ damage once it occurs. Clinicians should be aware of patients with compatible clinical syndromes suggestive of amyloidosis and elicit testing with IFE and FLC testing, followed by BM and abdominal fat biopsy, to confirm the diagnosis. Once a diagnosis of amyloidosis is confirmed, subtyping of the amyloid protein is essential to determine the appropriate treatment protocol. The management is multidisciplinary, including a specialized cardiologist, nephrologist, dietary support, etc. The current treatment protocol is the combination of daratumumab, cyclophosphamide, bortezomib and dexamethasone. Novel therapy options, including targeted immunotherapy and anti-amyloid antibodies, are under investigation with promising results.

References

1. Merlini G, Bellotti V. Molecular mechanisms of amyloidosis. N Engl J Med. 2003;349(6).
2. De Larrea CF, Verga L, Morbini P, Klersy C, Lavatelli F, Foli A, et al. A practical approach to the diagnosis of systemic amyloidoses. Blood. 2015;125(14).
3. Benson MD, Buxbaum JN, Eisenberg DS, Merlini G, Saraiva MJM, Sekijima Y, et al. Amyloid nomenclature 2018: recommendations by the International Society of Amyloidosis (ISA) nomenclature committee. Amyloid. 2018;25(4).
4. Weiss BM, Hebreo J, Cordaro DV, Roschewski MJ, Baker TP, Abbott KC, et al. Increased serum free light chains precede the presentation of immunoglobulin light chain amyloidosis. J Clin Oncol. 2014;32(25).
5. Basset M, Defrancesco I, Milani P, Nuvolone M, Rattotti S, Foli A, et al. Nonlymphoplasmacytic lymphomas associated with light-chain amyloidosis. Blood. 2020;135.
6. Marin-Argany M, Lin Y, Misra P, Williams A, Wall JS, Howell KG, et al. Cell damage in light chain amyloidosis fibril internalization, toxicity and cell-mediated seeding. J Bio Chem. 2016;291(38).
7. Palladini G, Kastritis E, Maurer MS, Zonder J, Minnema MC, Wechalekar AD, et al. Daratumumab plus CyBorD for patients with newly diagnosed AL amyloidosis: safety run-in results of ANDROMEDA. Blood. 2020;136(1).
8. Minnema MC, Dispenzieri A, Merlini G, Comenzo RL, Kastritis E, Wechalekar AD, et al. Outcomes by cardiac stage in patients with newly diagnosed AL amyloidosis: phase 3 ANDROMEDA trial. JACC CardioOncol. 2022;4(4).
9. Bal S, Gertz MA. Autologous stem cell transplantation in the age of ANDROMEDA. Br J Haematol. 2021;193.

10. Quock TP, Yan T, Chang E, Guthrie S, Broder MS. Epidemiology of AL amyloidosis: a real-world study using US claims data. Blood Adv. 2018;2(10).
11. Kumar N, Zhang NJ, Cherepanov D, Romanus D, Hughes M, Faller DV. Global epidemiology of amyloid light-chain amyloidosis. Orphanet J Rare Dis. 2022;17(1).
12. Shimazaki C, Hata H, Iida S, Ueda M, Katoh N, Sekijima Y, et al. Nationwide survey of 741 patients with systemic amyloid light-chain amyloidosis in Japan. Intern Med. 2018;57(2).
13. D'Souza A, Pezzin L, Laud P, Singh A. Racial disparities in patients diagnosed with light chain (AL) amyloidosis. Blood Cancer J. 2021;11
14. Kyle RA, Larson DR, Therneau TM, Dispenzieri A, Kumar S, Cerhan JR, et al. Long-term follow-up of monoclonal gammopathy of undetermined significance. N Engl J Med. 2018;378(3).
15. Madan S, Dispenzieri A, Lacy MQ, Buadi F, Hayman SR, Zeldenrust SR, et al. Clinical features and treatment response of light chain (AL) amyloidosis diagnosed in patients with previous diagnosis of multiple myeloma. Mayo Clin Proc. 2010;85(3).
16. Rajkumar SV, Gertz MA, Kyle RA. Primary systemic amyloidosis with delayed progression to multiple myeloma. Cancer. 1998;82(8).
17. Chakraborty R, Gertz MA, Dispenzieri A, Gonsalves WI, Zeldenrust SR, Russell SJ, et al. Natural history of amyloidosis isolated to fat and bone marrow aspirate. Br J Haematol. 2017;179.
18. Milani P, Basset M, Russo F, Foli A, Merlini G, Palladini G. Patients with light-chain amyloidosis and low free light-chain burden have distinct clinical features and outcome. Blood. 2017;130(5).
19. Staron A, Kataria Y, Murray DL, Sloan JM, Sanchorawala V. Systemic AL amyloidosis with an undetectable plasma cell dyscrasia: a zebra without stripes. Am J Hematol. 2020;95.
20. Muchtar E, Gertz MA, Kyle RA, Lacy MQ, Dingli D, Leung N, et al. A modern primer on light chain amyloidosis in 592 patients with mass spectrometry–verified typing. Mayo Clin Proc. 2019;94(3).
21. Wechalekar AD, Schonland SO, Kastritis E, Gillmore JD, Dimopoulos MA, Lane T, et al. A European collaborative study of treatment outcomes in 346 patients with cardiac stage III AL amyloidosis. Blood. 2013;121(17).
22. Gertz MA, Comenzo R, Falk RH, Fermand JP, Hazenberg BP, Hawkins PN, et al. Definition of organ involvement and treatment response in immunoglobulin light chain amyloidosis (AL): a consensus opinion from the 10th international symposium on amyloid and amyloidosis. Am J Hematol. 2005.
23. Agis H, Krauth MT. Immunoglobulin light chain amyloidosis: short tutorial in screening, early detection, risk assessment and response evaluation. Memo—Mag Eur Med Oncol. 2021;14.
24. Long TE, Indridason OS, Palsson R, Rognvaldsson S, Love TJ, Thorsteinsdottir S, et al. Defining new reference intervals for serum free light chains in individuals with chronic kidney disease: Results of the iStopMM study. Blood Cancer J. 2022;12(9).
25. Diao X, Li J, Ouyang J, Liu J, Huang B, Chen M, et al. Flow cytometry-based immunophenotypic analysis of primary systemic light chain amyloidosis. Oncol Lett. 2017;13(4).
26. Muchtar E, Dispenzieri A, Lacy MQ, Buadi FK, Kapoor P, Hayman SR, et al. Overuse of organ biopsies in immunoglobulin light chain amyloidosis (AL): the consequence of failure of early recognition. Ann Med. 2017;49(7).
27. Suzuki T, Kusumoto S, Yamashita T, Masuda A, Kinoshita S, Yoshida T, et al. Labial salivary gland biopsy for diagnosing immunoglobulin light chain amyloidosis: a retrospective analysis. Ann Hematol. 2016;95(2).
28. Chiu A, Dasari S, Kurtin PJ, Theis JD, Vrana JA, Dispenzieri A, et al. Bone marrow amyloid: a comprehensive analysis of 1,469 samples, including amyloid type, clinical features, and morphologic distribution. Amyloid. 2022;29(3).
29. Geller HI, Singh A, Mirto TM, Padera R, Mitchell R, Laubach JP, et al. Prevalence of monoclonal gammopathy in wild-type transthyretin amyloidosis. Mayo Clin Proc. 2017;92(12).
30. Murray DL, Dasari S. Clinical mass spectrometry approaches to myeloma and amyloidosis. Clin Lab Med. 41;2021.

31. Kumar S, Dispenzieri A, Lacy MQ, Hayman SR, Buadi FK, Colby C, et al. Revised prognostic staging system for light chain amyloidosis incorporating cardiac biomarkers and serum free light chain measurements. J Clin Oncol. 2012;30(9).
32. Sanchorawala V, Wright DG, Rosenzweig M, Finn KT, Fennessey S, Zeldis JB, et al. Lenalidomide and dexamethasone in the treatment of AL amyloidosis: results of a phase 2 trial. Blood. 2007;109(2).
33. Cibeira MT, Oriol A, Lahuerta JJ, Mateos MV, de la Rubia J, Hernández MT, et al. A phase II trial of lenalidomide, dexamethasone and cyclophosphamide for newly diagnosed patients with systemic immunoglobulin light chain amyloidosis. Br J Haematol. 2015;170(6).
34. Sanchorawala V, Shelton AC, Lo S, Varga C, Sloan JM, Seldin DC. Pomalidomide and dexamethasone in the treatment of AL amyloidosis: results of a phase 1 and 2 trial. Blood. 2016;128(8).
35. Palladini G, Milani P, Foli A, Basset M, Russo F, Perlini S, et al. A phase 2 trial of pomalidomide and dexamethasone rescue treatment in patients with AL amyloidosis. Blood. 2017;129(15).
36. Palladini G, Perfetti V, Perlini S, Obici L, Lavatelli F, Caccialanza R, et al. The combination of thalidomide and intermediate-dose dexamethasone is an effective but toxic treatment for patients with primary amyloidosis (AL). Blood. 2005;105(7).
37. Wechalekar AD, Goodman HJB, Lachmann HJ, Offer M, Hawkins PN, Gillmore JD. Safety and efficacy of risk-adapted cyclophosphamide, thalidomide, and dexamethasone in systemic AL amyloidosis. Blood. 2007;109(2).
38. Dispenzieri A, Dingli D, Kumar SK, Rajkumar SV, Lacy MQ, Hayman S, et al. Discordance between serum cardiac biomarker and immunoglobulin-free light-chain response in patients with immunoglobulin light-chain amyloidosis treated with immune modulatory drugs. Am J Hematol. 2010;85(10).
39. Basset M, Kimmich CR, Schreck N, Krzykalla J, Dittrich T, Veelken K, et al. Lenalidomide and dexamethasone in relapsed/refractory immunoglobulin light chain (AL) amyloidosis: results from a large cohort of patients with long follow-up. Br J Haematol. 2021;195(2).
40. Zhang Y, Godara A, Pan S, Toskic D, Mann H, Sborov D, et al. Belantamab mafodotin in patients with relapsed/refractory AL amyloidosis with myeloma. Ann Hematol. 101;2022.
41. Leung N, Chapman JA, Bhatia S. First report of teclistamab in a patient with relapsed AL amyloidosis and multiple myeloma. EJHaem. 2023;4(4).
42. Kfir-Erenfeld S, Asherie N, Grisariu S, Avni B, Zimran E, Assayag M, et al. Feasibility of a novel academic BCMA-CART (HBI0101) for the treatment of relapsed and refractory AL amyloidosis. Clin Cancer Res. 2022;28(23).
43. Muchtar E, Gertz MA, Lacy MQ, Go RS, Buadi FK, Dingli D, et al. Ten-year survivors in AL amyloidosis: characteristics and treatment pattern. Br J Haematol. 2019;187(5).
44. Muchtar E, Gertz MA, Kumar SK, Lacy MQ, Dingli D, Buadi FK, et al. Improved outcomes for newly diagnosed AL amyloidosis between 2000 and 2014: cracking the glass ceiling of early death. Blood. 2017;129(15).

Genetic Testing in Hereditary Transthyretin Amyloidosis

Smadar Horowitz-Cederboim and Ronen Durst

Abstract Hereditary transthyretin amyloidosis (ATTRv) is a multisystem disorder caused by pathogenic variants in the *TTR* gene, increasingly recognized for its impact on cardiac function. This review explores the genetic underpinnings of ATTRv and their implications for clinical care, including the complexities of diagnosis, family screening, and management. The importance of genetic testing and variant interpretation is emphasized, alongside the critical role of genetic counseling in patient care. Current and emerging targeted therapies, as well as strategies for monitoring asymptomatic carriers, are discussed. By integrating genetic evaluation into clinical practice and fostering collaboration between geneticists and cardiologists, early diagnosis, personalized treatment, and the identification of at-risk individuals can be achieved, ultimately enhancing the management of ATTRv.

Keywords Cardiac amyloidosis · Transthyretin amyloidosis (ATTR) · Genetic testing for cardiac amyloidosis · *TTR* gene mutation · Genetic counseling in ATTRv · Penetrance in hereditary amyloidosis · Cascade genetic screening · CRISPR for amyloidosis treatment

Introduction

Hereditary cardiac amyloidosis, particularly transthyretin amyloidosis (ATTR), is increasingly recognized as a significant cause of heart failure. Cardiac amyloidosis results from the deposition of misfolded proteins in the heart, leading to cardiomyopathy. The main types include light chain amyloidosis (AL) and ATTR, which is further classified as hereditary [ATTRv (v stands for variant)] and wild-type [ATTRwt (wt stands for wild type)] amyloidosis. This review provides a comprehensive analysis of the genetic aspects of hereditary cardiac amyloidosis, focusing on its clinical

---

S. Horowitz-Cederboim (✉) · R. Durst
Department of Cardiology, Hadassah Medical Center, Hebrew University of Jerusalem, Jerusalem, Israel
e-mail: Smadarho@hadassah.org.il

E. Herzog (ed.), *Cardiac Amyloidosis*, https://doi.org/10.1007/978-3-031-88342-2_9

implications for diagnosis, family screening, and management strategies. It emphasizes the crucial role of genetic evaluation and provides practical tools for its implementation, aiming to equip cardiologists and geneticists with the tools needed to deliver personalized care and improve outcomes for patients and their families.

Prevalence and Types of Cardiac Amyloidosis

ATTRwt is the more prevalent form of transthyretin amyloidosis, primarily affecting older adults, and accounts for approximately 13% of heart failure cases in individuals over 60 years old [1]. Despite its rarity overall, ATTRv accounts for up to 21% of ATTR-CM cases in elderly patients [2, 3].

Complementing these clinical observations, data from the Genome Aggregation Database (gnomAD), indicate that the global prevalence of ATTRv is estimated to be 57.4 per 100,000 individuals, which is much higher than previously estimated using classical methods. Genomic databases provide a large sample size and an unbiased approach to estimating the prevalence of rare diseases, highlighting the potential underestimation of the actual burden of the disease [4]. Low prevalence estimates from traditional methods may be due to factors such as penetrance variability, misdiagnosis, or delayed diagnosis rather than a true reflection of the disease prevalence. Higher prevalence estimates underscore the need for increased ATTRv awareness among healthcare providers.

Clinical Manifestations and Impact of Hereditary ATTR

ATTRv is a complex multisystem disease that primarily affects the heart, nervous system, kidneys, and eyes. Cardiac involvement frequently manifests as progressive cardiomyopathy, which may lead to heart failure and conduction abnormalities, often years before diagnosis. Neurologic features include both peripheral and autonomic dysfunction, commonly presenting with sensorimotor impairment and carpal tunnel syndrome [5]. The cumulative burden of these manifestations leads to a progressive decline in functional autonomy and significantly impacts quality of life. These considerations underscore the importance of early recognition and multidisciplinary management to improve patient outcomes [6].

Genetic Basis of ATTRv

Terminology

In the context of genetic disorders, it is appropriate to note that the terminology for describing DNA alterations has evolved. The term *mutation* has largely been replaced by *pathogenic variant* for a more accurate clinical depiction. However, for simplicity, *mutation* will be used in this chapter. Genetic variants can be described at both DNA (e.g., c.267G > A) and protein (e.g., p. Gly89Ser) levels; in this text, we will primarily refer to pathogenic variants using protein-level notation. To avoid ambiguity, the gene name *TTR* will be presented in italics, while the protein name TTR will appear in regular font.

Mechanism and Inheritance

The *TTR* gene, which exhibits an autosomal dominant inheritance pattern in ATTRv, encodes transthyretin, a homotetrameric protein responsible for thyroxine and retinol-binding protein transport. An affected individual has a 50% probability of transmitting the mutation to their offspring.

Mutations in this gene are predominantly gain-of-function (GOF), typically missense mutations resulting in single amino acid substitutions. These GOF mutations destabilize the normally stable transthyretin homotetramer, leading to its dissociation into monomers prone to misfolding and aggregation. The resultant amyloid fibrils accumulate in various tissues, notably the heart and neuronal fibers, manifesting as cardiac amyloidosis, cardiomyopathy, and neuropathy [7–9]. In contrast, loss-of-function (LOF) mutations, such as nonsense mutations, are rarely reported in ATTRv. This predominance of GOF over LOF mutations elucidates the pathogenic mechanism in ATTRv, where aberrant protein function, rather than its absence, drives disease progression. Rare cases of homozygosity and compound heterozygosity in the *TTR* gene have been documented, generally resulting in more severe cardiac amyloidosis phenotypes compared to heterozygous individuals, emphasizing the dose-dependent nature of the GOF effect [10, 11].

Diversity and Phenotypic Variability of TTR Mutations

Over 140 distinct *TTR* gene mutations have been identified, each often associated with specific clinical presentations broadly categorized as predominantly cardiac, neurological, or mixed. The phenotypic expression and penetrance of these mutations can vary based on geographical location. For example, the Val30Met variant causes a rapidly progressing, early-onset, highly penetrant disease dominated by neuropathy in Portugal, while in Sweden, it results in a slowly progressing, late-onset disease with low penetrance. Specific *TTR* variants, such as Val122Ile in North America and Ile68Leu in Italy, are known to be "cardiogenic," causing clinical manifestations that closely resemble ATTRwt, including a high prevalence of carpal tunnel syndrome and a similar age of onset in the seventh or eighth decade of life. These cardiac forms also exhibit male predominance, unlike mixed forms caused by variants like Phe64Leu or Glu89Gln, where the gender disparity is less pronounced or absent [12]. ATTR is often diagnosed using bone scintigraphy, where cardiac uptake of the tracer exceeds that of the bone. However, certain mutations, such as V30M and Y114C, predominantly lead to the deposition of full-length TTR protein fibrils (type B), which can result in false-negative scintigraphy findings.

Clinical Variability and Phenotypic Diversity

Partial Penetrance and Variable Expressivity

ATTRv typically demonstrates partial penetrance, meaning that not all individuals carrying the genetic variant will manifest amyloidosis clinically. Several factors influence the risk of developing cardiac amyloidosis in ATTRv, including the specific *TTR* variant, geographical location, gender, and the transmitting parent. The penetrance of ATTRv is age-dependent and further influenced by factors such as gender and parent-of-origin effects. For example, the Val30Met mutation exhibits a penetrance of less than 10% by age 40, rising to approximately 71% by age 90 [13]. Women carrying pathogenic variants are less likely to develop cardiac involvement, and asymptomatic carriers show a higher proportion of females, suggesting lower penetrance in women. Inheriting the pathogenic *TTR* variant from the mother has been associated with earlier disease onset and higher penetrance [12]. Hence, males and those with maternal inheritance show higher penetrance rates.

Environmental and Genetic Modifiers

ATTRv also exhibits significant clinical variability influenced by environmental factors, phenotypic diversity across populations, and genetic modifiers. Environmental factors such as diet, lifestyle, as well as accompanying comorbidities like hypertension, obesity, and diabetes impact disease expression and progression, affecting penetrance and severity [14]. Different mutations exhibit varied clinical outcomes across populations, for example, the Val122Ile mutation is linked to cardiac conditions in individuals of African descent, while the His90Asn mutation is associated with dermatologic outcomes in Central-South Asian populations and neoplasms in European populations [15]. This evidence implies that both population-specific genetic factors and environmental influences contribute to the diverse clinical manifestations of ATTRv.

Genetic modifiers, such as the *TTR* stabilizing variant T119M, can result in a milder disease phenotype when present alongside pathogenic mutations by stabilizing the TTR tetramer and slowing amyloid fibril formation [14]. Non-coding variants also contribute significantly to the clinical heterogeneity of ATTRv by regulating *TTR* gene expression and influencing the distribution and accumulation of TTR-derived fibrils across different tissues, leading to diverse clinical outcomes [16].

Diagnosis and Genetic Evaluation

Indications for Genetic Testing

Genetic testing is recommended for individuals presenting with clinical signs suggestive of a TTR-related phenotype, particularly those with unexplained heart failure. Key red-flag symptoms include cardiac hypertrophy, peripheral neuropathy, carpal tunnel syndrome, or a family history of amyloidosis [17].

The first family member identified with the condition is called *proband* or *index patient*. Upon identification of a pathogenic or likely pathogenic variant in the proband, genetic testing extends to first-degree relatives and subsequently to other family members through a process called *Cascade Screening*. This approach facilitates the identification of carriers among both symptomatic patients and asymptomatic family members, enabling personalized monitoring and early intervention strategies.

Molecular Diagnosis Through Cardiomyopathy Panels and Secondary Findings

Both hereditary and wild type ATTR can mimic the presentation of hypertrophic cardiomyopathy (HCM). The prevalence of ATTR amyloidosis prevalence among HCM patients ranges between 0.5% and 3.5%. Genetic evaluation is routinely recommended for individuals with HCM, employing gene panels that typically include the *TTR* gene alongside other HCM-associated genes. Consequently, some patients may receive an unexpected molecular diagnosis of ATTRv through what was initially intended as an HCM-focused genetic test [10, 18].

In addition to cardiomyopathy panels, the *TTR* gene was included in the American College of Medical Genetics and Genomics (ACMG) recommendations for reporting secondary findings (SF) in clinical exome and genome sequencing. The ACMG SF list is a curated set of genes associated with medically actionable hereditary conditions. These genes are reported during genetic testing even when unrelated to the primary reason for the test, allowing for the identification of potentially serious but preventable or treatable health risks that might otherwise go undetected. The ACMG included *TTR* in the latest SF v3.1 update in 2022 based on its population prevalence and the availability of FDA-approved treatments [19].

Adherence to existing guidelines for genomic investigation in HCM patients, along with the ACMG's recommendations, enhances the detection of *TTR* amyloidosis. This approach enables diagnosis in both phenotypically suggestive cases and asymptomatic individuals who may otherwise be missed.

Selecting Genetic Testing Method

When selecting an appropriate genetic test for suspected ATTRv, the options range from targeted mutation testing, which focuses on known *TTR* mutations, to comprehensive approaches:

1. **Targeted mutation testing:** Most efficient when a specific *TTR* mutation is strongly suspected based on factors such as ethnicity or family history.
2. **Whole TTR gene sequencing:** Useful when ATTRv is highly probable but no specific mutation is suspected.
3. **Gene panel testing:** *TTR* is commonly included in panels for various cardiomyopathy phenotypes and neuropathies, hence offering a balance between the breadth of sequencing and targeted relevance in cardiac amyloidosis.
4. **Whole Exome Sequencing (WES):** Captures all protein-coding regions (exons, about 1–2% of the genome), encompassing about 85% of disease-causing mutations.
5. **Whole Genome Sequencing (WGS):** Sequences the entire genome, including introns and intergenic regions, offering the most comprehensive genetic analysis.

WES and WGS may be considered for more comprehensive analyses, mainly when targeted testing is negative despite high clinical suspicion. These approaches offer the opportunity to investigate genetic factors for other hereditary disorders and the possibility of detecting secondary findings, which should be discussed with patients during pre-test counseling. The different genetic testing methods available each have distinct advantages and limitations that can influence their suitability for specific clinical scenarios. A detailed comparison is provided in Table 1.

Genetic counseling is essential both before and after testing to help patients understand the implications of the results for themselves and their families. This comprehensive approach ensures that individuals are fully aware of the possible outcomes and are supported in making informed decisions about their genetic testing options.

Table 1 Comparison of genetic testing methods for hereditary transthyretin amyloidosis (ATTRv)

Testing method	Genome coverage	Availability	Advantages	Disadvantages
Targeted mutation testing	Single mutation	Widely available	• High accuracy for specific known mutations • Cost-effective when the mutation is known	• Only detects known mutations • Not useful if the mutation is unknown • Misses other mutations
Whole *TTR* gene sequencing	Single gene (TTR)	Widely available	• Detects all mutations within the *TTR* gene • Suitable for definite diagnosis of ATTR	• Does not detect mutations in other genes • Limited scope (only *TTR* gene) • May identify VOUS
Gene panel testing	Multiple genes (panel-dependent)	Widely available	• Covers multiple genes, providing broader diagnostic coverage • Suitable for both cardiomyopathy and neuropathy cases	• May identify VOUS • Higher data complexity compared to single-gene tests
Whole exome sequencing (WES)	All exons (~1–2% of the genome)	Increasing availability	• Comprehensive analysis of all coding regions (exons) • Can identify both known and novel mutations • Useful for complex, undiagnosed cases	• Does not cover non-coding regions • Requires significant resources for data interpretation • May identify VOUS and SF
Whole genome sequencing (WGS)	Entire genome	Limited availability	• Most comprehensive genetic analysis covering both coding and non-coding regions • Detects complex variants, including regulatory mutations • Useful for research purposes and undiagnosed cases	• Very high data complexity • Requires significant resources for data interpretation • High probability of identifying VOUS and SF

This table provides a comparison of different genetic testing methods used for diagnosing ATTRv. The table includes information on genome coverage, availability, advantages, and disadvantages of each method. **VOUS**: variant of uncertain significance—a genetic variant whose clinical significance is unclear. **SF**: secondary findings—incidental genetic findings unrelated to the original reason for genetic testing, which may still have clinical significance

TTR Variant Interpretation

The ACMG guidelines [20] classifies variants into five classes: Pathogenic (P), Likely Pathogenic (LP), Variant of Uncertain Significance (VOUS), Likely Benign (LB), and Benign (B).

This classification is crucial for determining the clinical significance of genetic findings, with only pathogenic or likely pathogenic variants leading to a definitive genetic diagnosis. The advent of large-scale genomic databases, such as gnomAD, has revolutionized this process by providing frequency data on genetic variants in diverse populations. These resources, along with computational predictions, functional data, and evidence from literature on variant occurrence in affected individuals, help distinguish rare pathogenic variants from benign polymorphisms, significantly enhancing the accuracy of variant interpretation.

VOUS poses unique challenges in genetic diagnosis, as their clinical implications remain unresolved. As a result, they cannot be used to establish a definitive diagnosis or guide cascade screening—unless additional evidence, such as segregation studies or functional assays, eventually clarifies their significance. This cautious approach is designed to prevent misclassification, avoiding both false reassurance and unwarranted medicalization. In the absence of a definitive genetic diagnosis, clinical guidelines recommend regular clinical monitoring for all first-degree relatives, ensuring that potential disease manifestations are not missed due to genetic uncertainty.

ATTRv Targeted Management

Distinguishing between hereditary and wild-type forms of ATTR amyloidosis is crucial, as they may present with different disease onset, progression, and response to treatment [21]. Tafamidis, a TTR protein stabilizer and the only approved treatment for ATTR-CM, has demonstrated reduced all-cause mortality and cardiovascular-related hospitalizations in both ATTRv and ATTRwt subgroups [22]. However, *TTR* gene silencers, such as Patisiran and Inotersen, are currently approved only for ATTRv polyneuropathy with cardiac involvement [23, 24]. Recent research also suggests that standard heart failure therapy (HFT) with ACE inhibitors and beta-blockers may be potentially detrimental in ATTRv patients, particularly those with a mixed phenotype, emphasizing the importance of diagnosis and individualized treatment strategies [25]. As research advances, targeted therapies for specific genetic variants may emerge, highlighting the importance of genetic testing in determining the most effective treatment strategies for patients with ATTRv-CM.

Potential Future Treatments

Gene editing, particularly CRISPR-Cas9, shows great promise for ATTRv treatment. This innovative approach targets specific genomic locations to correct pathogenic *TTR* mutations at the DNA level, thereby preventing protein misfolding and amyloid formation. Notably, a recent phase 1 clinical trial of the CRISPR-Cas9-based therapy Nexiguran Ziclumeran (nex-z) for ATTR-CM demonstrated transient infusion-related reactions alongside consistent, rapid, and durable reductions in serum TTR levels [26]. Nevertheless, these therapies are still in the early stages of development, necessitating further research, large-scale clinical trials, and extended follow-up studies to fully evaluate their potential benefits and risks.

Monitoring and Care for Asymptomatic Carriers

Monitoring genotype-positive, phenotype-negative individuals is essential for early disease detection and timely treatment initiation. Minimal clinical testing includes screening ECG, cardiac biomarkers (natriuretic peptide and troponin), and echocardiogram with strain imaging. Further cardiac imaging (scintigraphy or MRI) may be warranted if symptoms arise or initial tests show abnormalities. Neurological assessments are recommended if there's evidence of neurological involvement. Regular screening is advised every three to five years, with more frequent evaluations as predicted disease onset approaches or if symptoms develop [17].

Presymptomatic therapy for ATTR amyloidosis lacks published clinical trials addressing efficacy and safety. While earlier intervention with ATTR-directed therapies has shown improved outcomes, most treatments are not recommended for asymptomatic carriers without clinical evidence of disease.

Patient-Specific Challenges in Genetic Counseling for ATTRv

Genetic counseling plays a crucial role in helping individuals and families navigate the complexities of ATTRv. Beyond the clinical aspects, genetic counselors must ensure the process is responsive to the specific needs of each individual, as people at different life stages may face distinct and evolving challenges that require personalized approaches.

Knowledge of carrying a pathogenic variant may impact individuals and their families emotionally and socially. Symptomatic patients often struggle with feelings of guilt and worry about their offspring's well-being. They may face challenges in deciding how and when to communicate genetic information to their children without causing undue anxiety.

Asymptomatic family members may experience fear and anxiety about their future health, the well-being of affected family members, and the implications for their own children. Concerns may also arise regarding relationships and family planning decisions, such as whether to pursue prenatal testing or preimplantation genetic testing. In families with early-onset or severe phenotypes, these options may offer a meaningful path toward informed reproductive planning and risk reduction.

Genetic counselors should provide comprehensive support, combining expertise in genetics with psychosocial counseling. By offering a supportive environment counselors can help patients and their families navigate these challenges, enhancing overall well-being, patient satisfaction, adherence to surveillance and management recommendations, and psychological health [27].

Future Directions and Unmet Needs

Current research in hereditary cardiac amyloidosis highlights several critical areas for further investigation:

1. Extensive genotype–phenotype correlation studies to better predict disease courses and guide management based on specific *TTR* mutations.
2. Development of reliable biomarkers for early detection, onset prediction, and disease progression monitoring, particularly in asymptomatic carriers.
3. Research into factors influencing *TTR* mutation penetrance and expressivity, including genetic modifiers, epigenetic factors, and environmental influences.

Addressing these gaps can lead to enhanced predictive models, personalized treatment plans, and more effective interventions. Partnerships between basic research, clinical genetics, and cardiology are vital to accelerate the translation of research findings into clinical practice, potentially revolutionizing ATTRv management.

Concluding Remarks

Genetic evaluation is a critical component in managing hereditary cardiac amyloidosis, particularly ATTRv. This chapter provides compelling evidence and practical tools to support the incorporation of routine genetic evaluation into clinical care. Understanding the genetic basis of ATTRv enables cardiologists and geneticists to facilitate early diagnosis, family screening, and personalized management, ultimately improving patient outcomes and quality of life. As research advances, healthcare professionals must stay updated and integrate genetic evaluation into clinical practice to improve management of this complex disease, providing hope for affected patients and families.

References

1. Porcari A, Fontana M, Gillmore JD. Transthyretin cardiac amyloidosis. Cardiovasc Res. 2022;118:3517–3535. Preprint at https://doi.org/10.1093/cvr/cvac119.
2. Porcari A, Sinagra G, Gillmore JD. Editorial: proceedings and predictions in cardiac amyloidosis: unsolved mysteries and challenges for the future. Front Med. 2023;10. Preprint at https://doi.org/10.3389/fmed.2023.1232212.
3. Mussinelli R, et al. 632 prevalence of variant genotype in patients with suspected cardiac ATTR amyloidosis. Eur. Heart J Suppl. 2022;24.
4. Yongsheng Z, et al. Prevalence estimation of ATTRv in China based on genetic databases. Front Genet 2023;14.
5. Carroll A, et al. Novel approaches to diagnosis and management of hereditary transthyretin amyloidosis. J Neurol Neurosurg Psychiatry. 2022;93:668–78.
6. Llonch MV, et al. Cardiovascular disease burden prior to hereditary transthyretin amyloidosis diagnosis. J Card Fail. 2020;26.
7. Bezerra F, Saraiva MJ, Almeida MR. Modulation of the mechanisms driving transthyretin amyloidosis. Front Mol Neurosci. 2020;13. Preprint at https://doi.org/10.3389/fnmol.2020.592644.
8. Manganelli F, et al. Hereditary transthyretin amyloidosis overview. Neurol Sci. 2022;43:595–604.
9. Ton VK, Mukherjee M, Judge DP. Transthyretin cardiac amyloidosis: pathogenesis, treatments, and emerging role in heart failure with preserved ejection fraction. Clin Med Insights Cardiol. 2014;8:39–44.
10. Lopes LR, et al. Prevalence of TTR variants detected by whole-exome sequencing in hypertrophic cardiomyopathy. Amyloid. 2019;26:243–7.
11. Nehashi T, et al. Sporadic cardiac amyloidosis by amyloidogenic transthyretin V122I variant. Int Heart J. 2019;60:1441–3.
12. Scirpa R, et al. Risk stratification in transthyretin-related cardiac amyloidosis. Front. Cardiovasc. Med. 2023;10. Preprint at https://doi.org/10.3389/fcvm.2023.1151803.
13. Gorram F, et al. New data on the genetic profile and penetrance of hereditary Val30Met transthyretin amyloidosis in Sweden. Amyloid. 2021;28:84–90.
14. Arno S, Cowger J. The genetics of cardiac amyloidosis. Heart Fail Rev. 2022;27:1485–1492. Preprint at https://doi.org/10.1007/s10741-021-10164-z.
15. De Lillo A, et al. Clinical spectrum of Transthyretin amyloidogenic mutations among diverse population origins. Hum Genomics. 2024;18.
16. Iorio A, et al. Non-coding variants contribute to the clinical heterogeneity of TTR amyloidosis. Eur J Hum Genet. 2017;25.
17. Kittleson MM, et al. 2023 ACC expert consensus decision pathway on comprehensive multidisciplinary care for the patient with cardiac amyloidosis. J Am Coll Cardiol. 2023;81.
18. Maurizi N, et al. Prevalence of cardiac amyloidosis among adult patients referred to tertiary centres with an initial diagnosis of hypertrophic cardiomyopathy. Int J Cardiol. 2020;300:191–5.
19. Miller DT, et al. ACMG SF v3.1 list for reporting of secondary findings in clinical exome and genome sequencing: a policy statement of the American College of Medical Genetics and Genomics (ACMG). Genet Med. 2022;24. Preprint at https://doi.org/10.1016/j.gim.2022.04.006.
20. Richards S, et al. Standards and guidelines for the interpretation of sequence variants: a joint consensus recommendation of the American College of Medical Genetics and Genomics and the Association for Molecular Pathology. Genet Med. 2015;17.
21. Tomasoni D, et al. Treating amyloid transthyretin cardiomyopathy: lessons learned from clinical trials. Front Cardiovasc Med. 2023;10.
22. Rapezzi C, et al. Efficacy of Tafamidis in patients with hereditary and wild-type transthyretin amyloid cardiomyopathy further analyses from ATTR-ACT. (2021).https://doi.org/10.1016/j.jchf.2020.09.011

23. Adams D, et al. Patisiran, an RNAi therapeutic, for hereditary transthyretin amyloidosis. N Engl J Med. 2018;379:11–21.
24. Benson MD, et al. Inotersen treatment for patients with hereditary transthyretin amyloidosis. N Engl J Med. 2018;379:22–31.
25. aus dem Siepen F, et al. Prognostic value of standard heart failure medication in patients with cardiac transthyretin amyloidosis. J Clin Med. 2024;13:2257.
26. Fontana M, et al. CRISPR-Cas9 gene editing with nexiguran ziclumeran for ATTR cardiomyopathy. N Engl J Med. 2024. https://doi.org/10.1056/NEJMoa2412309.
27. Barker N, Judge DP. Counseling family members and monitoring for evidence of disease in asymptomatic carriers of amyloid transthyretin cardiac amyloidosis. Am J Cardiol. 2022;185:S43–50.

Management of Cardiac Amyloidosis

Management of Heart Failure in Cardiac Amyloidosis

Israel Gotsman

Abstract Cardiac amyloidosis (CA) is caused by extracellular deposition of misfolded protein fragments in the myocardium, chiefly due to plasma cell dysregulation (AL amyloidosis) or transthyretin (ATTR amyloidosis). Amyloid deposition leads to irreversible damage to the myocardium, causing diastolic dysfunction and restrictive cardiomyopathy. Progression of the disease can lead to advanced restrictive disease and progress to severe systolic dysfunction. Treatment should primarily focus on addressing the fundamental pathology, targeting the underlying disease responsible for the amyloid deposition. Efficient disease-specific therapies are available for delaying the progression of the disease by reducing the accumulation of abnormal proteins. As amyloid deposition is largely irreversible, *timely diagnosis and* specific *preventive therapy initiation at the earliest stages of disease progression are imperative.* The main secondary goal is alleviation of clinical consequences of the failing myocardium leading to clinical heart failure (HF). The combination of restrictive physiology with increased filling pressures causes fluid accumulation and the restricted, fixed stroke volume as well as low heart rate leads to low cardiac output. Patients develop autonomic neuropathy with blunted sympathetic compensatory response. This makes regulation of volume status quite challenging and neurohormonal blockage not well tolerated**.** Alleviation of congestion includes salt restriction and judicial usage of loop diuretics and aldosterone antagonists with close monitoring of volume status. Neurohormonal blockage of the renin-angiotensin axis is contraindicated. Amyloid deposition in the atrium leads to significant atrial pathology and patients have a high risk of developing atrial fibrillation and embolic events. Treatment of rate or rhythm control is best managed with amiodarone. Beta blockers can be challenging but can be used in specific cases. Digoxin may be considered with low-dose and careful monitoring. Midodrine is very effective to increase blood pressure in patients that develop autonomic neuropathy. Syncope and sudden death due to conduction disease or pulseless activity can occur. Careful consideration to this should be given before initiating medications that effect the conduction system. Pacemaker implantation is indicated in appropriate cases and a defibrillator is indicated for secondary prevention of ventricular arrythmias. Patients often progress

I. Gotsman (✉)
Heart Institute, Hadassah Hebrew University Medical Center, Jerusalem, Israel
e-mail: igotsman@hadassah.org.il

E. Herzog (ed.), *Cardiac Amyloidosis*, https://doi.org/10.1007/978-3-031-88342-2_10

from restrictive cardiomyopathy to systolic dysfunction and develop advanced HF. Management of these patients is extremely challenging. Patients often develop renal failure and low cardiac output state with multi-organ failure and cardiogenic shock. Therapeutic options are very limited and prognosis is poor. Heart transplantation is an option in very select appropriate patients if extracardiac involvement is limited. Palliative therapy with alleviation of dyspnea and pain, should be offered.

Keywords Cardiac amyloidosis · AL amyloidosis · ATTR amyloidosis · Restrictive cardiomyopathy · Heart failure · Autonomic neuropathy · Digoxin toxicity · Neurohormonal blockage

Introduction

In this chapter, the management of the cardiac complications of cardiac amyloidosis are described. A detailed description of the management of heart failure (HF) and other related complications that can exacerbate HF and make the treatment of HF very challenging are provided. This includes the treatment of atrial and ventricular arrythmias and conduction system disorders.

Management of Cardiac Involvement in Cardiac Amyloidosis

Cardiac amyloidosis (CA) is caused by extracellular deposition of misfolded protein fragments (fibrils) in the myocardium, originating from a variety of serum proteins. The two most common proteins are gamma-globulins from plasma cell dysregulation (AL amyloidosis) or excessive breakdown of transthyretin (ATTR amyloidosis). Amyloid deposition can lead to irreversible damage to the myocardium causing diastolic dysfunction and restrictive cardiomyopathy. Progression of the disease, if not specifically treated, can lead to advanced restrictive disease and progress to severe systolic dysfunction. Goals in the management of cardiac involvement include primarily with disease-specific therapy for the underlying amyloid deposition disease and secondarily with alleviation of clinical consequences of the failing myocardium.

Disease-Specific Therapy

Treatment should primarily focus on addressing the fundamental pathology, targeting the underlying disease responsible for the amyloid deposition. Specific and efficient therapies are available for delaying the progression of the disease by reducing the accumulation of abnormal proteins [1–3]. In AL amyloidosis, treatment focuses on addressing the underlying hematologic disorder with recommended therapeutic regimens. In ATTR amyloidosis, treatment focuses on fibril stabilization with medications such as tafamidis [4] or acoramidis [5]. A detailed description of these therapies can be found in the other chapters of this book. It is crucial to emphasize that, at present, there are no proven therapies available for significant regression of the disease once amyloid deposition has occurred. Therefore, *timely diagnosis is of utmost importance, and initiating preventive therapy at the earliest stages of disease progression is imperative.*

Heart Failure Therapy

Heart failure (HF) symptoms and signs are the main clinical manifestation of cardiac amyloidosis. Diastolic dysfunction that can progress to restrictive physiology and classical restrictive cardiomyopathy or evolution to systolic dysfunction. These pathophysiological changes cause elevated filling pressures in the ventricles with the accumulation of fluid and reduced cardiac output, leading to overt clinical HF. The restrictive physiology primarily restricts ventricular filling causing accumulation of fluid. It can also reduce significantly stroke volume due to reduced myocardial compliance and limited ventricular volume. This may be aggravated by chronotropic incompetence and low heart rate and lead to low cardiac output. In addition, patients tend to develop autonomic neuropathy with blunted sympathetic compensatory response. This combination makes neurohormonal blockage problematic in most patients and regulation of volume status quite challenging in more advanced patients. Figure 1 gives a schematic outline of the central pathological processes involved in development of HF in CA. It also outlines the relevant clinical manifestations of the disease and recommended management and available therapies for HF.

The management of HF focuses primarily on alleviating congestion by salt restriction and the addition of diuretics including aldosterone antagonists as needed in conjunction with compressive stockings. Additional HF medications are generally not well tolerated and should only be added if there is a definite specific need and only after careful consideration of the pros and cons of each medication in these patients. For the development of autonomic neuropathy and low blood pressure, midodrine, an alpha agonist can be given. Table 1 summarizes the available medications for the management of heart failure and cardiac complications in CA.

Diuretics

Salt restriction is generally recommended in most CA patients that develop HF as part of a regiment to control fluid accumulation and prevent congestion. The mainstream

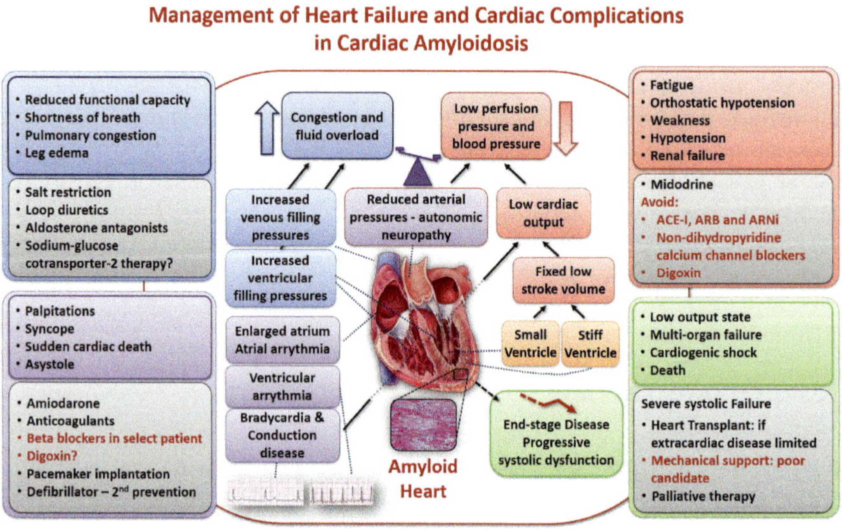

Fig. 1 Management of heart failure in cardiac amyloidosis

therapy to further alleviate congestion are loop diuretics and these are recommended by all cardiac scientific societies [2, 3, 6]. While this therapy alleviates congestion, this also reduces venous return, further reduces the limited stroke volume, and can lead to a low perfusion state and renal failure. Therefore, diuretic therapy should be carefully used to avoid hypotension and depletion of intravascular volume. Judicial usage of diuretics with a close surveillance of volume status and renal function is paramount in more advanced patients. Furthermore, thiazide diuretics such as metazolone should be used with caution, as they may cause over diuresis with detrimental effect on the already constrained volume balance status. Advanced patients often require frequent hospitalizations for intravenous diuresis to manage volume overload. A recent study [7] demonstrated that ambulatory intravenous diuresis as part of a multidisciplinary HF disease management clinic reduced hospitalization rate and may be a safe alternative to recurrent hospitalization, thus reducing hospitalization rates in CA.

Aldosterone Antagonists

Aldosterone antagonists (MRA) may be used in adjunctive with loop diuretics in patients with preserved blood pressure and renal function. No hard data is available regarding its safety and efficacy in cardiac amyloidosis. Hypothetically, the antifibrotic effect of aldosterone antagonist should be beneficial in CA. A recent retrospective sub analysis of the TOPCAT study in patients with HF with preserved ejection fraction using significantly abnormal diastolic indices as a surrogate marker

Table 1 Medication for the management of heart failure and cardiac complications in cardiac amyloidosis

Medication	Usage	Recommendation	Comments
Loop diuretics	First-line medication to alleviate congestion	Yes	May cause volume depletion and low cardiac output. Close monitoring recommended
Aldosterone antagonists	Alleviate congestion	Yes	Well tolerated. Follow renal function
Metazolone	Alleviate congestion	May consider	May cause over diuresis, carefully monitor
Midodrine	Treat autonomic neuropathy	Yes	Increase dosage according to response
Sodium-glucose cotransporter-2 therapy	Alleviate Congestion, additional benefits?	Can consider	Further evidence needed
ACE-I, ARB and ARNi	Neurohormonal blockage	No	Poorly tolerated. Avoid
Beta-adrenergic blockers	Rate control	May be considered in select patients	Can cause hypotension, reduce functional capacity and worsen fatigue
Digoxin	Improve contractility, rate control	May be considered cautiously in select patients	Use low doses, frequent monitoring of drug concentration, electrolytes and renal function
Non-dihydropyridine calcium channel blockers	Rate control	No	Worsening of systolic function and exacerbate heart failure
Amiodarone	Rhythm or rate control	Yes	Well tolerated

of CA suggested that spironolactone was associated with a similar clinical benefit of reduction in HF hospitalization and cardiovascular mortality as the whole cohort of HF patients [8]. A large retrospective observation study [9] in patients with ATTR-CA demonstrated that ~40% of these patients received MRA and discontinuation occurred infrequently; occurring in only 7.5% of patients receiving the medication in the study. Treatment with an MRA was associated with reduced mortality after adjustment for multiple covariates as well with propensity score matching. Based on the limited clinical evidence, it would appear the MRA are relatively tolerated and are recommended for the treatment of CA.

Neurohormonal Blockage

Neurohormonal blockage is the core therapeutic avenue in the treatment of heart failure, particularly in HF with reduced ejection fraction (HFREF). This constitutes of renin–angiotensin–aldosterone system (RAAS) blockade with angiotensin converting enzyme inhibition (ACE-I), angiotensin receptor blocker (ARB), angiotensin receptor-neprilysin inhibitor (ARNi) as well as beta-adrenergic blockers (BB). Well established data demonstrate that this blockade has significant clinical benefit in HFREF and are a class I indication in patients with HFREF [10]. However, there is limited data regarding neurohormonal blockage in CA.

ACE-I, ARB and ARNi

Patients with cardiac amyloidosis often develop autonomic neuropathy. The low blood pressure, low cardiac output due to myocardial disease and blunted sympathetic response limit significantly the utility of neurohormonal blockage in CA. Specifically, neurohormonal blockade with ACE-I, ARB or ARNi are very poorly tolerated in CA and are generally not recommended. In a small observation study, low dose ACE-I/ARB with slow-up titration in appropriate CA patients was reported to be tolerated without major side-effects or significant discontinuation over a 16-month follow-up [11]. However, a large observational study [9] demonstrated that ATTR-CA patients on ACE-I/ARB treatment (57% of the cohort), most were treated with low-dose therapy and approximately a third discontinued therapy due to low blood pressure. No difference was seen in prognosis with the therapy. There is a consensus within the majority of scientific societies [2, 6] that neurohormonal blockage with ACE-I/ARB/ARNi should not be given routinely in patients with CA and in most cases should be avoided due to its intolerance in these patients.

Beta-Adrenergic Blockers

Beta-adrenergic blockers (BB) are one of the cornerstones of treatment of HFREF and have been proven to improve prognosis. BB beneficial effects include ability to reverse the detrimental neurohumoral effects of the sympathetic nervous system, upregulation of adrenergic receptors with improved contractile reserve and systolic function, induce reverse ventricular remodeling, prevention of atrial and life-threatening ventricular arrhythmias and improves coronary flow. It also permits rate control in atrial fibrillation. The beneficial clinical effects have been proven in patients with HFREF in sinus rhythm [12] and are part of the guideline-recommended medical management of these patients. However, data regarding its effect in patients with diastolic dysfunction and in HFPEF are equivocal and have failed to demonstrate consistent beneficial effect [12]. Moreover, there is accumulating data to suggest that it may be clinically detrimental, predominantly in patients with advanced diastolic HF [13]. This is particularly a problem in patients with CA that have restrictive cardiomyopathy. Due to the small ventricle size in CA and fixed stroke volume, these patients are dependent on the heart rate to maintain cardiac output. The patients also develop conduction system disease and chronotropic incompetence and often suffer from bradycardia that can further compromise cardiac output and hemodynamic status. BB can lead to hypotension, reduce functional capacity and worsen fatigue. Therefore, BB are poorly tolerated in the majority of patients with CA. There are no definitive studies demonstrating a BB beneficial effect in patients with CA and reduced EF. These patients often have autonomic dysfunction and are prone to hypotension. In these patients, BB are also poorly tolerated. Therefore, BB are considered to be relatively contraindicated in the management of cardiac amyloidosis with either preserved or reduced EF. The consensus of most scientific societies is that BB therapy should be generally avoided in CA [6]. The European Society of Cardiology Working Group on Myocardial and Pericardial Diseases go further and recommend discontinuing BB therapy [3].

Despite this, BB may be considered in select patients with milder disease with diastolic or systolic dysfunction that may tolerate BB, if there is a specific need for the therapy, for example, the treatment of rate control in AF. A recent study [14] demonstrated that approximately a quarter of patients with AL cardiac amyloidosis received treatment with BB and the majority were initiated prior to CA diagnosis, mainly due to atrial fibrillation and coronary disease. Half discontinued BB due to hypotension and HF exacerbation. Notably, patients with advanced disease tolerated BB poorly. Intolerance to BB in this study was independently associated with increased all-cause mortality. Another small study on 135 patients demonstrated that 80% received BB but half discontinued due to intolerance mainly due to hypotension [15]. In a large retrospective analysis of patients with ATTR-CA, more than half of these patients received BB and less than half of these received target recommended dosages. A fifth discontinued BB therapy mainly due to low blood pressure and heart rate. Propensity score matching demonstrated an improved prognosis in patients with an EF <40% on BB therapy [9]. However, this was an observational study and does not prove that this therapy improves prognosis on its own. In another small observational study, discontinuing BB was associated with improved survival it ATTR-CA [16].

Based on emerging clinical practice data from the above observational studies, it may be reasonable to consider or continue therapy with BB in very select patients with particular specific needs for the medication, primarily heart rate control, with close monitoring for side effects and continuation if tolerated.

Sodium-Glucose Cotransporter-2 Therapy

Limited data exist regarding the use of sodium-glucose cotransporter-2 (SGLT2) inhibitors in patients with CA. SGLT2 inhibitors have demonstrated efficacy in reducing cardiovascular death or hospitalization in heart failure HF with reduced as well as preserved ejection fraction. However, data specific to patients with amyloidosis are limited. Nevertheless, given the diuretic properties associated with SGLT2 inhibitors, it appears reasonable to consider their use in individuals with CA and clinical HF. Emerging data from a small observational study in ATTR-CA [17] suggested that dapagliflozin was well tolerated. The study was underpowered to give definitive data regarding efficacy. A recent observational study utilizing propensity score matching demonstrated that SGLT2 inhibitors were well-tolerated in patients with ATTR-CA. The study observed improvements in HF symptoms, and a reduced risk of heart failure hospitalization, cardiovascular death, and all-cause mortality [18]. Based on the limited emerging data, it seems reasonable to consider this medication in select patients, but further definitive data is required.

Digoxin

Digoxin, one of the oldest cardiac medications is used for additional support in the treatment of systolic heart failure. It improves cardiac function by augmenting contractility due to increased entry of calcium in the heart. Digoxin also has parasympathomimetic effects and is used to control ventricular rate in atrial fibrillation. However, its use in CA is limited as it has been reported that there is an increased risk of digoxin sensitivity and toxicity in CA. Digoxin binds to amyloid fibrils in-vitro [19] and may predispose CA patients to digoxin toxicity. This finding suggests that there may be an increased risk of digoxin toxicity in amyloidosis, even with normal serum drug levels. Two recent observation studies with clinical usage of digoxin in patients CA including AL-amyloidosis did not show increased frequency of toxicity compared to expected [20, 21]. Based on this, digoxin may be considered cautiously in select patients with CA [6]. Rigorous patient selection is recommended, with close monitored during digoxin administration. Low doses should be used with frequent monitoring of drug concentration, electrolytes and renal function.

Calcium Channel Blockers

Non-dihydropyridine calcium channel blockers such as verapamil and diltiazem are used to control rate response in atrial fibrillation. These medications have been shown to bind avidly to amyloid fibrils [22] and may augment the physiological effects of these medications. This may cause exaggerated negative chronotropic and inotropic effects leading to worsening systolic function and exacerbate heart failure and thus are contraindicated in CA [23]. These medications should be avoided in patients with cardiac amyloidosis.

Amiodarone

Amiodarone is a very efficient class III anti-arrhythmic drug for the treatment of atrial as well as ventricular arrhythmias. Amiodarone has various electrophysiological effects, with its primary action being the blockade of potassium channels. It also blocks sodium and calcium channels and has beta receptor antagonist properties. Despite the numerous cardiac effects of the medication, it is relatively well tolerated in patients with CA. Amiodarone is the first drug choice for the treatment of atrial fibrillation in CA [6].

Midodrine

Patients with CA tend to develop autonomic neuropathy particularly in Al-amyloidosis, with diminished sympathetic response. This can lead to life disabling orthostatic hypotension and low blood pressure. This is aggravated by HF medications prescribed, that further reduce sympathetic response and venous return. Midodrine is an alpha-1 adrenoceptor agonist, resulting in arterial and venous constriction which increases venous return and arterial tone. Midodrine is very helpful in alleviating this issue and helps increase blood pressure in patients that develop autonomic neuropathy.

Cardiac Complications in CA Patients with HF

Atrial Fibrillation

Patients with CA are at increased risk of developing atrial arrythmias, mainly atrial fibrillation (AF). Amyloid fibrils deposit and accumulate in the extracellular compartment of the atriums as well as the ventricles causing significant atrial pathology. This predisposes to abnormal atrial contractility and causes electrical abnormalities leading to atrial arrythmia, primarily atrial fibrillation. Furthermore, increased ventricular filling pressures due to the development of restrictive physiology, leads to increased atrial pressure and causes additional atrial pathology, increasing the risk of developing atrial arrythmias. Therefore, patients that develop HF due to CA are at a high risk of developing AF. Due to the underlying cardiomyopathy, AF is often highly symptomatic and poorly tolerated [24].

Treatment of AF includes the treatment of the arrythmia with rate or rhythm control and prevention of embolic sequel. Ventricular rate control can be quite challenging due to the limited available therapeutic options in these patients due to the risk of bradycardia and conduction disease, low cardiac output and low blood pressure. Non-dihydropyridine calcium channel blockers are contraindicated in CA due to increased sensitivity and should not be used. Digoxin is also historically contradicted due to increased risk of toxicity in CA. However, recent data suggests that it may be safe when started in low doses with frequent monitoring. Current European and American guidelines suggest that it may be used cautiously in select patients [2, 3]. Beta blockers although problematic in CA, may be considered in specific cases after careful consideration of the risk profile of the specific patient. The best tolerated medication is amiodarone for rate as well as rhythm control. The choice of control strategy, either with rhythm or rate control, should depend on the extent of atrial pathology, clinical tolerability of AF and ability to achieve rate control, as there is no sound evidence to demonstrate superiority of one of these strategies. Data suggests that a rhythm control strategies are substantially more effective when performed earlier in the disease course as a large proportion fail to stay in sinus rhythm [25]. In specific cases, pulmonary vein isolation may be considered [26]. In extreme case, pacemaker implantation and atrioventricular node ablation may be considered.

Atrial pathology is usually quite extensive in patients that develop CA with significant restrictive cardiomyopathy. Therefore, their risk of developing atrial thrombi is very high in these patients, particularly in AL-amyloidosis [27]. Despite this, there is no consensus on anticoagulation therapy in patients with sinus rhythm. In patients that develop AF, anticoagulation should be give regardless of the CHA_2DS_2-VASc risk score as their embolic risk is high in any case [28]. There are limited data on which anticoagulant is most appropriate in these patients. Based on observational data, direct oral anticoagulants appear to be safe and efficient in this population [29].

Ventricular Arrythmia

Damage to the myocardium due to amyloid deposition increases the risk of ventricular arrythmia's in patients with CA. Ventricular arrythmia can be life threating, although the most common reason for sudden cardiac death in CA patients is pulseless electrical activity. Anti-arrhythmic drug of choice is amiodarone as it is generally tolerated in CA. Implantation of an implantable cardiac defibrillator is recommended by the European guidelines for secondary prevention only, after careful discussion of the competing risks of non-arrhythmic death and non-cardiac death [30]. The benefit of ICD implantation for primary prevention is uncertain and there is currently no recommendation regarding this.

Bradycardia and Conduction Disorders

Amyloid depositions accumulate in the heart of CA patients including the electrical conduction system causing conduction disturbances. In addition, autonomic neuropathy can further aggravate the problem due to the impaired sympathetic response in these patients. Therefore, these patients are at increased to suffer from bradycardia and more advanced conduction disorders. Syncope and sudden death due to conduction disease or pulseless activity can occur. Careful consideration to this should be given before initiating medications that effect the conduction system. Pacemaker implantation is indicated in appropriate cases and is not different from the standard indications for device therapy in other patients. There is limited clinical data regarding cardiac resynchronization therapy (CRT) in these patients. However, if a patient is expected to have a high percentage of paced and has systolic HF, CRT probably should be considered, as right ventricular pacing is detrimental in these patients [31], as it is with other HFREF patients.

Advanced Systolic Heart Failure

Patients with CA often progress from restrictive cardiomyopathy to systolic dysfunction and develop advanced HF. Management of these patients is extremely challenging as these patients suffer not only for severe systolic dysfunction, they also may have extracardiac disease with additional organ failure, further compounding the problem. At this stage, most patients have developed autonomic neuropathy and treatment options are very limited. Neurohormonal therapy is very poorly tolerated and is contraindicated. Management of volume is also challenging, with frequent accumulation of fluid and volume overload state, requiring frequent hospitalizations due to HF exacerbation. Diuretic therapy with increasing need for intravenous therapy and increasing dosages is required. Patients often develop renal failure and may progress to end stage renal failure that may require dialysis. Low cardiac output state may develop with multi-organ failure and cardiogenic shock. Therapeutic options are very limited and prognosis is poor. Heart transplantation is an option is select appropriate patients if extracardiac involvement is limited. Recent data suggest that in the current era, outcomes in patients with CA undergoing heart transplant are comparable to other heart transplant recipients [32, 33]. Mechanical circulatory support with a left ventricular assist device (LVAD) is usually not relevant as most patients have significant right ventricular disease, and are not candidates for an LVAD. Centers that have experience with biventricular assist devices or total artificial hearts may consider this therapy in very select patients, although outcomes are poor.

Palliative Therapy

In advanced patients with limited options and poor prognosis, palliative therapy with alleviation of dyspnea and pain, should be initiated [34]. It is recommended to discuss end-of-life preferences with the patient and family. Social support, spiritual counseling (if relevant), and legal assistance in dealing with end-of-life issues should be offered.

References

1. Palladini G, Milani P, Merlini G. Management of AL amyloidosis in 2020. Blood. 2020;136(23):2620–7.
2. Kittleson MM, Maurer MS, Ambardekar AV, Bullock-Palmer RP, Chang PP, Eisen HJ, et al. Cardiac amyloidosis: evolving diagnosis and management: a scientific statement from the American heart association. Circulation. 2020;142(1):e7–22.
3. Garcia-Pavia P, Rapezzi C, Adler Y, Arad M, Basso C, Brucato A, et al. Diagnosis and treatment of cardiac amyloidosis: a position statement of the ESC working group on myocardial and pericardial diseases. Eur Heart J. 2021;42(16):1554–68.
4. Maurer MS, Schwartz JH, Gundapaneni B, Elliott PM, Merlini G, Waddington-Cruz M, et al. Tafamidis treatment for patients with transthyretin amyloid cardiomyopathy. N Engl J Med. 2018;379(11):1007–16.
5. Gillmore JD, Judge DP, Cappelli F, Fontana M, Garcia-Pavia P, Gibbs S, et al. Efficacy and safety of acoramidis in transthyretin amyloid cardiomyopathy. N Engl J Med. 2024;390(2):132–42.
6. Rapezzi C, Aimo A, Serenelli M, Barison A, Vergaro G, Passino C, et al. Critical comparison of documents from scientific societies on cardiac amyloidosis: JACC state-of-the-art review. J Am Coll Cardiol. 2022;79(13):1288–303.
7. Vaishnav J, Hubbard A, Chasler JE, Lepley D, Cuomo K, Riley S, et al. Management of heart failure in cardiac amyloidosis using an ambulatory diuresis clinic. Am Heart J. 2021;233:122–31.
8. Sperry BW, Hanna M, Shah SJ, Jaber WA, Spertus JA. Spironolactone in patients with an echocardiographic HFpEF phenotype suggestive of cardiac amyloidosis: results from TOPCAT. JACC Heart Fail. 2021;9(11):795–802.
9. Ioannou A, Massa P, Patel RK, Razvi Y, Porcari A, Rauf MU, et al. Conventional heart failure therapy in cardiac ATTR amyloidosis. Eur Heart J. 2023;44(31):2893–907.
10. McDonagh TA, Metra M, Adamo M, Gardner RS, Baumbach A, Bohm M, et al. 2021 ESC guidelines for the diagnosis and treatment of acute and chronic heart failure. Eur Heart J. 2021;42(36):3599–726.
11. Aimo A, Vergaro G, Castiglione V, Rapezzi C, Emdin M. Safety and tolerability of neurohormonal antagonism in cardiac amyloidosis. Eur J Intern Med. 2020;80:66–72.
12. Cleland JGF, Bunting KV, Flather MD, Altman DG, Holmes J, Coats AJS, et al. Beta-blockers for heart failure with reduced, mid-range, and preserved ejection fraction: an individual patient-level analysis of double-blind randomized trials. Eur Heart J. 2018;39(1):26–35.
13. Palau P, Seller J, Dominguez E, Sastre C, Ramon JM, de La Espriella R, et al. Effect of beta-blocker withdrawal on functional capacity in heart failure and preserved ejection fraction. J Am Coll Cardiol. 2021;78(21):2042–56.
14. Briasoulis A, Stamatelopoulos K, Petropoulos I, Patras R, Theodorakakou F, Gavriatopoulou M, et al. Utilization and tolerance of beta-blockers among patients with AL amyloidosis. Amyloid. 2022;29(1):31–7.
15. Ramsell S, Arias Bermudez C, Takem Baiyee CAM, Rodgers B, Parikh S, Almaani S, et al. Beta-Adrenergic antagonist tolerance in amyloid cardiomyopathy. Front Cardiovasc Med. 2022;9: 907597.

16. Cheng RK, Vasbinder A, Levy WC, Goyal P, Griffin JM, Leedy DJ, et al. Lack of association between neurohormonal blockade and survival in transthyretin cardiac amyloidosis. J Am Heart Assoc. 2021;10(24): e022859.
17. Dobner S, Bernhard B, Asatryan B, Windecker S, Stortecky S, Pilgrim T, et al. SGLT2 inhibitor therapy for transthyretin amyloid cardiomyopathy: early tolerance and clinical response to dapagliflozin. ESC Heart Fail. 2023;10(1):397–404.
18. Porcari A, Cappelli F, Nitsche C, Tomasoni D, Sinigiani G, Longhi S, et al. SGLT2 inhibitor therapy in patients with transthyretin amyloid cardiomyopathy. J Am Coll Cardiol. 2024;83(24):2411–22.
19. Rubinow A, Skinner M, Cohen AS. Digoxin sensitivity in amyloid cardiomyopathy. Circulation. 1981;63(6):1285–8.
20. Donnelly JP, Sperry BW, Gabrovsek A, Ikram A, Tang WHW, Estep J, et al. Digoxin use in cardiac amyloidosis. Am J Cardiol. 2020;133:134–8.
21. Muchtar E, Gertz MA, Kumar SK, Lin G, Boilson B, Clavell A, et al. Digoxin use in systemic light-chain (AL) amyloidosis: contra-indicated or cautious use? Amyloid. 2018;25(2):86–92.
22. Gertz MA, Skinner M, Connors LH, Falk RH, Cohen AS, Kyle RA. Selective binding of nifedipine to amyloid fibrils. Am J Cardiol. 1985;55(13 Pt 1):1646.
23. Pollak A, Falk RH. Left ventricular systolic dysfunction precipitated by verapamil in cardiac amyloidosis. Chest. 1993;104(2):618–20.
24. Giancaterino S, Urey MA, Darden D, Hsu JC. Management of arrhythmias in cardiac amyloidosis. JACC Clin Electrophysiol. 2020;6(4):351–61.
25. Donnellan E, Wazni OM, Hanna M, Elshazly MB, Puri R, Saliba W, et al. Atrial fibrillation in transthyretin cardiac amyloidosis: predictors, prevalence, and efficacy of rhythm control strategies. JACC Clin Electrophysiol. 2020;6(9):1118–27.
26. Donnellan E, Wazni O, Kanj M, Elshazly MB, Hussein A, Baranowski B, et al. Atrial fibrillation ablation in patients with transthyretin cardiac amyloidosis. Europace. 2020;22(2):259–64.
27. Feng D, Syed IS, Martinez M, Oh JK, Jaffe AS, Grogan M, et al. Intracardiac thrombosis and anticoagulation therapy in cardiac amyloidosis. Circulation. 2009;119(18):2490–7.
28. Donnellan E, Elshazly MB, Vakamudi S, Wazni OM, Cohen JA, Kanj M, et al. No association between CHADS-VASc score and left atrial appendage thrombus in patients with transthyretin amyloidosis. JACC Clin Electrophysiol. 2019;5(12):1473–4.
29. Mentias A, Alvarez P, Chaudhury P, Nakhla M, Moudgil R, Kanj M, et al. Direct oral anticoagulants in cardiac amyloidosis-associated heart failure and atrial fibrillation. Am J Cardiol. 2022;164:141–3.
30. Zeppenfeld K, Tfelt-Hansen J, de Riva M, Winkel BG, Behr ER, Blom NA, et al. 2022 ESC guidelines for the management of patients with ventricular arrhythmias and the prevention of sudden cardiac death. Eur Heart J. 2022;43(40):3997–4126.
31. Donnellan E, Wazni OM, Saliba WI, Baranowski B, Hanna M, Martyn M, et al. Cardiac devices in patients with transthyretin amyloidosis: Impact on functional class, left ventricular function, mitral regurgitation, and mortality. J Cardiovasc Electrophysiol. 2019;30(11):2427–32.
32. Kristen AV, Kreusser MM, Blum P, Schonland SO, Frankenstein L, Dosch AO, et al. Improved outcomes after heart transplantation for cardiac amyloidosis in the modern era. J Heart Lung Transplant. 2018;37(5):611–8.
33. Griffin JM, Chiu L, Axsom KM, Bijou R, Clerkin KJ, Colombo P, et al. United network for organ sharing outcomes after heart transplantation for al compared to ATTR cardiac amyloidosis. Clin Transplant. 2020;34(10): e14028.
34. Tsukanov J, Fabbro ED. Palliative care and symptom management in amyloidosis: A review. Curr Probl Cancer. 2016;40(5–6):220–8.

Management of Advanced Heart Failure in Cardiac Amyloidosis

Rabea Asleh and Offer Amir

Abstract Cardiac amyloidosis (CA), encompassing transthyretin amyloidosis (ATTR) and light-chain amyloidosis (AL), poses significant challenges in managing advanced heart failure (HF). This chapter explores the role of mechanical circulatory support (MCS) devices and heart transplantation (HT) in treating CA, emphasizing recent advancements that have improved outcomes. MCS devices, including durable left ventricular assist devices (LVADs) and temporary mechanical support, have limited utility in CA due to restrictive cardiac physiology and systemic involvement. While durable LVADs are rarely used, they may serve as a bridge to HT in selected ATTR cases. Temporary MCS devices can stabilize cardiogenic shock but are often constrained by high complication rates and poor outcomes. HT remains the only curative option for end-stage HF in CA. For AL CA, achieving a durable hematologic response to chemotherapy is critical to prevent recurrent amyloid deposition post-transplant. Combining HT with autologous stem cell transplantation (ASCT) has significantly improved survival, with five-year rates exceeding 60% in carefully selected patients. ATTR CA patients demonstrate excellent post-HT outcomes, with five-year survival rates surpassing 70%. In hereditary ATTR (ATTRv), combined heart and liver transplantation may be required, whereas isolated HT is typically sufficient for wild-type ATTR (ATTRwt). Advances in disease-modifying therapies, including transthyretin stabilizers and gene-silencing agents, have further enhanced survival and reduced recurrence. Recent policy changes have improved prioritization for CA patients requiring HT, reducing waitlist mortality and wait times. Post-transplant outcomes in CA patients now parallel those in non-CA populations, with comparable survival rates and complications. As systemic therapies evolve and patient selection criteria refine, integrating MCS and HT with disease-targeted treatments provides a multidisciplinary strategy for optimizing outcomes in advanced HF secondary to CA.

Keywords Cardiac amyloidosis · Advanced heart failure · Heart transplantation · Mechanical circulatory support · LVAD · Outcomes

---

R. Asleh (✉) · O. Amir
Heart Institute, Hadassah Medical Center, Faculty of Medicine, Hebrew University of Jerusalem, Jerusalem, Israel
e-mail: rasleh@hadassah.org.il

E. Herzog (ed.), *Cardiac Amyloidosis*, https://doi.org/10.1007/978-3-031-88342-2_11

Introduction

Cardiac Amyloidosis (CA) is a progressive disease caused by the deposition of amyloid fibrils in the heart, generally leading to heart failure (HF) with restrictive physiology. The two main forms of amyloid cardiomyopathy are light-chain amyloidosis (AL) and transthyretin amyloidosis (ATTR), which can either be hereditary/variant (ATTRv) or acquired/wild type (ATTRwt). These misfolded proteins accumulate in the myocardium, causing both structural and functional abnormalities in the heart, which can lead to HF [1, 2]. While the disease was once considered rare, it is now increasingly recognized as a significant cause of HF, and advances in diagnostic tools and therapies have made early diagnosis more feasible [3]. Early diagnosis is pivotal since new therapies can delay the disease progression and improve outcomes [3–5]. Unfortunately, diagnosis is often made in advanced stages, when HF has already significantly progressed, limiting treatment options. As the disease progresses, advanced therapeutic options such as left ventricular assist devices (LVAD), orthotopic heart transplantation (HT), and temporary mechanical circulatory support (tMCS) devices in the acute setting, may be considered. This chapter reviews these modalities, including their applicability, outcomes, and limitations within the context of CA.

Mechanical Circulatory Support (MCS) Devices

CA presents unique challenges in the management of advanced HF due to its infiltrative nature and associated biventricular dysfunction. In this condition, amyloid fibril deposition leads to restrictive cardiomyopathy, characterized by small left ventricular (LV) cavity size, thickened walls, and increased myocardial stiffness [2]. These pathophysiological changes complicate the use of MCS devices, which play a crucial role in bridging patients to HT or serving as destination therapy in advanced HF. MCS devices can be broadly categorized into tMCS and durable MCS (dMCS). tMCS devices, such as intra-aortic balloon pumps (IABP), Impella systems, and venoarterial extracorporeal membrane oxygenation (VA-ECMO), are typically used for short-term stabilization, allowing patients to recover or be bridged to definitive therapies, such as HT. dMCS devices, including LVADs, biventricular assist devices (BiVAD) or total artificial heart (TAH), are designed for long-term support but present significant challenges in CA due to the small LV cavity size, increased risk of suction events, incomplete unloading, and biventricular involvement [6].

In CA, the decision between LV support and biventricular support is critical, as many patients exhibit significant right ventricular (RV) dysfunction secondary to biventricular infiltration and chronically elevated LV end-diastolic pressures (LVEDP). While LVADs are commonly used in other cardiomyopathies, they may not provide adequate support in CA due to the frequent coexistence of RV failure. In these cases, biventricular support with TAH or temporary strategies, such as

ECMO or tMCS with biventricular unloading, may be required. This highlights the complexity of selecting and managing MCS devices in patients with CA, emphasizing the need for careful patient selection, individualized device choice, and consideration of disease-specific challenges. The use of tMCS and dMCS, as well as the balance between LV and biventricular support, underscores the importance of multidisciplinary expertise and high-volume centers in optimizing outcomes for this unique patient population.

Temporary Mechanical Circulatory Support (tMCS)

In centers with experience using tMCS, this strategy has shown promise as a bridge to HT. Axillary intra-aortic balloon pump (IABP) support is often used in these cases, as it allows patients to mobilize and engage in cardiac rehabilitation before undergoing HT [7]. This approach is increasingly being utilized following the 2018 United Network for Organ Sharing (UNOS) policy change, which raised the priority status of patients using tMCS to a higher listing level. Retrospective studies from single centers indicate that tMCS is a safe and feasible strategy for bridging CA patients to HT, particularly in the absence of overt and refractory RV failure [8, 9].

VA-ECMO provides tMCS for patients in cardiogenic shock, offering a bridge to recovery, decision-making, or definitive therapy such as HT. Its application in CA requires careful consideration. ECMO may be used in refractory cardiogenic shock secondary to CA. However, its role is primarily limited to short-term stabilization in patients who are potential candidates for HT or other interventions. The use of ECMO in CA is not intended as destination therapy in patients who are ineligible for HT or dMCS due to the progressive and multisystemic nature of the disease. Amyloidosis-associated vascular fragility increases the risk of bleeding during ECMO support. Additionally, systemic involvement in AL amyloidosis—including renal, hepatic, and neurological dysfunction—often limits the feasibility of prolonged ECMO use. The anticoagulation required for ECMO further exacerbates bleeding risks. Some studies have documented higher rates of intracranial hemorrhage and gastrointestinal bleeding in amyloidosis patients receiving ECMO compared to other populations. Case reports have described the successful use of ECMO as a bridge to HT in selected patients with CA. These cases emphasize the importance of rapid patient selection and aggressive management of extracardiac organ dysfunction [6, 8, 10].

Left Ventricular Assist Devices (LVAD)

HF management in amyloid cardiomyopathy remains a challenge due to the limited medical therapies available for restrictive cardiomyopathies. Traditional HF treatments are often ineffective or poorly tolerated in these patients [3]. Unlike other forms of HF, guideline-directed medical therapy (GDMT), including beta-blockers, angiotensin-converting enzyme inhibitors (ACEi), or angiotensin II receptor blockers (ARBs), has shown limited efficacy in CA patients. These treatments, aimed at reducing afterload or controlling neurohormonal pathways, frequently result in clinical deterioration rather than improvement. The absence of definitive evidence supporting GDMT use in this population highlights the unique challenges posed by CA. Expert consensus currently advises against routine use of these therapies, emphasizing the need for alternative strategies tailored to the underlying amyloid pathology [11]. Moreover, HT, which could provide a life-saving intervention for some patients, is not always feasible. The systemic nature of amyloid deposition complicates HT eligibility, as the disease affects multiple organs beyond the heart. Additionally, the long wait times associated with HT and the irreversible pulmonary hypertension that often develops in CA make it difficult to pursue this option for many patients. Therefore, LVADs have emerged as a potential therapeutic option for patients with advanced HF due to CA.

LVADs are durable mechanical pumps that assist the LV in pumping blood to the rest of the body, and they have been shown to improve survival and quality of life in patients with advanced HF of various etiologies. Initial studies focused on durable continuous flow LVADs in ATTR and AL CA patients demonstrated feasibility but poor long-term survival for those who survived the index hospitalization. LV unloading with these devices resulted in reduced LV end-diastolic dimension (LVEDD) and LV end-systolic dimension (LVESD), but RV failure was common, occurring in 39–50% of patients. An LVEDD ≤4.6 cm was correlated with significantly reduced survival post-LVAD implantation [12, 13]. These early studies highlighted that while LV dMCS is feasible in CA, outcomes were poor when compared to non-amyloid restrictive cardiomyopathies or dilated cardiomyopathies. A comprehensive analysis from the Interagency Registry for Mechanically Assisted Circulatory Support (INTERMACS) between 2005 and 2017 showed increased mortality for CA patients receiving solitary LV durable support compared to those with non-CA restrictive or dilated cardiomyopathies. CA patients more frequently required biventricular support, and for those who received it, mortality outcomes were similar to those of non-CA patients. However, CA patients experienced higher rates of early device complications, including major bleeding, neurologic dysfunction, hemorrhagic stroke, and renal dysfunction. This large registry analysis provided valuable insights into dMCS outcomes in CA but had limitations, such as small sample sizes and device heterogeneity [14].

New-generation LVADs, with HeartMate 3 being the only currently available device in the market, have demonstrated significant improvements in safety, survival, and complication rates across different INTERMACS scales, making them an increasingly viable option for HF patients [15]. Though LVADs have demonstrated promise for improving outcomes in end-stage restrictive and hypertrophic cardiomyopathies, including CA, their use in this population is complicated by several challenges. The restrictive physiology and myocardial stiffness characteristic of CA, along with anatomical issues such as a small LV cavity and increased myocardial wall thickness, complicate LVAD implantation and function.

Restrictive cardiomyopathies, including CA, are typically characterized by a small LV cavity and restrictive diastolic function. These features are particularly pronounced in CA, where amyloid deposits lead to increased LV wall thickness and RV involvement. The combination of small LV size, increased wall thickness, and RV dysfunction creates significant challenges for LVAD implantation [16]. LVADs are preload-dependent and afterload-sensitive, meaning that their function depends on the volume of blood entering the LV and the pressure in the arteries. In CA, the small LV cavity, along with the thickened myocardial walls, increases the risk of suction events, where the septum may encroach on the LVAD inflow cannula. This can result in a reduction of LVAD output, leading to severe complications such as cardiogenic shock or ventricular arrhythmias. These complications can undermine the efficacy of the LVAD and pose a significant risk to patient survival [17, 18].

Given these anatomical issues, imaging assessment plays a critical role in selecting appropriate candidates for LVAD implantation in CA. Echocardiography is a central diagnostic tool for assessing heart function, including LV and RV size, function, and the degree of tricuspid regurgitation. Echocardiographic parameters such as the LVEDD and LV mass index are valuable for predicting postoperative outcomes in CA patients undergoing LVAD implantation. In restrictive cardiomyopathies, a smaller LVEDD of less than 46 mm is associated with poorer survival after LVAD implantation, underscoring the importance of preoperative imaging in identifying suitable candidates [13, 19]. Additionally, RV dysfunction is a major predictor of postoperative complications, including RV failure, which is a leading cause of mortality after LVAD implantation. Assessing RV function is therefore crucial for evaluating LVAD candidacy in CA. Echocardiographic parameters such as the tricuspid annular plane systolic excursion (TAPSE) and RV free wall longitudinal strain are useful for predicting RV dysfunction. RV free wall longitudinal strain has proven to be a more sensitive marker for RV dysfunction than other echocardiographic measures, enabling earlier detection of RV dysfunction and better prognostication in patients with CA [20]. Importantly, cardiac magnetic resonance (CMR) has gained importance in the evaluation of RV function in CA patients. CMR offers detailed structural and functional assessment of the heart and has been shown to provide accurate myocardial characterization. CMR-derived RV parameters, including RV-late gadolinium enhancement (LGE) and RV end-systolic volume index, have been associated with worse outcomes and higher mortality in CA. These advanced imaging techniques are valuable in providing a more comprehensive picture of the heart's structural and functional state and can help guide clinical decision-making regarding LVAD implantation in CA patients [17, 21].

Endomyocardial biopsy and histopathological analysis is also important for the diagnosis and risk stratification in specific LVAD candidates with CA. Amyloid burden has been shown to correlate with echocardiographic parameters of cardiac function, and capillary density can provide additional prognostic information. Studies have demonstrated that assessment of capillary density and amyloid deposits by endomyocardial biopsy can help predict LV function and long-term prognosis. The correlation between the extent of amyloid deposits and RV function parameters derived from echocardiography and CMR, could provide an additional tool for predicting RV failure post-LVAD implantation [22].

Although both types of amyloidosis (AL and ATTR) involve the deposition of misfolded proteins in the myocardium, they exhibit distinct differences in clinical presentation, disease progression, and treatment response. The type of amyloidosis is particularly important when considering LVAD implantation, as it can affect the timing and pattern of cardiac involvement by amyloid deposits, which in turn influences postoperative outcomes. In AL amyloidosis, the RV is typically spared in the early stages of the disease, with RV involvement occurring later in the disease process. By contrast, ATTRwt amyloidosis often involves both the LV and RV early on, with RV dysfunction being a prominent feature. These differences in the pattern of disease progression should be considered when evaluating patients for LVAD implantation. In AL, RV function tends to be less affected, and LV parameters such as LVEDD and global longitudinal strain are more predictive of outcomes. In ATTRwt, RV function is more strongly correlated with disease severity, and RV parameters such as RV free wall longitudinal strain are crucial for predicting prognosis [17, 20].

The timing of LVAD intervention is a critical factor in improving patient outcomes. Early referral for LVAD evaluation is essential for CA patients, as advanced disease with significant RV involvement and small LV cavity size complicates LVAD implantation. Preoperative imaging and functional assessments can help determine the optimal timing for surgery, ensuring that patients who will benefit most from LVAD therapy are identified early in the disease course. Delayed intervention increases the likelihood of RV involvement and further diminishes the LV cavity size, making implantation more difficult and less effective [23].

Technical challenges also play a significant role in the feasibility of LVAD implantation in CA patients. The small LV cavity and thickened myocardial walls often complicate the placement of the LVAD inflow cannula. In some cases, surgical modifications such as LV myomectomy may be necessary to create adequate space for the cannula. Ensuring proper alignment of the cannula with the long axis of the LV, directed towards the mitral valve, helps reduce the risk of suction events and improves the overall success of the procedure.

Postoperative complications such as bleeding and thromboembolic events are common in CA patients and represent a significant risk following LVAD implantation. The bleeding tendency in CA is multifactorial, including amyloid deposits in perivascular tissue, coagulation abnormalities, and liver involvement. Gastrointestinal bleeding is particularly common, as the non-pulsatile flow of modern LVADs increases shear stress, which can lead to endothelial dysfunction, oxidative stress, and vascular abnormalities. Thromboembolic events, particularly cerebrovascular accidents, are relevantly more frequent in CA patients, exacerbated by the inflammatory response induced by LVAD implantation [24, 25].

Hemodynamic ramp tests, conducted invasively via right heart catheterization or non-invasively through echocardiography, are particularly important in CA patients for guiding LVAD speed adjustment and optimizing medical therapy. The ramp test aims to optimize LV unloading, maintain LV septum alignment, minimize mitral regurgitation, and allow intermittent aortic valve opening. Given the unique characteristics of CA, ramp tests may be particularly useful in optimizing hemodynamic outcomes post-LVAD implantation.

Emerging disease-modifying therapies for ATTR, such as RNA/oligonucleotide inhibition and small molecule stabilizers, offer promising avenues for reducing amyloidogenesis and improving outcomes in CA patients. These therapies could potentially mitigate RV dysfunction and enhance the efficacy of LVADs by reducing amyloid deposition in the myocardium. Combining medical therapy with LVAD implantation may slow disease progression and reduce the risk of late RV failure, ultimately improving the long-term success of LVAD therapy in CA patients.

Collectively, LVAD therapy is a feasible and potentially beneficial option for selected patients with advanced CA, but its use remains limited by several challenges. These include anatomical issues, such as small LV cavity size, increased LV wall thickness, and RV involvement, as well as the pathophysiological modifications induced by amyloid deposition. These factors increase the risk of post-implant complications, including bleeding and thromboembolic events. However, advances in disease-modifying therapies that reduce amyloid deposition provide hope for improving LVAD outcomes in this patient population. Further investigation is needed to determine the optimal timing for LVAD implantation in CA and to optimize surgical techniques and management strategies to overcome the unique challenges posed by this disease.

Durable Biventricular MCS Devices

In advanced HF due to CA, where biventricular dysfunction is prominent, durable biventricular MCS devices are occasionally necessary. These devices, such as TAH and BiVAD, can provide critical hemodynamic support as a bridge to decision-making or HT [17, 26]. However, the infiltrative and restrictive nature of CA poses unique challenges to the utilization of dMCS, necessitating specialized expertise and high-volume centers to optimize outcomes.

The TAH offers a complete replacement of native cardiac function, providing support for both ventricles and eliminating the need for residual myocardial function, which is often severely impaired in CA. Data from Cedars-Sinai Medical Center demonstrate the feasibility of TAH as a bridge to HT in patients with CA, including both ATTR and AL types [26]. In this cohort, a subset of patients successfully transitioned from TAH to HT, highlighting its potential as a life-saving strategy for biventricular HF. However, patients with ATTR amyloidosis awaiting heart-liver transplantation were excluded due to the high risk of bleeding complications associated with liver transplantation and the technical challenges of TAH explantation in this setting. The outcomes of TAH support in CA are heavily dependent on institutional expertise and procedural volume. High-volume centers with established TAH programs report superior survival and fewer complications, emphasizing the need for experienced multidisciplinary teams when considering this advanced therapy.

Despite these advantages, the adoption of TAH for CA patients remains limited due to the complexity of patient selection, procedural risks, and the availability of suitable donor hearts for subsequent transplantation [6, 17].

In situations where the right ventricle (RV) cannot compensate despite LV unloading, a BiVAD may be necessary to provide simultaneous support to both ventricles. BiVADs use two ventricular assist pumps to manage the unique hemodynamic needs of CA patients with biventricular dysfunction as a bridge to HT. However, BiVAD implantation in CA poses technical challenges due to the restrictive LV cavity size, stiff myocardial walls, and increased risk of pump thrombosis or suction events. Evidence from retrospective studies indicates that BiVADs can achieve comparable outcomes in carefully selected CA patients. Nonetheless, BiVAD use is often limited by the potential for complications, including bleeding, infection, and thromboembolic events, as well as the high cost and resource intensity associated with long-term biventricular support [26, 27].

Consequently, both TAH and BiVAD strategies are associated with substantial challenges in CA. The restrictive myocardial phenotype, systemic vascular remodeling, and underlying multi-organ involvement in amyloidosis increase the risk of adverse events during and after device implantation. Patients with CA often present with coexisting renal dysfunction, gastrointestinal amyloid deposition, or bleeding diathesis, all of which complicate perioperative management and long-term device function. Additionally, the infiltrative nature of CA and its impact on the vascular and systemic circulation necessitate a meticulous, multidisciplinary approach to care. Proper patient selection, tailored perioperative strategies, and close post-implantation monitoring are crucial to minimizing complications and maximizing the benefits of durable biventricular MCS.

Selection of the Type of MCS Device

Given the challenges and the evolving landscape of MCS for CA patients with advanced HF, a treatment approach for these patients should incorporate considerations for both tMCS and dMCS options, depending on the patient's specific clinical circumstances. The use of biventricular support may be required upfront in patients with significant RV dysfunction or other contraindications to LVAD use. In addition, tMCS strategies should be considered in centers with expertise in these techniques, with close monitoring for any potential complications, particularly in the post-implantation phase. This selection of the type of MCS should consider factors like LV cavity size, RV function, the presence of extra-cardiac amyloid involvement, and the patient's candidacy for heart or multi-organ transplantation. As experience with new MCS devices continues to grow, ongoing assessment of clinical outcomes will be essential in optimizing patient selection and treatment strategies for CA patients requiring MCS [17, 28].

Heart Transplantation

HT remains the only curative option for end-stage HF in cardiac amyloidosis. Advances in patient selection, perioperative management, and post-HT therapies have significantly improved outcomes in recent years [6, 29]. Historically, HT was contraindicated in AL amyloidosis due to poor post-HT survival. However, the advent of effective chemotherapy has transformed the treatment landscape. Achieving a durable hematologic response is now a prerequisite for HT in AL amyloidosis, as uncontrolled plasma cell dyscrasia leads to recurrent amyloid deposition. Post-HT outcomes in AL amyloidosis have improved significantly when HT is combined with autologous stem cell transplantation (ASCT). This sequential approach addresses both cardiac and systemic disease, with studies reporting 5-year survival rates exceeding 60% in carefully selected patients. A UNOS registry study from 1988 to 2013 reported lower 5-year and 10-year survival rates for amyloid patients compared to non-amyloid counterparts (56% vs. 71% and 31% vs. 51%) [30]. However, newer chemotherapeutic agents for AL amyloidosis (e.g., bortezomib, lenalidomide, daratumumab) and therapies for ATTR (e.g., RNA silencers, TTR stabilizers) have significantly improved outcomes [1, 31, 32]. Strict selection criteria now identify optimal candidates for HT, further enhancing survival in this challenging population.

In ATTRv amyloidosis, a combined heart and liver transplant may be required to halt transthyretin production. Conversely, ATTRwt amyloidosis typically involves isolated cardiac involvement and is managed with HT alone. The development of disease-modifying therapies, such as transthyretin stabilizers (tafamidis) and gene-silencing therapies (patisiran and inotersen), has further improved outcomes by slowing amyloid deposition and enhancing post-HT survival. Five-year survival rates after HT in ATTR amyloidosis exceed 70%, underscoring the efficacy of this approach in selected patients.

Post-HT management in amyloidosis includes vigilant monitoring for recurrent amyloid deposition, particularly in AL amyloidosis. Immunosuppressive regimens must be carefully tailored to minimize infection risk while ensuring graft survival. Emerging therapies targeting amyloid fibrils may further enhance post-HT outcomes.

In the past, patients with AL CA had significantly worse outcomes following HT compared to those with other forms of cardiac amyloidosis. Outcomes were notably worse for patients with extracardiac amyloid involvement at the time of HT listing, compared to those with isolated cardiac amyloidosis. The International Symposium on Amyloid and Amyloidosis (ISAA) has since established consensus definitions for extracardiac involvement, which now play a pivotal role in patient selection for HT [33]. The presence and severity of extracardiac involvement often determine HT eligibility. Common contraindications for HT in AL CA include symptomatic gastrointestinal amyloid deposits (e.g., diarrhea, gastric dysmotility, malnutrition), significant proteinuria (>2–2.5 g/day), advanced renal dysfunction (GFR < 30 ml/min), severe autonomic dysfunction, advanced multiple myeloma with hypercalcemia or bone lesions, and severe peripheral neuropathy impairing functional recovery. Additionally, poor hematological response to pre-HT chemotherapy, defined as less than a

50% reduction in serum free light chains or monoclonal protein, is often considered unfavorable for HT eligibility. Some centers may consider partially treated patients in urgent cases of cardiogenic shock, where time does not permit full assessment of hematological response. Recent studies highlight that minimizing extracardiac involvement is crucial for improving long-term survival in AL CA patients [28]. For instance, the University of Heidelberg's "DANGER" criteria prioritize stringent screening of extracardiac organ involvement, demonstrating significant mortality benefits in carefully selected patients. This refined approach underscores the importance of individualized assessment and multidisciplinary collaboration in managing HT candidates with AL CA [34].

Despite careful selection and inclusion in the UNOS registry for heart transplantation (HT), patients with AL cardiac amyloidosis (CA) have higher waitlist mortality compared to non-CA patients. One study found a 35% waitlist mortality rate in AL CA patients, mostly due to cardiac causes. Multivariate analyses identified waitlist time as a key predictor of survival to HT, and a UNOS registry study confirmed that CA patients face significantly higher risks of waitlist mortality and delisting. This disparity was most notable in those listed as Status 1B under the 2006 classification, although Status 1A patients did not show the same trend, highlighting the need for earlier listing and prioritization for CA patients [35].

To address these disparities, UNOS updated its listing criteria in 2018, allowing patients with restrictive cardiomyopathies, including AL CA, to achieve higher listing status if they required continuous inotropic support or invasive hemodynamic monitoring. A comparison of the pre-2018 and post-2018 HT periods showed improvements in waitlist times and HT rates, with reduced waitlist mortality. Importantly, six-month post-HT survival rates remained stable (~91% vs. ~92%). Recent data indicate that CA patients are more often transplanted under high urgency status, experience shorter wait times, and are more frequently bridged to HT with tMCS or inotropic therapy compared to non-CA patients, suggesting recent policy changes have modestly improved outcomes [36].

Studies also show that well-selected AL CA patients experience similar short-term outcomes to non-AL CA patients post-HT, with comparable 1-year survival rates, incidences of cardiac allograft vasculopathy, acute rejection, and infectious complications. The risk of infections related to chemotherapy or immunosuppression is not significantly higher in these patients. Finally, a recent study from Mayo Clinic that evaluated 55 cardiac amyloidosis (CA) patients who underwent heart transplantation (HT) between 2007 and 2020), including 8 with light chain amyloidosis (AL, 14.5%), 28 with hereditary transthyretin amyloidosis (ATTRv, 50.9%), 17 with wild-type transthyretin amyloidosis (ATTRwt, 30.9%), and 2 with hereditary apolipoprotein A1 amyloidosis (AApoA1, 3.6%). Post-transplant survival was similar between CA and non-amyloid patients. Following the introduction of the new allocation system in 2018, median wait times significantly decreased from 174 to 45 days. Additionally, the use of multiorgan transplantation in hereditary amyloidosis declined over time, driven by increased utilization of disease-targeted therapies, highlighting improved access and outcomes for CA patients undergoing HT.

Role of Bone Marrow Transplant in AL CA HT

ASCT after high-dose melphalan has been explored in AL amyloidosis treatment. Initially, patients with decompensated CA were excluded from ASCT studies due to high morbidity. ASCT is typically performed 6 months to 1 year post-HT. In a Mayo Clinic cohort, 56% of patients underwent ASCT with a median time of 8 months after HT. These patients had a longer median survival (6.3 years) compared to those who did not undergo ASCT (2.4 years). Similarly, the Heidelberg cohort reported that ASCT was performed a median of 3.8 months after HT, though no data on long-term outcomes between the two groups was provided.

Studies have also examined ASCT in patients receiving modern therapies like bortezomib and daratumumab. In a Stanford cohort, 5 of 13 AL amyloidosis patients who underwent ASCT 6 months after HT had no deaths due to amyloid progression. Although mortality rates did not differ between those receiving medical therapy or ASCT, the increased efficacy of modern treatments has reduced the necessity of ASCT. The role of ASCT is being questioned considering newer treatments like proteasome inhibitors, which offer improved hematological responses and reduced toxicity. A study showed that ASCT performed 12 months after HT resulted in long-term outcomes comparable to earlier ASCT. Some centers have ceased routine ASCT following HT, reflecting the effectiveness of these modern treatments.

Temporal Trends in HT for AL CA and Future Considerations

In recent years, HT outcomes for AL CA patients have improved, largely due to the more rigorous patient selection criteria and advancements in treating AL amyloidosis. Previously, HT for AL amyloidosis was associated with poorer outcomes, mainly due to disease recurrence in the transplanted heart and complications from systemic chemotherapy. However, the introduction of proteasome inhibitors has led to more durable disease responses, improving long-term HT outcomes [28].

As early recognition of CA increases and therapies like daratumumab become more widely used, further improvements in patient outcomes are anticipated. The recent Phase III ANDROMEDA trial demonstrated that daratumumab treatment significantly improved hematological and cardiac responses, offering hope for improved outcomes in pre-HT patients [37]. However, the impact of pre-HT daratumumab on post-HT survival remains uncertain, and ongoing studies will need to evaluate potential risks, particularly regarding infection. Patients receiving daratumumab have a heightened risk of respiratory infections and CMV reactivation, which may complicate the post-HT recovery phase. Future research will be crucial in determining the role of daratumumab and other novel therapies in improving post-HT outcomes and managing infectious complications.

Heart Transplantation for ATTR CA

ATTR CA is characterized by a slower disease progression compared to AL amyloidosis, making ATTR patients more favorable candidates for HT. Advances in diagnostic tools, such as technetium pyrophosphate and DPD scintigraphy as well as free genetic testing, have enabled earlier recognition of ATTR CA, allowing for better patient selection and improved outcomes. In the contemporary era, post-HT survival for ATTR patients has significantly improved, with 1-year survival rates ranging from 75 to 100% and 3-year survival rates increasing from 50–67% in earlier cohorts to 75–100% in recent years [28, 38]. Importantly, ATTR CA patients now experience survival outcomes similar to those of non-amyloid HT recipients, with no significant differences in rates of graft rejection, cardiac allograft vasculopathy, or infection.

ATTR patients generally exhibit fewer extracardiac manifestations than AL CA patients, further enhancing their suitability for HT. The most common extracardiac features include carpal tunnel syndrome, peripheral neuropathy, and spinal stenosis. In contemporary cohorts, the frequency of significant extracardiac involvement has declined markedly, with reported rates dropping from 17.7–37.5% in earlier eras to 6.7–12.5% currently [29]. For patients with ATTR CA and significant organ involvement, multiorgan transplantation offers a viable option. Heart-liver and heart-kidney combinations are commonly performed in such cases, yielding outcomes comparable to single-organ HT. For instance, patients with advanced kidney dysfunction (e.g., GFR < 30 mL/min or severe proteinuria) may benefit from heart-kidney transplantation, while heart-liver transplantation in ATTRv can be curative by eliminating the mutant TTR production [39, 40].

Despite these advancements, ATTR recurrence in the transplanted heart or systemically remains a challenge. This phenomenon, attributed to the "seeding hypothesis," occurs when residual ATTR deposits act as a nidus for further amyloid fibril deposition, even after liver transplantation. Clinical reports document systemic ATTR progression post-HT in both ATTRwt and ATTRv patients, manifesting as worsening peripheral neuropathy, gastrointestinal symptoms, or lumbar stenosis. In some cases, amyloid deposition in the cardiac graft has also been observed, though this remains rare.

Emerging ATTR-targeted therapies, such as patisiran (an RNA interference agent), offer promise in mitigating disease progression and managing systemic symptoms post-HT. Case reports highlight their feasibility and effectiveness in treating symptomatic neuropathy and reducing systemic amyloid burden in post-HT patients. These findings underscore the importance of close post-HT monitoring for ATTR progression and the potential role of continued ATTR-directed therapies, particularly in patients with ATTRv who did not undergo liver transplantation. Future research is needed to determine optimal post-transplant management strategies, including the routine use of disease-modifying therapies to prevent systemic progression and improve long-term outcomes in ATTR CA patients.

Taken together, the literature highlights the significant improvement in survival outcomes for patients with AL and ATTR CA following HT and multi-organ transplants. In AL amyloidosis, the introduction of newer generation chemotherapies, coupled with careful patient selection, has led to markedly improved post-HT survival. Similarly, ATTR CA patients have shown enhanced outcomes due to more stringent selection criteria. There may also be a role for post-transplant targeted therapies, specifically those aimed at ATTR, to reduce disease progression and potentially avoid the need for heart-liver transplantation. Future research should focus on identifying optimal indications and contraindications for HT. Additionally, further trials are needed to evaluate the efficacy and safety of ATTR-targeted therapies in the post-HT setting, for both patients who have received concomitant liver transplants and those who have not. These efforts will be crucial in refining treatment strategies and improving the long-term management of CA patients requiring heart or multi-organ transplants.

Conclusions

The management of advanced HF in CA has evolved significantly in recent years, driven by advancements in both pharmacologic and mechanical therapies. Despite its unique challenges, outcomes in CA are improving, particularly through a combination of refined patient selection, multidisciplinary care, and the integration of novel therapeutic approaches.

The use of MCS in CA, historically limited due to concerns about bleeding complications, pump thrombosis, and poor outcomes, has seen incremental progress. Contemporary LVAD offers a viable bridge to transplantation or destination therapy in selected patients with CA and limited extracardiac involvement. However, challenges remain, particularly in AL amyloidosis, where systemic disease recurrence and bleeding diatheses continue to limit broader application. Emerging evidence suggests that tailored anticoagulation strategies, enhanced patient selection, and technological advancements in device design may expand the role of MCS in CA management.

HT remains the cornerstone of therapy for end-stage HF in CA, offering long-term survival and improved quality of life for appropriately selected patients. Advances in chemotherapeutic agents for AL amyloidosis and disease-modifying therapies for ATTR amyloidosis have significantly transformed the treatment landscape, enabling better systemic disease control and improving post-transplant outcomes. Five-year survival rates for well-selected CA patients now approach those of non-amyloid HF patients. The 2018 revisions to the UNOS allocation system have further enhanced access to HT by prioritizing patients with restrictive cardiomyopathies and inotropic dependence, resulting in reduced waitlist times and improved transplant rates.

Future Directions

Future directions in the management of advanced HF in CA will focus on improving MCS strategies, with the development of smaller, more biocompatible devices and further research on anticoagulation management to optimize outcomes. Additionally, more studies are needed to explore the role of MCS in bridging patients to HT, particularly for those with advanced forms of amyloidosis. In terms of systemic therapies, advancements in gene-editing technologies for ATTR amyloidosis, as well as enhanced plasma cell therapies for AL amyloidosis, hold the potential for more effective disease control and improved post-transplant outcomes.

Further progress in patient selection will involve integrating advanced imaging techniques, such as CMR and nuclear scintigraphy, along with biomarkers to better assess the extent of disease and predict outcomes. Additionally, refining risk assessment models will help ensure that only the most suitable candidates are selected for HT, optimizing survival rates and quality of life. Innovations in immunosuppressive regimens will aim to minimize the risk of infection and rejection while preventing recurrent amyloid deposition in the graft. Targeted therapies designed to address amyloid fibril recurrence post-transplant will also be a key area of research. As the transplant allocation system continues to evolve, particularly in response to the growing number of eligible CA patients, it is crucial to foster multidisciplinary collaboration to ensure that treatment strategies are tailored to individual patient needs, ultimately leading to improved survival and quality of life for those affected by cardiac amyloidosis.

Authors Disclosures The authors have no conflicts of interest to disclose.

References

1. Ruberg FL, Maurer MS. Cardiac amyloidosis due to transthyretin protein. JAMA. 2024;331:778. Available from: https://jamanetwork.com/journals/jama/fullarticle/2815711
2. Griffin JM, Rosenblum H, Maurer MS. Pathophysiology and therapeutic approaches to cardiac amyloidosis. Circ Res. 2021;128:1554–75. Available from: https://www.ahajournals.org/doi/10.1161/CIRCRESAHA.121.318187
3. Garcia-Pavia P, Rapezzi C, Adler Y, Arad M, Basso C, Brucato A, Burazor I, Caforio ALP, Damy T, Eriksson U, Fontana M, Gillmore JD, Gonzalez-Lopez E, Grogan M, Heymans S, Imazio M, Kindermann I, Kristen AV., Maurer MS, Merlini G, Pantazis A, Pankuweit S, Rigopoulos AG, Linhart A. Diagnosis and treatment of cardiac amyloidosis: a position statement of the ESC working group on myocardial and pericardial diseases. European Heart Journal. 2021;42:1554–68. Available from: https://academic.oup.com/eurheartj/article/42/16/1554/6212698
4. Falk RH, Alexander KM, Liao R, Dorbala S. AL (Light-Chain) cardiac amyloidosis: a review of diagnosis and therapy. J Am College Cardiol. 2016;68:1323–41. Available from: https://linkinghub.elsevier.com/retrieve/pii/S0735109716346046
5. Ruberg FL, Grogan M, Hanna M, Kelly JW, Maurer MS. Transthyretin amyloid cardiomyopathy. J Am College Cardiol. 2019;73:2872–2891. Available from: https://linkinghub.elsevier.com/retrieve/pii/S0735109719347291

6. Witteles RM. Cardiac transplantation and mechanical circulatory support in amyloidosis. JACC: cardioOncology. 2021;3:516–521. Available from: https://linkinghub.elsevier.com/retrieve/pii/S2666087321001538
7. Bhimaraj A, Agrawal T, Duran A, Tamimi O, Amione-Guerra J, Trachtenberg B, Guha A, Hussain I, Kim J, Kassi M, Xu J, Suarez E, Ngo UQ, Torre-Amione G, Estep JD. Percutaneous left axillary artery placement of intra-aortic balloon pump in advanced heart failure patients. JACC: Heart Failure. 2020;8:313–323. Available from: https://linkinghub.elsevier.com/retrieve/pii/S2213177920300846
8. Bhimaraj A, Cordero-Reyes AM, Trachtenberg BH, Ashrith G, Loza LP, Loebe M, Suarez EE, Bruckner BA, Torre-Amione G, Estep JD. Use of various mechanical circulatory support strategies in end stage amyloidosis—a single center experience from an amyloid heart transplant center. J Heart Lung Transplant. 2014;33:S210–11. Available from: https://linkinghub.elsevier.com/retrieve/pii/S1053249814009383
9. Randhawa VK, Lee R, Ives L, Soltesz EG, Tong MZ, Starling RC, Hernandez-Montfort J, Hanna M, Estep JD. An analysis of cardiac amyloidosis patients in cardiogenic shock bridged with temporary mechanical circulatory support to durable left ventricular assist device and heart transplant. J Heart Lung Transplant. 2021;40:S405. Available from: https://linkinghub.elsevier.com/retrieve/pii/S1053249821011517
10. Mancio Silva J, Fontes-Carvalho R, Valente D, Almeida C, Cruz AJ, Tente D, Coelho H, Oliveira M, Albuquerque A, Ribeiro VG. Extracorporeal membrane oxygenation as bridge-to-decision in acute heart failure due to systemic light-chain amyloidosis. Am J Case Rep . 2015;16:174–81. Available from: http://www.amjcaserep.com/abstract/index/idArt/892772
11. Heidenreich PA, Bozkurt B, Aguilar D, Allen LA, Byun JJ, Colvin MM, Deswal A, Drazner MH, Dunlay SM, Evers LR, Fang JC, Fedson SE, Fonarow GC, Hayek SS, Hernandez AF, Khazanie P, Kittleson MM, Lee CS, Link MS, Milano CA, Nnacheta LC, Sandhu AT, Stevenson LW, Vardeny O, Vest AR, Yancy CW. 2022 AHA/ACC/HFSA guideline for the management of heart failure: executive summary: a report of the american college of cardiology/american heart association joint committee on clinical practice guidelines. Circulation. 2022;145:E876–94. Available from: https://www.ahajournals.org/doi/10.1161/CIR.0000000000001062
12. Swiecicki PL, Edwards BS, Kushwaha SS, Dispenzieri A, Park SJ, Gertz MA. Left ventricular device implantation for advanced cardiac amyloidosis. J Heart Lung Transplant. 2013;32:563–568. Available from: https://linkinghub.elsevier.com/retrieve/pii/S1053249813010243
13. Grupper A, Park SJ, Pereira NL, Schettle SD, Gerber Y, Topilsky Y, Edwards BS, Daly RC, Stulak JM, Joyce LD, Kushwaha SS. Role of ventricular assist therapy for patients with heart failure and restrictive physiology: improving outcomes for a lethal disease. J Heart Lung Transplant: Official Publication International Society for Heart Transplantation. 2015;34:1042–9. Available from: https://linkinghub.elsevier.com/retrieve/pii/S1053249815011080
14. Michelis KC, Zhong L, Tang WHW, Young JB, Peltz M, Drazner MH, Pandey A, Griffin J, Maurer MS, Grodin JL. Durable mechanical circulatory support in patients with amyloid cardiomyopathy: insights from INTERMACS. Circ Heart Failure. 2020;13:e007931. Available from: https://www.ahajournals.org/doi/10.1161/CIRCHEARTFAILURE.120.007931
15. Mehra MR, Uriel N, Naka Y, Cleveland JC, Yuzefpolskaya M, Salerno CT, Walsh MN, Milano CA, Patel CB, Hutchins SW, Ransom J, Ewald GA, Itoh A, Raval NY, Silvestry SC, Cogswell R, John R, Bhimaraj A, Bruckner BA, Lowes BD, Um JY, Jeevanandam V, Sayer G, Mangi AA, Molina EJ, Sheikh F, Aaronson K, Pagani FD, Cotts WG, Tatooles AJ, Babu A, Chomsky D, Katz JN, Tessmann PB, Dean D, Krishnamoorthy A, Chuang J, Topuria I, Sood P, Goldstein DJ. A fully magnetically levitated left ventricular assist device—final report. New England J Med. 2019;380:1618–27. Available from: http://www.nejm.org/doi/10.1056/NEJMoa1900486
16. Arvidsson S, Henein MY, Wikström G, Suhr OB, Lindqvist P. Right ventricular involvement in transthyretin amyloidosis. Amyloid Int J Exp Clin Inv Official J Int Soc Amyloidosis. 2018;25:160–6. Available from: https://www.tandfonline.com/doi/full/10.1080/13506129.2018.1493989
17. Sciaccaluga C, De Carli G, Fusi C, Stefanini A, Mandoli GE, Giacomin E, D'Ascenzi F, Focardi M, Valente S, Cameli M. Left ventricular assist device in cardiac amyloidosis: friend or foe?

Heart Fail Rev. 2022;28:359–65. Available from: https://link.springer.com/10.1007/s10741-022-10288-w
18. Topilsky Y, Pereira NL, Shah DK, Boilson B, Schirger JA, Kushwaha SS, Joyce LD, Park SJ. Left ventricular assist device therapy in patients with restrictive and hypertrophic cardiomyopathy. Circ Heart Fail. 2011;4:266–75. Available from: https://www.ahajournals.org/doi/10.1161/CIRCHEARTFAILURE.110.959288
19. Imamura T, Kinugawa K, Kato N, Muraoka H, Fujino T, Inaba T, Maki H, Kinoshita O, Hatano M, Kyo S, Ono M. Late-onset right ventricular failure in patients with preoperative small left ventricle after implantation of continuous flow left ventricular assist device. Circulation J Official J Japanese Circ Soc. 2014;78:625–33. Available from: https://www.jstage.jst.go.jp/article/circj/78/3/78_CJ-13-1201/_article
20. Fine NM, White JA, Jimenez-Zepeda V, Howlett JG. Determinants and prognostic significance of serial right heart function changes in patients with cardiac amyloidosis. Canadian J Cardiol. 2020;36:432–40. Available from: https://linkinghub.elsevier.com/retrieve/pii/S0828282X20300568
21. Wan K, Lin J, Guo X, Song R, Wang J, Xu Y, Li W, Cheng W, Sun J, Zhang Q, Han Y, Chen Y. Prognostic value of right ventricular dysfunction in patients with AL amyloidosis: comparison of different techniques by cardiac magnetic resonance. J Magn Reson Imag JMRI. 2020;52:1441–8. Available from: https://onlinelibrary.wiley.com/doi/10.1002/jmri.27200
22. Mehta P, Chapel DB, Goyal N, Yu DB, Mor-Avi V, Narang A, Addetia K, Sarswat N, Lang RM, Husain AN, Patel AR. A histopathologic schema to quantify the burden of cardiac amyloidosis: Relationship with survival and echocardiographic parameters. Echocardiography (Mount Kisco, NY). 2019;36:285–91. Available from: https://onlinelibrary.wiley.com/doi/10.1111/echo.14245
23. Asleh R, Hasin T, Briasoulis A, Schettle SD, Borlaug BA, Behfar A, Pereira NL, Edwards BS, Clavell AL, Joyce LD, Maltais S, Stulak JM, Kushwaha SS. Hemodynamic assessment of patients with and without heart failure symptoms supported by a continuous-flow left ventricular assist device. Mayo Clinic Proc. 2018
24. Nicol M, Siguret V, Vergaro G, Aimo A, Emdin M, Dillinger JG, Baudet M, Cohen-Solal A, Villesuzanne C, Harel S, Royer B, Arnulf B, Logeart D. Thromboembolism and bleeding in systemic amyloidosis: a review. ESC Heart Failure. 2022;9:11–20. Available from: https://onlinelibrary.wiley.com/doi/10.1002/ehf2.13701
25. Khalil F, Asleh R, Perue RK, Weinstein J-M, Solomon A, Betesh-Abay B, Briasoulis A, Alnsasra H. Vascular function in continuous flow LVADs: implications for clinical practice. Biomedicines. 2023;11:757. Available from: https://www.mdpi.com/2227-9059/11/3/757
26. Kittleson MM, Cole RM, Patel J, Ramzy D, Passano E, Chang DH, Geft DR, Czer L, Vescio R, Chung J, Kobashigawa JA, Arabia F, Esmailian F, Moriguchi JD. Mechanical circulatory support for cardiac amyloidosis. Clinical Transpl. 2019;33:e13663. Available from: https://onlinelibrary.wiley.com/doi/10.1111/ctr.13663
27. Arabía FA, Cantor RS, Koehl DA, Kasirajan V, Gregoric I, Moriguchi JD, Esmailian F, Ramzy D, Chung JS, Czer LS, Kobashigawa JA, Smith RG, Kirklin JK. Interagency registry for mechanically assisted circulatory support report on the total artificial heart. J Heart Lung Transpl. 2018;37:1304–12. Available from: https://linkinghub.elsevier.com/retrieve/pii/S1053249818314347
28. Kumar S, Li D, Joseph D, Trachtenberg B. State-of-the-art review on management of end-stage heart failure in amyloidosis: transplant and beyond. Heart Failure Reviews. 2022;27:1567–78. Available from: https://link.springer.com/10.1007/s10741-021-10209-3
29. Kristen A V., Kreusser MM, Blum P, Schönland SO, Frankenstein L, Dösch AO, Knop B, Helmschrott M, Schmack B, Ruhparwar A, Hegenbart U, Katus HA, Raake PWJ. Improved outcomes after heart transplantation for cardiac amyloidosis in the modern era. J Heart Lung Transpl Official Publication Int Soc Heart Transpl. 2018;37:611–18. Available from: https://linkinghub.elsevier.com/retrieve/pii/S1053249817321162
30. DePasquale EC, Nasir K, Jacoby DL. Outcomes of adults with restrictive cardiomyopathy after heart transplantation. J Heart Lung Transpl Official Publication Int Soc Heart Transpl.

2012;31:1269–75. Available from: https://linkinghub.elsevier.com/retrieve/pii/S1053249812012995

31. Maurer MS, Schwartz JH, Gundapaneni B, Elliott PM, Merlini G, Waddington-Cruz M, Kristen A V., Grogan M, Witteles R, Damy T, Drachman BM, Shah SJ, Hanna M, Judge DP, Barsdorf AI, Huber P, Patterson TA, Riley S, Schumacher J, Stewart M, Sultan MB, Rapezzi C. Tafamidis treatment for patients with transthyretin amyloid cardiomyopathy. New England J Med. 2018;379:1007–16. Available from: http://www.nejm.org/doi/10.1056/NEJMoa1805689
32. Adams D, Gonzalez-Duarte A, O'Riordan WD, Yang C-C, Ueda M, Kristen A V., Tournev I, Schmidt HH, Coelho T, Berk JL, Lin K-P, Vita G, Attarian S, Planté-Bordeneuve V, Mezei MM, Campistol JM, Buades J, Brannagan TH, Kim BJ, Oh J, Parman Y, Sekijima Y, Hawkins PN, Solomon SD, Polydefkis M, Dyck PJ, Gandhi PJ, Goyal S, Chen J, Strahs AL, Nochur S V., Sweetser MT, Garg PP, Vaishnaw AK, Gollob JA, Suhr OB. Patisiran, an RNAi therapeutic, for hereditary transthyretin amyloidosis. New England J Med. 2018;379:11–21. Available from: http://www.nejm.org/doi/10.1056/NEJMoa1716153
33. Gertz MA, Comenzo R, Falk RH, Fermand JP, Hazenberg BP, Hawkins PN, Merlini G, Moreau P, Ronco P, Sanchorawala V, Sezer O, Solomon A, Grateau G. Definition of organ involvement and treatment response in immunoglobulin light chain amyloidosis (AL): a consensus opinion from the 10th international symposium on amyloid and amyloidosis, tours, France, 18–22 April 2004. Am J Hematol. 2005;79:319–28. Available from: https://onlinelibrary.wiley.com/doi/10.1002/ajh.20381
34. Kristen A V., Sack F, Schonland SO, Hegenbart U, Helmke BM, Koch A, Schnabel PA, Röcken C, Hardt S, Remppis A, Goldschmidt H, Karck M, Ho AD, Katus HA, Dengler TJ. Staged heart transplantation and chemotherapy as a treatment option in patients with severe cardiac light-chain amyloidosis. European J Heart Fail. 2009;11:1014–20. Available from: https://onlinelibrary.wiley.com/doi/10.1093/eurjhf/hfp121
35. Panhwar MS, Al-Kindi SG, Tofovic D, Oliveira GH, Ginwalla M. Waitlist mortality of patients with amyloid cardiomyopathy who are listed for heart transplantation and implications for organ allocation. J Card Fail. 2019;25:767–71. Available from: https://linkinghub.elsevier.com/retrieve/pii/S107191641930421X
36. Griffin JM, Chiu L, Axsom KM, Bijou R, Clerkin KJ, Colombo P, Cuomo MO, De Los Santos J, Fried JA, Goldsmith J, Habal M, Haythe J, Helmke S, Horn EM, Latif F, Hi Lee S, Lin EF, Naka Y, Raikhelkar J, Restaino S, Sayer GT, Takayama H, Takeda K, Teruya S, Topkara V, Tsai EJ, Uriel N, Yuzefpolskaya M, Farr MA, Maurer MS. United network for organ sharing outcomes after heart transplantation for al compared to ATTR cardiac amyloidosis. Clin Transpl. 2020;34:e14028. Available from: https://onlinelibrary.wiley.com/doi/10.1111/ctr.14028
37. Kastritis E, Palladini G, Minnema MC, Wechalekar AD, Jaccard A, Lee HC, Sanchorawala V, Gibbs S, Mollee P, Venner CP, Lu J, Schönland S, Gatt ME, Suzuki K, Kim K, Cibeira MT, Beksac M, Libby E, Valent J, Hungria V, Wong SW, Rosenzweig M, Bumma N, Huart A, Dimopoulos MA, Bhutani D, Waxman AJ, Goodman SA, Zonder JA, Lam S, Song K, Hansen T, Manier S, Roeloffzen W, Jamroziak K, Kwok F, Shimazaki C, Kim J-S, Crusoe E, Ahmadi T, Tran N, Qin X, Vasey SY, Tromp B, Schecter JM, Weiss BM, Zhuang SH, Vermeulen J, Merlini G, Comenzo RL. Daratumumab-Based treatment for immunoglobulin light-chain amyloidosis. New England J Med. 2021;385:46–58. Available from: http://www.nejm.org/doi/10.1056/NEJMoa2028631
38. Griffin JM, DeFilippis EM, Rosenblum H, Topkara VK, Fried JA, Uriel N, Takeda K, Farr MA, Maurer MS, Clerkin KJ. Comparing outcomes for infiltrative and restrictive cardiomyopathies under the new heart transplant allocation system. Clin Transpl. 2020;34:e14109. Available from: https://onlinelibrary.wiley.com/doi/10.1111/ctr.14109
39. Rosenbaum AN, AbouEzzeddine OF, Grogan M, Dispenzieri A, Kushwaha S, Clavell A, Daly RC, Edwards BS. Outcomes after cardiac transplant for wild type transthyretin amyloidosis. Transplantation. 2018;102:1909–13. Available from: https://journals.lww.com/00007890-201811000-00028

40. Barrett CD, Alexander KM, Zhao H, Haddad F, Cheng P, Liao R, Wheeler MT, Liedtke M, Schrier S, Arai S, Weisshaar D, Witteles RM. Outcomes in patients with cardiac amyloidosis undergoing heart transplantation. JACC Heart Fail. 2020;8:461–8. Available from: https://linkinghub.elsevier.com/retrieve/pii/S2213177920300755

Management of Arrythmias in Cardiac Amyloidosis

Yotam Kolben, Eyal Herzog, and Yitschak Biton

Abstract Cardiac amyloidosis presents a diverse spectrum of electrical disturbances that significantly impact patient outcomes and management. This chapter comprehensively reviews the three main categories of electrical manifestations in cardiac amyloidosis. The prevalence and characteristics of these disturbances vary notably between amyloid subtypes, with AL cardiac amyloidosis showing higher rates of arrhythmias (up to 60%) compared to ATTR cardiac amyloidosis (20–40%). Atrial fibrillation, the most common arrhythmia, presents unique challenges in management, including high thrombotic risk regardless of conventional risk scores and limited tolerance to standard rate-control medications. Ventricular arrhythmias, more prevalent in AL amyloidosis, pose significant mortality risk with one-year mortality rates of 50% in affected patients, though the role of ICD therapy remains controversial due to high rates of electromechanical dissociation. Conduction system disorders, particularly affecting the His-Purkinje system, are highly prevalent and often necessitate pacing, with evidence suggesting potential adverse effects from high right ventricular pacing burden and possible benefits from biventricular pacing. The chapter explores the pathophysiology, clinical implications, and management strategies for each type of electrical disturbance, incorporating emerging evidence and evolving treatment approaches. The complex interplay between the restrictive physiology of cardiac amyloidosis and its electrical manifestations necessitates careful individualization of management strategies, as conventional anti-arrhythmic approaches often prove poorly tolerated. Understanding these electrical manifestations and their management challenges is crucial for optimizing outcomes in this unique patient population.

Keywords Cardiac amyloidosis · Atrial arrythmias · Ventricular arrythmias · Conduction disorders

---

Y. Kolben (✉) · E. Herzog · Y. Biton
Heart Institute, Hadassah Medical Center, Hebrew University of Jerusalem, Jerusalem, Israel
e-mail: yotamkol@hadassah.org.il

E. Herzog (ed.), *Cardiac Amyloidosis*, https://doi.org/10.1007/978-3-031-88342-2_12

Introduction

Cardiac amyloidosis presents a complex spectrum of electrical disturbances that significantly impact patient outcomes. Arrhythmias and conduction abnormalities are not only common manifestations of the disease but also contribute substantially to its morbidity and mortality. The prevalence and type of arrhythmias vary notably between amyloid subtypes, with AL cardiac amyloidosis showing arrhythmias in up to 60% of patients, while ATTR cardiac amyloidosis demonstrates a lower prevalence of 20–40% [1, 3].

The electrical manifestations span across three main categories: supraventricular arrhythmias (predominantly atrial fibrillation), ventricular arrhythmias, and conduction system disease. Each presents unique challenges in diagnosis and management, often requiring individualized treatment approaches. The underlying restrictive physiology of cardiac amyloidosis adds complexity to these electrical disturbances, as patients often demonstrate poor tolerance to conventional anti-arrhythmic strategies [2, 4].

Notably, electrocardiographic changes are nearly universal in cardiac amyloidosis, with normal ECGs being exceedingly rare—present in only 5% of AL-CA cases, 10% in ATTRv-CA, and completely absent in ATTRwt-CA [1]. The historical underrepresentation of cardiac amyloidosis patients in clinical trials, particularly due to historically short life expectancy in AL amyloidosis, has resulted in limited evidence-based guidance for managing these complex electrical manifestations. This chapter explores the full spectrum of electrical disturbances in cardiac amyloidosis, their mechanisms, clinical implications, and management considerations, incorporating emerging evidence and evolving treatment strategies.

Atrial Arrythmias

Atrial fibrillation (AF) is the most common arrhythmia in CA patients, with a prevalence ranging from 16 to 80% depending on the CA subtype and stage [1, 4]. Due to the high amyloid protein deposition, the left atrium (LA) presents significant structural and electrical remodeling, and thromboembolic events are also frequent in these patients. Amyloid fibril deposition and infiltration of the myocardium have been shown to cause atrial and ventricular wall thickening, impaired relaxation, and restrictive filling [2]. Elevated filling pressure leads to atrial dilation, predisposing to AF and other atrial arrhythmias such as atrial flutter (Fig. 1). In addition, amyloid deposition in the atria is thought to promote myocardial fibrosis and structural remodeling, again predisposing to AF. Pathologic atrial amyloid deposition has been positively correlated with clinical AF in multiple studies. It is thought that AF, in turn, potentiates further amyloid deposition, thereby leading to a vicious cycle [3, 5].

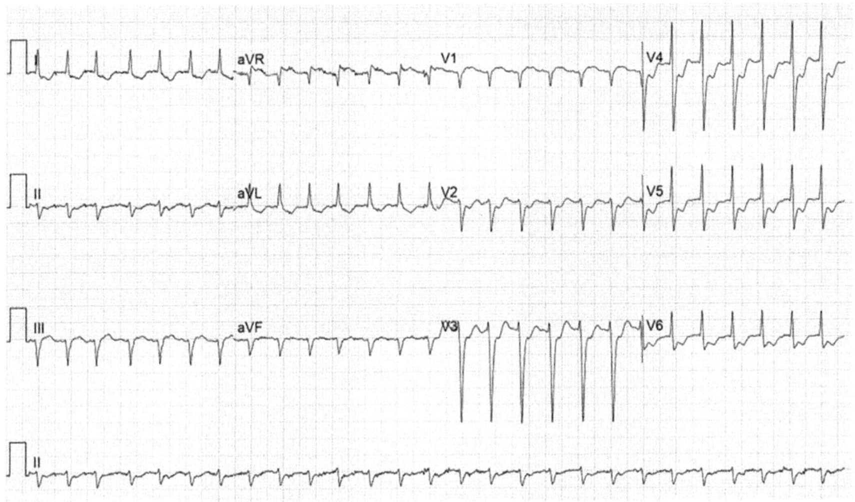

Fig. 1 ECG recording from an 81-year-old male patient with ATTR amyloidosis showing a regular narrow complex tachycardia with small, visible flutter waves representing atypical atrial flutter. The tracing demonstrates left axis deviation along with characteristically low QRS voltage and a pseudoinfarct pattern in leads V1-V3

Thromboembolic Risk and Anticoagulation

Cardiac amyloidosis has been associated with a high risk of intracardiac thrombus, stroke, and systemic embolism compared with the general population [1, 5]. The presence of AF or subtype of AF has not been associated with differences in overall survival in cardiac amyloid. Myocardial amyloid infiltration involving both the right and left atria has been suggested as a pathophysiologic mechanism leading to reduced atrial contractility, blood stasis, endothelial dysfunction, and relative hypercoagulability predisposing to thrombus formation [2]. AL amyloidosis as a single entity may increase thrombogenicity and thromboembolism without the presence of AF [3].

Notably, there is no association between the CHADS-VASc score and LAA thrombus in subjects with ATTR-CA on transesophageal echocardiogram (TEE). Therefore, systemic anticoagulation therapy should be considered in ATTR-cardiac amyloidosis patients with AF regardless of their CHADS-VASc score [4].

Left atrial thrombi visualized by TEE have been reported in up to 30% of patients with cardiac amyloidosis before planned direct current cardioversion (DCCV) for AF [5]. Studies found that of those discovered to have intracardiac thrombus, 46% had either a therapeutic level of anticoagulation for >3 weeks or arrhythmia onset <48 h before the planned cardioversion [2]. Other research found that 88% of those with intracardiac thrombus were therapeutically anticoagulated for at least 3 weeks prior. In light of these findings, authors propose that all patients with cardiac amyloidosis have a TEE performed before DCCV to ensure no intracardiac thrombus is present.

Management Considerations

An understanding of the hemodynamics underlying cardiac amyloidosis is essential in management of atrial arrhythmias in this population. Patients with cardiac amyloidosis often have restrictive physiology with a low, fixed stroke volume that requires: (1) high filling pressures to preserve stroke volume; and (2) a faster heart rate to maintain adequate cardiac output [3]. The benefit of rhythm control may be ineffective in those who are asymptomatic with restrictive physiology, as ventricular filling occurs during early diastole with negligible filling with the atrial kick as suggested by the Doppler mitral inflow velocity waveforms [2].

Rate Control

Rate control is traditionally the primary treatment strategy in many patients. Beta-blockers and non-dihydropyridine calcium channel blockers (CCBs) are the preferred agents for rate control in non-CA patients. However, rate control strategy poses a great challenge in CA patients. CCBs are contraindicated for their negative inotropic/chronotropic effect and the high risk of hypotension. In addition, postural hypotension in the setting of dysautonomia related to systemic amyloidosis and impaired vasomotor function is further exacerbated by the negative inotropic effects of medications like CCBs [1].

Avoidance of aggressive heart rate control is necessary, and pharmacologic therapy for rate control can be challenging. In general, beta-blockers, calcium-channel blockers, and digoxin are considered to be poorly tolerated and should be used with caution in cardiac amyloidosis because of depression of compensatory heart rate response, which is a main driver of cardiac output [2]. The risk of decompensation is perhaps highest with calcium-channel blockers and digoxin. Beta-blockers may also be poorly tolerated; however, low doses may be an option to achieve rate control in AF with a rapid ventricular response. It is important to note that most of the time, AF in CA patients is not related to rapid ventricular rate due to concomitant conduction system disease [3].

Digoxin remains controversial in amyloidosis due to the high risk of toxicity. Digoxin binds avidly to amyloid fibrils in vitro [4]. Investigators have proposed this binding leads to increased tissue and serum drug levels, prolonged exposure of digoxin receptors, and high risk of digoxin toxicity. Interestingly, toxicity may be precipitated by an ability of amyloid fibrils to bind pharmacotherapies and thus enhanced concentration of the drug available to receptors within the myocardium. In any case of AF refractory to medical therapy, atrioventricular nodal ablation and permanent pacemaker implant can be considered.

Rhythm Control and Cardioversion

Rhythm control strategy is more effective when introduced earlier during the disease course. However, it is not associated with improved survival. The data on the safety of antiarrhythmics are insufficient in this population. Many antiarrhythmic agents cannot be used in CA either due to cardiomyopathy (such as flecainide and propafenone) or due to concomitant advanced kidney disease (such as sotalol, dronedarone, and dofetilide). Amiodarone appears to be well tolerated in this population and may be the antiarrhythmic of choice. Because of the restrictive filling physiology and dependence on heart rate, expert consensus is that these patients are best maintained in sinus rhythm, though there is no mortality benefit from rhythm control with antiarrhythmic drugs, including amiodarone, sotalol, dofetilide, or propafenone versus rate control [1].

Direct current cardioversion (DCCV) in patients with AF and cardiac amyloidosis presents notable clinical challenges. Recurrence rates are substantial, with studies reporting up to 70% AF recurrence at one year. Procedural cancellations are significantly more frequent in cardiac amyloidosis patients, primarily due to intracardiac thrombus detection, occurring in 28% of cases compared to 7% in control groups. Notably, 81% of cancellations in the amyloidosis group were thrombus-related, despite appropriate anticoagulation. Initial DCCV success rates remain similar between amyloidosis and control groups, with no significant differences observed between AL and ATTR amyloidosis subtypes [2].

Complication rates are markedly higher in cardiac amyloidosis patients, reaching 14% versus 2% in control populations, encompassing risks of ventricular arrhythmia, bradyarrhythmia, hypoxemia, and stroke. Given these findings, clinicians are advised to perform transesophageal echocardiography before DCCV in all cardiac amyloidosis patients with AF, regardless of anticoagulation status [3].

Catheter Ablation

There are limited data on the safety and efficacy of catheter ablation for atrial arrhythmias in cardiac amyloid patients. Studies demonstrate significantly high rates of AF recurrence following catheter ablation in cardiac amyloid. The recurrence rate of atrial arrhythmia in CA patients undergoing ablation depends on the stage of the disease, ranging from 36% in stage 1 or 2 ATTR to 90% in stage 3 disease [1]. More studies are needed to determine if this is an effective rhythm control strategy. Hence, AF ablation may be considered early in the disease course for patients who are refractory to antiarrhythmic therapy [2].

Ventricular Arrhythmias

Ventricular arrhythmias (VA), such as ventricular tachycardia (VT) and ventricular fibrillation (VF), are less common in CA patients. They are more frequently observed in AL-CA (Fig. 2). The most frequent arrhythmia observed during peri-transplantation was NSVT. Studies have shown ventricular ectopy in 72% and NSVT in 18% of AL amyloid patients [1]. NSVT was present in 74%, and sustained ventricular tachycardia or any VF occurred in 19% of patients with cardiac amyloidosis [2]. Nonsustained ventricular arrhythmias commonly affect more than 60% of patients with ATTR cardiomyopathy who undergo monitoring for arrhythmias; however, their prognostic significance is unclear [3].

Multiple potential mechanisms can account for the occurrence of VAs in the CA population, including abnormal autonomic balance, reentry circuits, and myocardial ischemia due to amyloid infiltration of capillaries, as well as electromechanical dysfunction and autonomic dysregulation. VF may be caused by PVC originating from the Purkinje system. However, the precise cause of VF arising in CA is not well understood [4].

Numerous potential mechanisms drive ventricular arrhythmogenicity in CA. One proposal involves patchy amyloid fibril infiltration within the ventricular myocardium along with microvascular ischemia leading to the development of anatomical re-entrant circuits suitable for VA. Other mechanisms include preferential amyloid cytotoxicity to ventricular myocardial cells. This may explain the apparent higher prevalence of VAs in AL-CA over ATTR-CA [5].

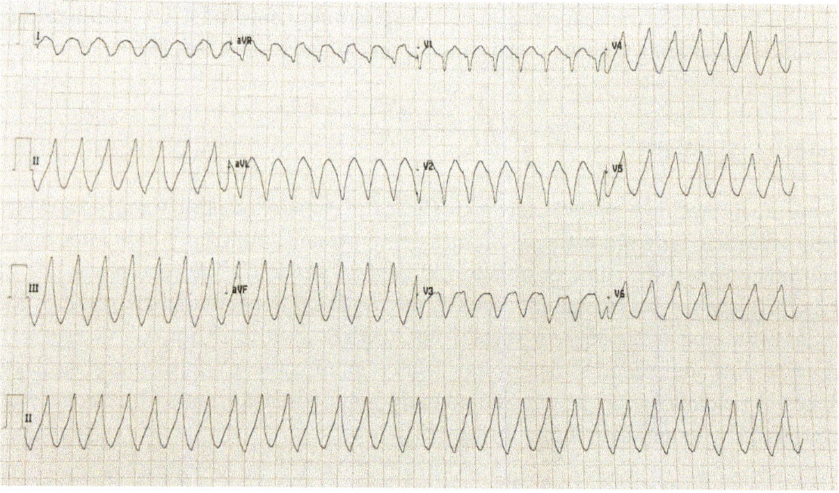

Fig. 2 ECG recording from a 67-years-olf female with AL amyloidosis showing monomorphic ventricular tachycardia

The presence of VAs is associated with a higher risk of SCD and overall mortality. In a study of patients with CA and VT/VF, the 1-year mortality rate was 50%, with SCD accounting for 60% of deaths [5].

Management of Ventricular Arrhythmias

In patients with frequent or sustained VA, antiarrhythmic drugs, such as amiodarone, may be used to suppress VA [1, 2]. Beta-blockers may be detrimental to CA patients, resulting in compromise of cardiac output [3, 4]. The management of VAs is mainly based on ICD therapy. One-half of patients with cardiac amyloid die suddenly; however, ICD placement for both primary and secondary prevention in cardiac amyloid has not been strongly supported by expert guidelines [5].

Reasons for this include: (1) the most common cause of sudden death has been historically thought to be secondary to electromechanical dissociation resulting in pulseless electrical activity rather than a lethal ventricular arrhythmia [3]; (2) suggestion that cardiac amyloidosis carries a higher defibrillation threshold that may be refractory to ICD therapy [2, 4]. The incidence of appropriate ICD therapies ranged from 6 to 32% in patients with cardiac amyloidosis [5]. Despite successful ICD therapies for ventricular arrhythmias, no studies have demonstrated a mortality benefit from ICD implantation in patients with cardiac amyloidosis [3, 5].

Patients with cardiac amyloidosis frequently show worse prognosis than other types of HF and, thus, strategies for primary prevention, such as ICDs, may not help in the advanced stages [4]. The choice between a conventional pacemaker and an ICD remains controversial in patients with cardiac amyloidosis. Usually, an individual decision should be made based on a patient's characteristics, the type of conduction disturbance or the arrhythmia, and the risk stratification according to the most updated guidelines [1, 5].

Although sudden death, ventricular arrhythmia, and conduction disease is common, timing of implantable cardioverter-defibrillator (ICD) or pacemaker implantation remain controversial among experts and society guidelines. Survival is often <1 year, which is generally a contraindication to ICD insertion [2, 3]. Second, SCD in these patients is often caused by PEA or asystole rather than VAs [3, 5].

It is likely ICD may be more efficacious in AL-CA over ATTR-CA. VAs are more common in the former, whereas SVTs are more common in the latter, resulting in higher rates of inappropriate ICD therapies [4]. Consideration for ICD insertion will become an increasingly common scenario faced by clinicians treating patients with CA, because CA survival improves through new disease modifying therapies [5]. The current data are conflicting and recommendations from major consensus guidelines are ambiguous. Further high-quality studies are necessary going forward to elucidate this potentially life-saving question [1, 4]. Consequently, shared decision making between the patient and the multidisciplinary team is critical when considering ICD insertion in CA [3, 5].

Conduction System Disorders

Conduction disease is highly prevalent in cardiac amyloidosis, and atrioventricular conduction delay involving the His-Purkinje system appears to be more common than pure sinus node disease [2, 4] (Fig. 3). Heart block is another type of arrhythmia that could occur in cardiac amyloidosis [1, 5] (Fig. 4). It can cause dizziness, fatigue, and fainting. Complete heart block can lead to agonal bradycardia, syncope, or even SCD [3, 4]. The prevalence of the need for pacemaker implantation at diagnosis ranges between 8.9 and 10% [4, 5].

Pathophysiology and Mechanisms

Cytotoxicity may play a role, because certain forms of amyloid precursor proteins are well-recognized noxious agents that induce apoptosis through oxidative stress [1, 3]. For instance, infusion of light chains from patients with AL-CA into isolated mouse hearts has been shown to induce diastolic dysfunction independent of amyloid deposition in vitro [2, 4].

Transthyretin is a well-known neurotoxic agent. The mechanism of cytotoxicity not only involves oxidative stress and apoptosis but also dysregulation of intracellular

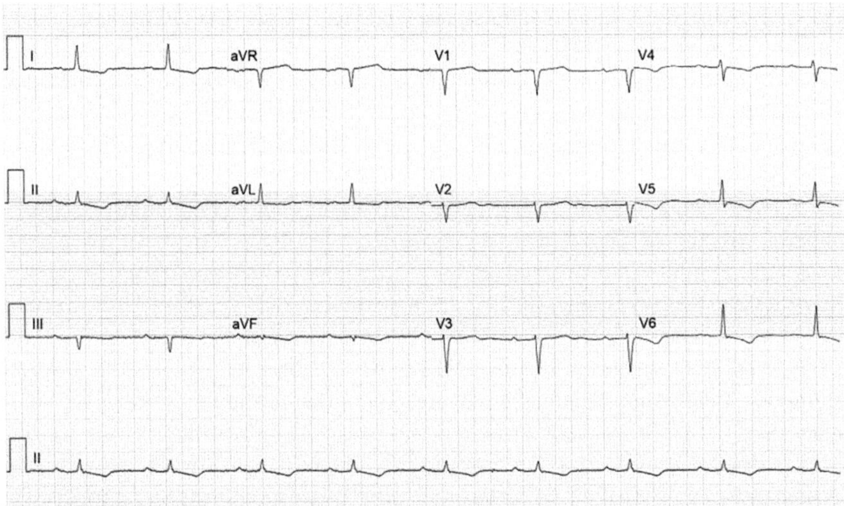

Fig. 3 ECG recording from an 88-year-old patient with ATTR amyloidosis. The tracing shows characteristically low voltage QRS complexes in both limb and precordial leads, anterior pseudoinfarct pattern, sinus bradycardia likely due to sick sinus syndrome, and first-degree AV block with a PR interval of 220 ms

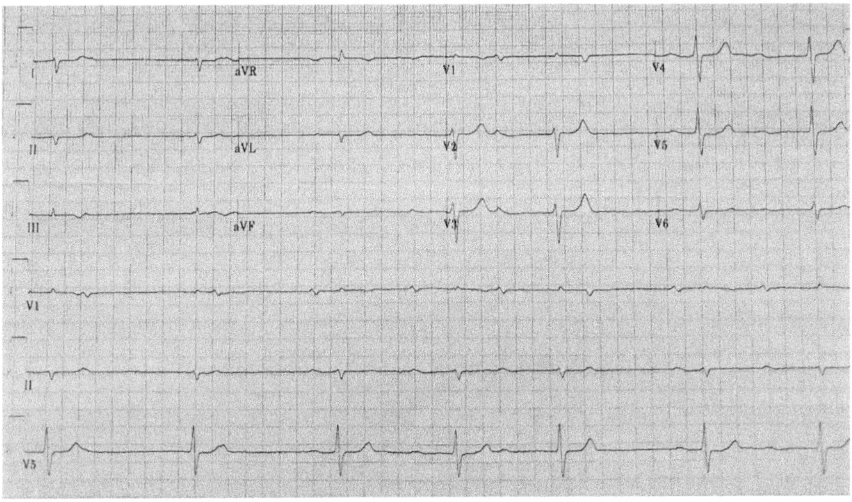

Fig. 4 ECG recording from an 83-year-old male patient with ATTR amyloidosis demonstrating characteristically low voltage QRS complexes throughout both limb and precordial leads, along with a second-degree Mobitz type I (Wenckebach) atrioventricular block

calcium signaling [3, 5]. Early cardiac sympathetic denervation may also contribute to arrhythmogenesis [4, 5].

Autopsy and Clinical Findings

Notably, autopsies of 23 patients with cardiac amyloidosis and clinical arrhythmias demonstrated only 3 of 23 patients had histologic evidence of amyloid involvement of the conduction system tissue [1, 4]. Electrophysiologic testing on 25 patients with AL cardiac amyloidosis found that infra-His (HV) conduction times were prolonged in 92% of patients, whereas 88% had normal sinus node function [2, 5].

Patients with CA present a prolonged His-ventricle (HV) conduction interval compared to patients without CA. The HV conduction delay is more profound in ATTR than in AL [3, 5]. HV interval prolongation with relatively narrow QRS duration may suggest frequent widespread involvement of both right and left bundle branches [4, 5]. There is possible evidence of narrow ECG QRS complexes despite demonstrated prolonged H-V intervals, likely due to equal and homogeneous infiltration of both bundle branches and the distal conduction system [2, 3]. Advanced AV block has been demonstrated to be associated with reduced left atrial contractile function in patients with ATTR CA [4, 5].

Pacing Considerations and Outcomes

Patients with ATTRwt have higher rates of pacemaker implantation compared with both AL and ATTRh, which is attributed to the older age and less aggressive disease course [1, 4]. They have a higher risk of complete AV blocks and SCD due to electromechanical dissociation [3, 5].

Progression of conduction system disease is common and often leads to increased right ventricular (RV) pacing burden with time. Studies from Duke University examined the longitudinal electrophysiology data from pacemaker interrogation in 34 patients with CA and cardiac implantable electronic devices. Pronounced dependence on RV pacing was evident over time, from an average pacing burden of 35.5% at 6 months postinsertion up to 96.2% 5 years later [4, 5].

In a retrospective observational cohort study of 78 patients with ATTR-CA and cardiac implantable electronic devices, a pacing burden >40% was shown to result in adverse structural and clinical consequences, including worsening NYHA functional class, left ventricular ejection fraction (LVEF), and an increased severity of mitral regurgitation [3, 5]. Patients with CA appear to be particularly vulnerable to the interventricular and intraventricular dyssynchrony brought about by RV pacing, given their restrictive physiology. As a corollary, biventricular pacing has been associated with improvements in NYHA functional class, LVEF, and mitral regurgitation severity [4, 5].

Summary

Cardiac amyloidosis presents complex electrical manifestations that pose significant challenges in clinical management. The disease demonstrates a spectrum of arrhythmias, with prevalence varying significantly between AL (up to 60%) and ATTR (20–40%) subtypes. Atrial fibrillation, the most common arrhythmia affecting 16–80% of patients, carries unique management challenges including high thrombotic risk irrespective of conventional risk scores and limited tolerance to rate-control medications. Cardioversion attempts face substantial recurrence rates and procedural risks, while catheter ablation shows diminishing success with advancing disease. Ventricular arrhythmias, more prevalent in AL-CA, significantly impact survival, though the role of ICD therapy remains controversial due to high rates of electromechanical dissociation. Conduction system disease, particularly affecting the His-Purkinje system, frequently necessitates pacing, with evidence suggesting potential adverse effects from high right ventricular pacing burden and possible benefits from biventricular pacing. Management strategies must carefully consider the unique pathophysiology of cardiac amyloidosis, as conventional anti-arrhythmic approaches often prove poorly tolerated, with amiodarone emerging as the most viable pharmacological option. The evolving landscape of disease-modifying therapies may influence the approach to device therapy, highlighting the need for individualized decision-making in this complex patient population. Understanding these electrical manifestations and their management challenges is crucial for optimizing outcomes in cardiac amyloidosis patients.

References

1. Donnellan E, Wazni OM, Hanna M, Kusumoto F, Jaber WA. Management of arrhythmias in cardiac amyloidosis. JACC Clin Electrophysiol. 2020;6(4):351–61. https://doi.org/10.1016/j.jacep.2019.10.018.
2. Garcia-Pavia P, Rapezzi C, Adler Y, et al. Electrophysiological manifestations of cardiac amyloidosis: JACC: cardiooncology state-of-the-art review. JACC CardioOncol. 2021;3(4):563–85. https://doi.org/10.1016/j.jaccao.2021.07.010.
3. Ruberg FL, Maurer MS. Cardiac amyloidosis due to transthyretin protein: a review. JAMA. 2024;331(9):778–91. https://doi.org/10.1001/jama.2024.0442.
4. Bukhari S, Khan SZ, Ghoweba M, Khan B, Bashir Z. Arrhythmias and device therapies in cardiac amyloidosis. J Clin Med. 2024;13(5):1300. https://doi.org/10.3390/jcm13051300.
5. Bianchi G, Tini G, Bencardino G, et al. Arrhythmias in patients with cardiac amyloidosis: a comprehensive review on clinical management and devices. J Clin Med. 2023;12(15):5095. https://doi.org/10.3390/jcm12155095.

Aortic Stenosis in Patients with Cardiac Amyloidosis

Jonathan Koslowsky, Batel Nissan, and Eyal Herzog

Abstract Aortic stenosis (AS), the most prevalent valvular heart disease, significantly impacts the lives of older adults, with over 4% of octogenarians affected. This condition, characterized by the narrowing of the aortic valve, imposes excessive pressure on the heart, leading to a cascade of detrimental effects. These include the thickening of the heart muscle (left ventricular hypertrophy), impaired heart function, and ultimately, heart failure. While severe, untreated AS carries a grave prognosis, timely aortic valve replacement offers a promising avenue for reversing these detrimental effects and restoring a patient's life expectancy to levels comparable to their healthy peers. Cardiac amyloidosis (CA), a condition characterized by the abnormal accumulation of protein deposits within the heart, affects a significant portion of the elderly population. While sharing some similarities with aortic stenosis (AS), CA carries a generally poorer prognosis. Recent studies have revealed a higher-than-expected incidence of AS and CA coexisting in patients. This co-occurrence presents unique challenges for diagnosis and treatment, as both conditions require distinct management strategies. The emergence of effective therapies for certain types of CA underscores the urgent need for improved diagnostic evaluation and optimized treatment approaches for patients with both AS and CA. In this chapter we comprehensively examine the pathophysiology and prevalence of CA in patients with AS and delve into the best practices for diagnosing and treating both conditions when they occur together. Our team has developed a novel algorithm for the management of aortic stenosis and cardiac amyloidosis.

Keywords Aortic stenosis · Cardiac amyloidosis · Transthyretin · Amyloid light chain · ATTR amyloidosis · AL amyloidosis · Low-flow low-gradient · Paradoxical aortic stenosis

J. Koslowsky (✉) · B. Nissan · E. Herzog
Department of Cardiology, Hadassah Medical Center, Hebrew University of Jerusalem, Jerusalem, Israel
e-mail: kyonathan@hadassah.org.il

E. Herzog (ed.), *Cardiac Amyloidosis*, https://doi.org/10.1007/978-3-031-88342-2_13

Introduction

Case Presentation

An 82-year-old woman presented with progressive dyspnea, initially on exertion and later at rest. Physical examination revealed a harsh systolic ejection murmur characteristic of aortic stenosis, but also notable signs of heart failure, including significant jugular venous distension, bibasilar crackles, and peripheral edema. Echocardiography confirmed severe aortic stenosis, however, other findings of normal systolic function alongside impaired diastolic function, and a restrictive filling pattern. The presence of "red flags" such as unexplained fatigue, weight loss, and mild lower extremity edema further suggested a more complex clinical picture than isolated aortic stenosis. These findings prompted a broader differential diagnosis, including the possibility of an underlying condition such as cardiac amyloidosis. Subsequent investigations confirmed the diagnosis of transthyretin-related cardiac amyloidosis, and appropriate treatment was initiated.

Aortic stenosis (AS), the most prevalent valvular heart disease, significantly impacts the lives of older adults, with over 4% of octogenarians affected. This condition, characterized by the narrowing of the aortic valve, imposes excessive pressure on the heart, leading to a cascade of detrimental effects. These include the thickening of the heart muscle (left ventricular hypertrophy), impaired heart function, and ultimately, heart failure. While severe, untreated AS carries a grave prognosis, timely aortic valve replacement offers a promising avenue for reversing these detrimental effects and restoring a patient's life expectancy to levels comparable to their healthy peers.

Cardiac amyloidosis (CA), a condition characterized by the abnormal accumulation of protein deposits within the heart, affects a significant portion of the elderly population [1]. While sharing some similarities with aortic stenosis (AS), CA carries a generally poorer prognosis. Recent studies have revealed a higher-than-expected incidence of AS and CA coexisting in patients [2]. This co-occurrence presents unique challenges for diagnosis and treatment, as both conditions require distinct management strategies. The emergence of effective therapies for certain types of CA underscores the urgent need for improved diagnostic evaluation and optimized treatment approaches for patients with both AS and CA. In this chapter we comprehensively examine the pathophysiology and prevalence of CA in patients with AS and delve into the best practices for diagnosing and treating both conditions when they occur together.

Pathophysiology of CA

Cardiac amyloidosis arises from the abnormal accumulation of amyloid fibrils, misfolded proteins, within the heart. Two primary proteins contribute to CA: transthyretin (TTR) and immunoglobulin light chains (AL). TTR-CA can manifest in two forms: wild-type TTR and hereditary TTR. Wild-type TTR-CA, more common in the elderly, involves the deposition of normally occurring TTR, although the exact cause of this abnormal deposition remains unclear. Hereditary TTR-CA, a genetic disorder, affects younger individuals. Among the numerous TTR mutations, some variants have been found to be more strongly associated with CA [3]. Depending on the specific mutation, the disease may primarily affect the heart or the nervous system. TTR-CA, particularly in older men, is the most common type of amyloidosis associated with aortic stenosis. In contrast, AL-CA, linked to the abnormal production of light chains by plasma cells, is rarely observed in patients with AS.

Cardiac amyloidosis can infiltrate various heart structures, including the myocardium, valves, atria, and pericardium [4]. Myocardial infiltration, often beginning at the base of the heart, leads to thickening and stiffening of the heart walls, resulting in a restrictive cardiomyopathy pattern. This severely impairs the heart's ability to fill with blood (diastolic dysfunction) and efficiently pump blood out (systolic dysfunction). While diastolic heart failure is most common in CA, a significant proportion of patients also experience reduced ejection fraction. These features can also be observed in severe AS, potentially masking the presence of concurrent CA. Amyloid deposition within the aortic valve may contribute to the development and progression of AS.

Prevalence of CA and AS

The true prevalence of CA in the general population, including those with AS, is likely underestimated due to several factors. These include the lack of widespread screening programs, the challenges associated with definitively diagnosing CA, and the overlap of its symptoms with other heart conditions. Previous studies have reported a wide range of CA prevalence in the general population, from 5 to 74%, largely attributed to variations in study populations and diagnostic methods. Importantly, the frequency of myocardial amyloid deposits increases significantly with age, reaching high rates in the very elderly. Recent advancements in diagnostic techniques, particularly non-invasive methods, have facilitated the identification of TTR-CA in patients with AS. Retrospective analyses have revealed that a substantial proportion (up to 29%) of patients with AS may have coexisting TTR-CA [5]. This suggests that the coexistence of AS and CA is more common than previously recognized, particularly in the elderly population.

Diagnosis of Amyloidosis in the Setting of Aortic Stenosis

Diagnosing amyloidosis in the presence of AS presents significant challenges, often leading to under-recognition in clinical practice. This underdiagnosis stems from several factors. Firstly, our understanding of the diverse cardiac manifestations of amyloidosis is continuously evolving. Secondly, definitive diagnosis often requires advanced imaging techniques like cardiac MRI or nuclear imaging, and potentially invasive procedures such as endomyocardial biopsy. In contrast, AS is a well-established valvular disorder, predominantly affecting the elderly. Its diagnosis and staging primarily rely on echocardiography, a readily available and widely utilized tool. This familiarity with AS can inadvertently mask the subtle signs of coexisting CA. The presence of AS may overshadow the distinctive features of CA, leading to missed diagnoses, particularly when advanced diagnostic tools are not readily accessible or utilized routinely.

Recognizing the possibility of CA in patients with AS requires a high index of suspicion. While numerous diagnostic algorithms focus on advanced imaging for isolated CA, it's crucial to emphasize the value of careful clinical assessment and routine investigations. These initial observations are pivotal, as they drive the need for further, more specialized investigations like cardiac MRI or scintigraphy. Early recognition of cardiac amyloidosis is vital, especially considering the availability of recent effective targeted treatments. This necessitates meticulous scrutiny of routine clinical assessments, such as past medical history, detailed physical assessment, ECGs and TTEs, in patients with AS to identify potential "red flags" that may indicate coexisting CA. By emphasizing this initial clinical evaluation, we can improve early suspicion and facilitate the timely implementation of advanced diagnostic modalities, ultimately leading to more accurate and timely diagnoses.

Screening and Diagnosis of CA in Patients with AS

Currently, there are no established guidelines for routine screening for CA in patients with aortic stenosis. While the screening and diagnostic approach for TTR-CA is generally similar in patients with AS and the general population, it presents unique challenges due to the overlap in clinical features between these two conditions. Therefore, CA screening should be considered in patients with AS who exhibit specific "red flags" or suggestive clinical features of CA.

Suspicion Criteria for CA

In patients with AS, TTR-CA occurs more commonly in men. Several clinical features should raise suspicion of TTR-CA in this population (Table 1). These include a history of carpal tunnel syndrome, lumbar spinal stenosis, hearing loss, the need for early pacemaker implantation, severe heart failure symptoms despite relatively mild AS, and evidence of right ventricular dysfunction. While less common in TTR-CA than in other types of amyloidosis, macroglossia (enlarged tongue) and other soft tissue manifestations may be present. Electrocardiogram findings in CA can be nonspecific, but certain abnormalities may suggest its presence. These include abnormal heart rhythms (conduction abnormalities), low voltage on the ECG despite thickened heart muscle, and Q waves in the absence of a previous heart attack.

Table 1 Suggestive features of cardiac amyloidosis "red flags" [9, 10]

Suspicion criteria—"red flags"	
Demographic	• Age >65 • Male • Black race
Cardiac features	• Heart failure with preserved ejection fraction (HFpEF) • Low-flow low-gradient pattern • RV heart failure signs and symptoms • Disproportionate HF symptoms
Non-cardiac clinical features	• Carpal tunnel syndrome (bilateral) • Lumber spinal stenosis • Deafness • Macroglossia • Dysautonomia
Biomarkers	• Troponin elevated without coronary heart disease • BNP elevated disproportionately to AS severity
ECG	• Discordance between low-voltage and LV wall thickness • Pseudo-infarction pattern (Q waves) without history of myocardial infarction • Atrioventricular conduction abnormalities
Echocardiography	• Disproportionate left ventricular hypertrophy (LVH) • Disproportionate diastolic dysfunction • Bilateral atrial dilatation • Reduced longitudinal strain with apical sparing • Pulmonary HTN • Myocardial granular sparkling • Pericardial effusion
CMR	• Circumferential and extensive late gadolinium enhancement (LGE) which starts subendocardialy and predominating at the basal segments • Elevated native T1 mapping • Extracellular volume (ECV) expansion

Echocardiography in patients with AS may reveal "red flags" suggestive of concomitant CA. These include disproportionate LV wall thickening and diastolic dysfunction relative to the severity of AS, RV wall thickening, pericardial effusion, bilateral atrial enlargement, myocardial "granular sparkling", and impaired LV longitudinal systolic function. A mitral annular S' velocity $\leq$6 cm/s has been identified as a useful screening tool for CA in AS patients with preserved left ventricular ejection fraction [6]. Furthermore, LV global longitudinal strain measured by speckle tracking echocardiography is often markedly reduced ($\geq -12\%$) in CA patients [7]. While apical sparing of LV longitudinal strain may sometimes occur in CA, it can also be observed in AS patients without amyloidosis. The presence of a paradoxical low-flow, low-gradient AS pattern (preserved LVEF despite hemodynamically significant AS) should strongly increase the suspicion of underlying CA.

Cardiac magnetic resonance (CMR) plays a valuable role in diagnosing and prognosticating CA, utilizing techniques such as late gadolinium enhancement (LGE), native T1 mapping, and extracellular volume (ECV) measurements. However, it's important to note that approximately 15% of CMR examinations may appear normal in patients with CA [8]. Characteristic CMR findings in CA include circumferential LGE within the entire LV sub-endocardium, often with varying degrees of myocardial extension and a base-to-apex gradient. Elevated native T1 and ECV values are also commonly observed. CMR is particularly useful in differentiating myocardial extracellular amyloid deposition from diffuse fibrosis in patients with aortic stenosis (AS). Additionally, CMR can aid in distinguishing between transthyretin (TTR)-type and immunoglobulin light chain (AL)-type amyloidosis.

Confirmation Criteria for CA

While suggestive, the findings mentioned alone are insufficient to definitively diagnose CA, and further investigations are necessary (Table 2). Bone scintigraphy with technetium-labeled bisphosphonates, combined with blood and urine tests for monoclonal light chains, play a crucial role in confirming the diagnosis. A specific pattern of cardiac uptake on scintigraphy, along with the absence of monoclonal proteins, strongly supports the diagnosis of TTR-CA. Genetic testing is then required to differentiate between wild-type and hereditary TTR-CA. The absence of both cardiac uptake on scintigraphy and monoclonal proteins in the blood or urine significantly reduces the likelihood of both TTR-CA and AL-CA. In patients with AS, most CA cases are of the TTR type. Therefore, bone scintigraphy can often be sufficient for diagnosis. However, due to the poor prognosis of AL-CA if left untreated, systematic screening for this type should be performed in all patients with suspected CA, including those with AS, using blood and urine tests for light chain proteins.

Table 2 Confirmation criteria for the diagnosis of cardiac amyloidosis [9, 10]

Confirmation criteria	
Bone scintigraphy (for TTR-CA)	• Strong cardiac uptake at bone scintigraphy Extracardiac fixation: lung or soft tissue
Serum/urine monoclonal free light chain protein (for AL-CA)	• Monoclonal free light chain in blood and/or urine
Histology on endomyocardial and/or extracardiac biopsies	• Positive Congo red staining Apple-green birefringence when viewed under polarizing microscopy

Aortic Stenosis Severity Assessment in Cardiac Amyloidosis

In patients with both CA and AS, accurately assessing the severity of AS presents unique challenges. Traditionally, severe AS is defined by echocardiographic findings of a peak aortic jet velocity greater than or equal to 4 m/s and/or a mean transvalvular pressure gradient exceeding 40 mmHg. However, patients with both conditions are more likely to exhibit a "low-flow, low-gradient" pattern, characterized by a reduced blood flow across the aortic valve resulting in low pressure gradients, compared with those without CA (30–80% vs. <30%) [5, 6]. This low-flow, low-gradient pattern is typically defined by an aortic valve area (AVA) less than or equal to 1.0 cm^2, a mean gradient below 40 mmHg, and a stroke volume index less than 35 ml/m^2.

Figure 1 compares echocardiographic findings in three scenarios: a normal aortic valve (left), classic severe AS (center), and low-flow low-gradient AS (right). The top row illustrates short-axis views on echocardiography. The normal valve (left) exhibits thin, flexible leaflets, while the diseased valves (center and right) show thickened, calcified leaflets obstructing valve opening, characteristic of severe AS. The middle row displays continuous-wave (CW) Doppler recordings. The normal valve (left) demonstrates physiological pressure gradients across the valve. Classic severe AS (center) is characterized by high gradients, with peak aortic jet velocities $\geq$4 m/s and mean transvalvular pressure gradients exceeding 40 mmHg. In contrast, low-flow low-gradient AS (right) exhibits lower gradients that do not fulfill the established criteria for diagnosing severe AS. The bottom row depicts pressure gradients across the left ventricular outflow tract (LVOT), which remain normal in all three cases.

Approximately 50% of patients with CA and low-flow low-gradient AS exhibit preserved LV ejection fraction, a phenomenon referred to as *paradoxical* low-flow, low-gradient pattern [2, 11]. This pattern shares similarities with the classic low-flow, low-gradient AS, including an aortic valve area (AVA) less than or equal to 1.0 cm^2 and a mean gradient below 40 mmHg. However, it is distinguished by a stroke volume index greater than 35 ml/m^2.

This phenomenon can be attributed to several factors, including severe LV concentric remodeling, impaired diastolic filling, LA remodeling and dysfunction, markedly reduced LV longitudinal systolic function (with LV global longitudinal strain typically more than 12%), and RV remodeling and dysfunction.

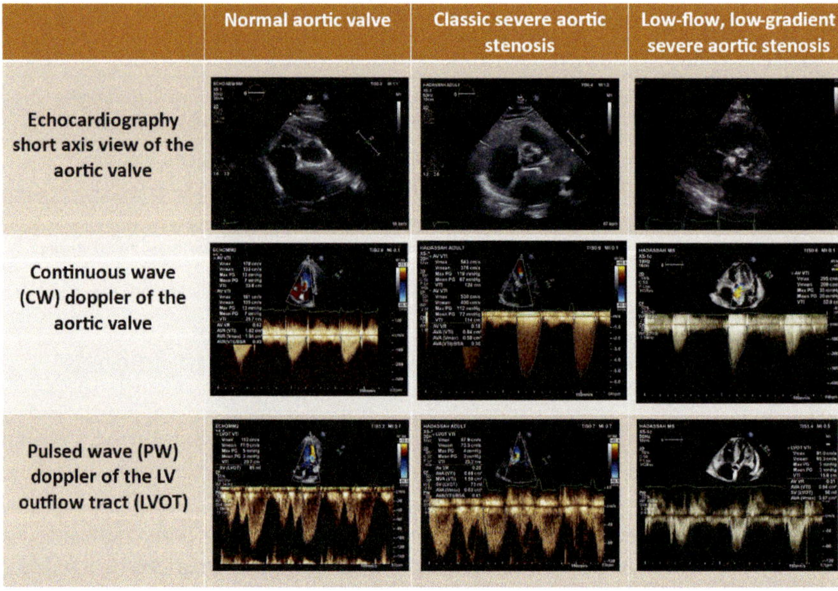

Fig. 1 Figure compares echocardiographic findings in three scenarios: a normal aortic valve (left), classic severe AS (center), and low-flow low-gradient AS (right). The top row illustrates short-axis views on echocardiography. The normal valve (left) exhibits thin, flexible leaflets, while the diseased valves (center and right) show thickened, calcified leaflets obstructing valve opening, characteristic of severe AS. The middle row displays continuous-wave (CW) Doppler recordings. The normal valve (left) demonstrates physiological pressure gradients across the valve. Classic severe AS (center) is characterized by high gradients, with peak aortic jet velocities $\geq$4 m/s and mean transvalvular pressure gradients exceeding 40 mmHg. In contrast, low-flow low-gradient AS (right) exhibits lower gradients that do not fulfill the established criteria for diagnosing severe AS. The bottom row depicts pressure gradients across the left ventricular outflow tract (LVOT), which remain normal in all three cases

The assessment of AS severity in patients with the low-flow, low-gradient pattern is particularly challenging, requiring careful differentiation between true severe AS and a pseudo-severe state. While dobutamine stress echocardiography may be used to confirm severe AS by demonstrating an increase in mean gradient to 40 mmHg or higher during stress, its utility is often limited in patients with CA due to an inadequate increase in LV outflow after dobutamine injection.

A non-contrast computed tomography (CT) for the quantification of aortic valve calcium burden has emerged as a more reliable method for assessing AS severity in patients with CA, regardless of their hemodynamic profile. By directly measuring the extent of aortic valve calcification, CT provides valuable insights into the severity of the stenotic process in CA patients, even in the presence of the low-flow, low-gradient pattern [12].

The Approach to Patient Care in Aortic Stenosis and Cardiac Amyloidosis

CA and AS frequently coexist in patients, making it challenging to determine which condition primarily influences the patient's prognosis. Some studies have observed comparable mortality rates in patients with either CA alone, AS alone, or both conditions together, suggesting that either condition could significantly impact survival [13]. However, a growing body of evidence indicates that the coexistence of CA and AS carries a poorer prognosis than either condition in isolation [14, 15]. This may be attributed to a complex interplay between the two diseases, potentially leading to a synergistic effect on cardiac remodeling and a worsening of overall cardiac function.

Clinical Management of CA in Patients with AS

The optimal management of CA in patients with AS remains an area of active investigation, with no established guidelines or randomized trials to guide clinical decision-making. The therapeutic approach typically involves a combination of general supportive measures and targeted therapies (Fig. 2) [6, 7].

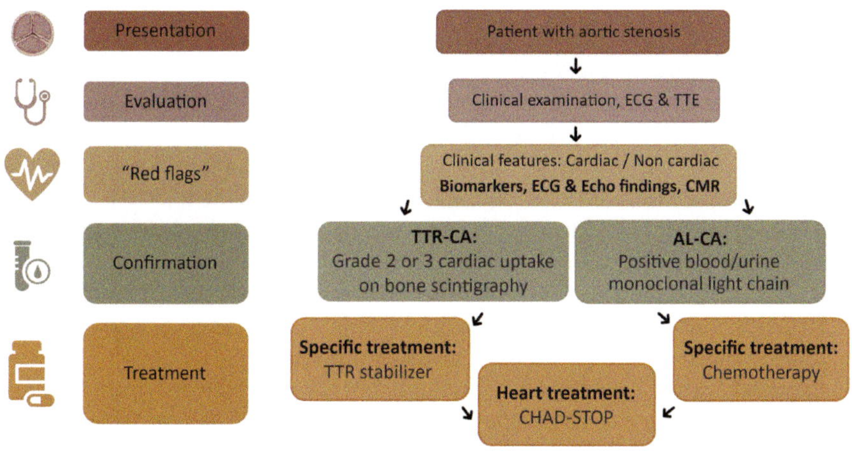

Fig. 2 Algorithm for the evaluation and management of aortic stenosis patients with suspected cardiac amyloidosis. TTR-CA—Transthyretin cardiac amyloidosis, AL-CA—amyloid light chain cardiac amyloidosis. CHAD-STOP—mnemonic for guiding clinical decision-making, encompassing strategies for Conduction and rhythm disorder prevention, High heart rate maintenance, Anticoagulation, Diuretic therapy, and STOP the use of Beta-blockers, Calcium channel blockers, Digoxin, and RAAS inhibitors

General management strategies aim to address the various manifestations of the disease while minimizing potential adverse effects of medications. The CHAD-STOP mnemonic provides a framework for guiding clinical decision-making, encompassing strategies for Conduction and rhythm disorder prevention, High heart rate maintenance, Anticoagulation, Diuretic therapy, and STOP the use of Beta-blockers, Calcium channel blockers, Digoxin, and RAAS inhibitors.

This general framework includes:

- **Optimizing heart failure medications**: Traditional heart failure medications may need to be adjusted due to the unique pathophysiology of CA. The restrictive nature of the cardiomyopathy often limits the ability to increase preload effectively. Therefore, medications that can lower heart rate, such as beta-blockers and calcium channel blockers, may need to be used with caution or even discontinued to avoid excessive slowing of the heart rate, which is the primary mechanism for maintaining cardiac output in this setting.
- **Renin–Angiotensin–Aldosterone System (RAAS) Inhibitors**: These medications, including angiotensin-converting enzyme (ACE) inhibitors and angiotensin receptor blockers (ARBs), should be used with caution due to the risk of severe hypotension, particularly in patients with autonomic nervous system dysfunction frequently observed in CA.
- **Managing fluid balance**: Diuretics are essential for managing fluid overload in symptomatic patients or during episodes of heart failure decompensation. However, excessive diuresis can significantly compromise cardiac output due to the limited preload reserve. Careful titration of diuretic doses is crucial to avoid significant volume depletion.
- **Addressing arrhythmias**: Antiarrhythmic medications like amiodarone may be necessary to control arrhythmias. The use of digoxin, which is given occasionally to control tachyarrhythmias, requires close monitoring due to the risk of accumulation within amyloid deposits, potentially leading to toxicity.
- **Anticoagulation**: Patients with CA are at increased risk of blood clots, even in the absence of atrial fibrillation. Anticoagulation therapy is recommended in patients with atrial fibrillation, a history of stroke, or evidence of intracardiac thrombi. However, routine anticoagulation for all patients with CA and AS is not currently recommended due to the risk of bleeding complications.
- **Pacemaker implantation**: Given the high risk of conduction disturbances, pacemaker implantation may be considered in patients with first-degree atrioventricular block, unexplained syncope, or abnormal conduction below the level of the His bundle. Pacemaker implantation may also be considered prior to aortic valve replacement procedures, particularly transcatheter aortic valve replacement (TAVR).
- **Defibrillator implantation**: The role of implantable cardioverter-defibrillators (ICDs) in patients with CA and AS is still under investigation.

Targeted therapies aim to address the underlying amyloid deposition. AL-CA, which is relatively uncommon in patients with AS, requires close cardiovascular monitoring during chemotherapy due to the risk of acute heart failure. In select cases, cardiac transplantation may be considered for young patients with advanced but stable heart failure who are at high risk of adverse outcomes and without significant extracardiac comorbidities.

For TTR-CA, significant therapeutic advancements have emerged in recent years. Two landmark clinical trials have demonstrated the efficacy and safety of novel medications:

- **Tafamidis**: This medication stabilizes the transthyretin protein, preventing its misfolding and promoting its clearance from the body. The ATTR-ACT trial, which included patients with severe TTR-CA encompassing both wild-type (75%) and hereditary (25%) forms, demonstrated that tafamidis significantly lowered the risk of all-cause mortality and cardiovascular-related hospitalizations at 30-month follow-up compared to placebo [16]. The benefits of tafamidis became significant after 18 months and were most pronounced when treatment was initiated early in the disease course (New York Heart Association functional class I and II).
- **Patisiran**: This RNA interference therapy targets the liver to reduce the production of both normal and mutated transthyretin [17]. While initially studied in patients with TTR-related neuropathy, sub-analyses have shown promising results in patients with TTR-CA, including improvements in cardiac function and biomarkers.

These novel therapies represent a significant breakthrough in the management of TTR-CA, offering hope for improved outcomes for patients with this challenging condition.

Important Considerations:

- **Individualized Treatment**: The optimal management of CA in patients with AS requires an individualized approach, considering the specific clinical presentation, disease severity, and patient comorbidities.
- **Multidisciplinary Care**: A multidisciplinary team approach involving cardiologists, hematologists, neurologists, and other specialists is crucial for optimal patient care.

Therapeutic Management of AS in Patients with CA

Data on the optimal management of AS in patients with concomitant CA is limited. Studies have reported a high risk of mortality and limited functional improvement following aortic valve replacement (AVR) in these patients. While small studies suggest that TAVR may offer potential advantages over surgical AVR in this population, further research is needed.

Patients with CA may be at increased risk of procedural complications during or after TAVR due to the fragility of amyloid-infiltrated tissues. Therefore, a multidisciplinary team approach, including cardiologists, geriatricians, and cardiomyopathy specialists, is crucial for evaluating and managing these complex cases (Fig. 3).

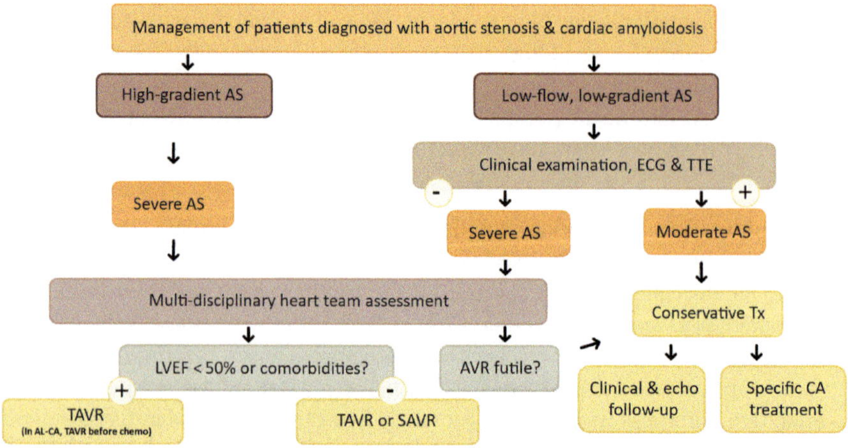

Fig. 3 Outlines for the management of patients with aortic stenosis and cardiac amyloidosis

Factors that may predict poor outcomes and limit the benefits of AVR (especially SVAR) in patients with AS and CA include:

- Reduced left ventricular ejection fraction (LVEF) (<50%)
- Severely impaired left ventricular systolic function (global longitudinal strain ≥ −10%)
- Restrictive cardiomyopathy (Grade III diastolic dysfunction) Moderate-to-severe low-flow, low-gradient AS (stroke volume index <30 ml/m^2)

These factors, along with patient comorbidities, functional status, frailty, and life expectancy, should be carefully considered when determining the most appropriate treatment strategy.

In cases where the multidisciplinary team deems AVR unlikely to provide significant benefit, the focus should shift towards optimizing medical management and initiating treatment with transthyretin (TTR) stabilizers, such as tafamidis, to address the underlying amyloid deposition.

When AVR is considered a viable option:

- **TAVR/SAVR**—TAVR may be preferred in patients with intermediate or high surgical risk, low-flow, low-gradient AS, depressed LVEF, markedly reduced global longitudinal strain, and/or severe low-flow state.
- **TTR stabilizer therapy**—Tafamidis should be initiated promptly upon confirmation of TTR-CA diagnosis.

Key Considerations:

- **Early Identification:** Screening for CA should be considered in patients with non-severe AS and unexplained heart failure symptoms to allow for early diagnosis and initiation of appropriate treatment, including TTR stabilizers.

- **Multidisciplinary Approach:** A comprehensive assessment and treatment plan require close collaboration among cardiologists, geriatricians, cardiomyopathy specialists, and other relevant healthcare professionals.

Conclusion

Cardiac amyloidosis occurs in up to 29% of patients with aortic stenosis. The presence of "red flags" during clinical evaluation should prompt suspicion of CA and trigger further investigations, including bone scintigraphy and serum free light chain assays, to confirm the diagnosis. Patients with AS and CA frequently exhibit a low-flow, low-gradient hemodynamic profile. Therefore, CT calcium scoring is crucial to accurately assess the severity of AS in these cases. A multidisciplinary "Heart Team" approach is essential for the comprehensive evaluation and management of symptomatic patients with severe AS and concomitant CA. Transcatheter aortic valve replacement (TAVR) is often favored over surgical aortic valve replacement (SAVR) in these patients due to their generally higher surgical risk. The recent advent of targeted therapies for transthyretin (TTR) amyloidosis holds the potential to revolutionize the treatment and prognosis of patients with AS and CA.

References

1. Cornwell GG 3rd, Murdoch WL, Kyle RA, et al. Frequency and distribution of senile cardiovascular amyloid. A clinicotholic correlation. Am J Med. 1983;75(4):618–23.
2. Galat A, Guellich A, Bodez D, et al. Aortic stenosis and transthyretin cardiac amyloidosis: the chicken or the egg? Eur Heart J. 2016;37:3525.
3. Garcia-Pavia P, Rapezzi C, Adler Y, et al. Diagnosis and treatment of cardiac amyloidosis: a position statement of the ESC working group on myocardial and pericardial diseases. Eur Heart J. 2021;42:1554–68.
4. Kristen AV, Schnabel PA, Winter B, et al. High prevalence of amyloid in 150 surgically removed heart valves—a comparison of histological and clinical data reveals a correlation to atheroinflammatory conditions. Cardiovasc Pathol. 2010;19:228–35.
5. Nietlispach F, Webb JG, Ye J, et al. Pathology of transcatheter valve therapy. JACC Cardiovasc Interv. 2012;5(5):582–90.
6. Castaño A, Narotsky DL, Hamid N, et al. Unveiling transthyretin cardiac amyloidosis and its predictors among elderly patients with severe aortic stenosis undergoing transcatheter aortic valve replacement. Eur Heart J. 2017;38:2879.
7. Ternacle J, Bodez D, Guellich A, et al. Causes and consequences of longitudinal LV dysfunction assessed by 2D strain echocardiography in cardiac amyloidosis. J Am Coll Cardiol Img. 2016;9:126.
8. Fontana M, Banypersad SM, Treibel TA, et al. Native T1 mapping in transthyretin amyloidosis. J Am Coll Cardiol Img. 2014;7:157.
9. Ternacle J, Krapf L, Mohty D, et al. Aortic stenosis and cardiac amyloidosis: JACC review topic of the week. JACC. 2019;74(21):2638–51.
10. Jaiswal V, Agrawal V, Khulbe Y et al. Cardiac amyloidosis and aortic stenosis: a state-of-the-art review. European Heart J Open. 3(6)

11. Longhi S, Lorenzini M, Gagliardi C, et al. Coexistence of degenerative aortic stenosis and wild-type transthyretin-related cardiac amyloidosis. J Am Coll Cardiol Img. 2016;9:325.
12. Clavel MA, Pibarot P, Messika-Zeitoun D, et al. Impact of aortic valve calcification, as measured by MDCT, on survival in patients with aortic stenosis: results of an international registry study. J Am Coll Cardiol. 2014;64:1202.
13. Sperry BW, Jones BM, Vranian MN, Hanna M, Jaber WA. Recognizing transthyretin cardiac amyloidosis in patients with aortic stenosis: impact on prognosis. JACC Cardiovasc Imaging. 2016;9:904–6.
14. Nitsche C, Aschauer S, Kammerlander AA, et al. Light-chain and transthyretin cardiac amyloidosis in severe aortic stenosis: prevalence, screening possibilities, and outcome. Eur J Heart Fail. 2020;22:1852–62.
15. Chacko L, Martone R, Bandera F, et al. Echocardiographic phenotype and prognosis in transthyretin cardiac amyloidosis. Eur Heart J. 2020;41:1439–47.
16. Maurer MS, Schwartz JH, Gundapaneni B, et al. Tafamidis treatment for patients with transthyretin amyloid cardiomyopathy. N Engl J Med. 2018;379:1007.
17. Adams D, Gonzalez-Duarte A, O'Riordan WD, et al. Patisiran, an RNAi therapeutic, for hereditary transthyretin amyloidosis. N Engl J Med. 2018;379:11.

Hematological Treatments and Disease Modifying Therapies in AL Cardiac Amyloidosis

Eyal Lebel, Noa Gross Even-Zohar, and Moshe E. Gatt

Abstract Light-chain AL amyloidosis (AL) is a rare plasma cell disorder (PCD) characterized by multi-organ damage due to misfolded immunoglobulin light chains (LC) secreted by clonal abnormal plasma cells (PC). In the last decade significant progress has been made in the care of this disease, with the use of efficacious novel agents that enable the eradication of the abnormal PC, leading to the cessation of toxic light chain secretion and eventually improvement in organ function. Treatment of AL has traditionally followed that of the much more common PCD multiple myeloma (MM), utilizing a combination of PC-targeted agents, while therapies directly targeting the amyloid fibrils formation and accumulation are only investigational. Discussed here are general concepts of AL treatment approaches, as well as revision of the data on approved therapies and investigational approaches. Alkylating agents and steroids are still utilized, but now accompanied in frontline therapy by bortezomib; a proteosome inhibitor, and an anti-CD38 antibody. Autologous stem-cell transplant is a valuable option for eligible patients. Though prospective data is scarce, other anti-PC agents like immune modulators and more recently venetoclax (utilized for patients with the translocation 11:14) and belantamab mafodotin are optional for relapsed/refractory disease. Following the pronounced advances in therapy for MM, immunotherapies such as bispecific antibodies and chimeric antigen receptor T-cell (CART) may become a valuable option for AL amyloidosis. Finally, antibodies targeting the amyloidogenic LC and promoting its clearance are under extensive investigation. In conclusion, AL patients may currently be treated by a variety of effective therapies. The landscape of this disease is rapidly changing, and it is likely that in the next few years further progress will be made in the care of these patients.

E. Lebel (✉) · N. G. Even-Zohar · M. E. Gatt
Department of Hematology, Hadassah Medical Center, Jerusalem, Israel
e-mail: eyal.lebel@gmail.com

Faculty of Medicine, The Hebrew University, Jerusalem, Israel

M. E. Gatt
e-mail: rmoshg@hadassah.org.il

E. Herzog (ed.), *Cardiac Amyloidosis*, https://doi.org/10.1007/978-3-031-88342-2_14

Keywords AL amyloidosis · Proteosome inhibitors · Anti-CD38 antibodies · Autologous stem-cell transplant · Immune therapies

Introduction

AL amyloidosis (light-chain amyloidosis; AL) is a rare plasma cell disorder (PCD) characterized by progressive multi-organ damage due to misfolded immunoglobulin light chains (LC) secreted by clonal abnormal plasma cells (PC). Treatment of AL has traditionally followed that of the much more common PCD multiple myeloma (MM), utilizing a combination of anti-PC agents [1, 2]. Therapies to target the amyloidogenic protein, protein stabilization and sedimentation have not been successful as yet. Although there is a growing interest in removing AL amyloid fibrils, which aim to promote the clearance of the amyloidogenic LC from affected organs rather than targeting the abnormal PC secreting the amyloidogenic LC, the mainstay of treatment is anti-PC therapy [3]. Mirroring improvements in MM survival over the last decades with the introduction of novel therapeutic agents [4–6] significant progress has also been made in the treatment of AL [7]. Nevertheless, the prognosis of many patients, especially those of older age or with advanced cardiac disease at diagnosis, remains dismal [8]. Moreover, improvement in organ function usually lags behind the cessation of further secretion of the toxic amyloidogenic LC [9]. Therefore, patients with advanced cardiac disease may succumb to pre-existing organ damage before gaining any benefit from therapy, as evidenced by high rates of early mortality (within 3–6 months of diagnosis) in this frail patient population [8, 10, 11].

Within this chapter, we discuss the current and future treatment approaches to AL, and review the various therapies available, as well as investigational approaches.

Treatment for AL Amyloidosis—General Concepts

Being a complex and challenging to treat disease, the general concepts of AL therapy are hereby presented (and highlighted in Table 1):

1. AL is a systemic disease, with multi-organ involvement in the majority of patients, including (in order of frequency) the heart, kidneys, liver, gastrointestinal (GI) tract, peripheral nervous system, soft-tissues and others [12]. For this reason, the care of this disease should be multidisciplinary, ideally with a specialized team in an experienced excellence center. This team should include the hematologist, cardiologist and other specialists according to the patient's organ involvement, nurses, nutritionists, physiotherapists and others.
2. Supportive care, particularly for heart failure and other cardiac complications cannot be overestimated. The prognosis is dependent mostly on the extent of

Table 1 Key principle in the management of AL amyloidosis

• Organ dysfunction depends on the extent of LC sedimentation and amyloidogenic LC toxicity, not just amyloid deposition
• Therapy aims to improve survival and quality of life by achieving an "organ response" monitored by biomarkers and functional capacity
• Achieving a "hematological response" is crucial, focusing on significant reductions in amyloidogenic LC levels. Deeper responses are critical in AL. The treatment goal is to achieve a deep hematological response
• Multidisciplinary care is crucial, involving a specialized team across various specialties, cardiologists in particular
• Supportive care, especially for cardiac complications is vital due to its impact on prognosis

cardiac involvement. As such, management of cardiac failure and other cardiac complications should be meticulously done on a frequent basis.

3. The goal of therapy, aiming to ultimately improve the survival and quality of life of these patients, is to achieve what is termed an "organ response"—a significant improvement in the function of involved organs. These may be measured and followed by cardiac biomarkers (e.g. proBNP and troponin levels), parallel to the patient's functional capacity.
4. Cardiac staging (Table 2) is based on the levels of biomarkers. The former Mayo Clinic staging [13] utilizes only troponin and proBNP, and the newer staging system [14] refines the old one and also includes FLC levels (Table 2).
5. Organ dysfunction is dependent not only on the extent of LC sedimentation with the damaged organ, but on the amyloidogenic LC toxicity. Examining the

Table 2 Prognostic MAYO staging systems [1–4]

Staging system	Markers	Stages	Median survival (months)
Cardiac markers based staging	NT-proBNP > 332 ng/L cTnT > 0.035 ng/mL or cTnI > 0.01 ng/mL	I. Zero markers above the cutoff II. One marker above the cutoff III. Two markers above the cutoff	I. 26.4–27.2 II. 10.5–11.1 III. 3.5–4.1
Revised mayo clinic staging	NT-proBNP > 1800 ng/L cTnT > 0.025 ng/mL dFLC > 180 mg/L	I. Zero markers above the cutoff II. One marker above the cutoff III. Two markers above the cutoff IV. Three markers above the cutoff	I. 94.1 II. 40.3 III. 14 IV.5.8

Abbreviations: *NT-proBNP* N-terminal prohormone brian natriuretic peptide; *cTnT* cardiac troponin T; *cTnT* cardiac troponin I; *dFLC* difference between involved (amyloidogenic) and uninvolved circulating free light chain cardiac function levels of patients with ATTR as compared with AL amyloidosis, reveals a profound difference for the same sized heart. Patients with AL, albeit suffering from the same hypertrophied heart, have a far worse functional cardiac capacity as manifested by proBNP levels [15], hence, implying the amyloid sediment itself is not the sole cause for the congestive heart failure. Moreover, the elimination of LC from the circulation translates directly into survival and organ responses. Consequently, the goal of therapy is the reduction of toxic amyloidogenic LC levels as fast and low as possible.

6. A crucial step toward the achievement of organ response is the achievement of what is termed "hematological response"—a significant drop in the serum level of the involved amyloidogenic LC. This key step is important for a few reasons: (a) It can prevent further formation of amyloid fibrils composed of misfolded LC, and subsequent further organ damage. (b) It can prevent the above-mentioned toxicity to target organs formed by the toxic LC, which is independent of the mechanical damage of the amyloid fibrils [16]. (c) It can deflect the balance between amyloid fibrils formation and clearance, towards the clearance of fibrils from target organs.
7. In MM, while very deep hematological responses correlate with better clinical outcomes, commonly the approach is <u>not</u> to switch therapy as long as the disease is not progressing. In contrast, in AL the achievement of deeper responses (= maximal reduction of the involved LC) is crucial for the subsequent achievement of organ responses. Thus, partial responses (PR) are not satisfactory and are frequently a reason to switch therapy.
8. The achievement of hematological response is dependent on the successful elimination of the amyloidogenic aberrant PC which secretes the LC, which is done through PC-directed therapies. As expected, and mentioned above, the armamentarium of such therapies stems from the much more common PCD: MM.
9. Measurements of hematological response are based on the delta between the involved and the uninvolved LC (dFLC, i.e. subtracting the uninvolved from the involved to assess response). A sufficient response is considered when the dFLC is below 40 mg/L (very good partial response—VGPR) and normalization of FLC levels is the desired level of complete response (CR) (Table 3). Moreover, it has been shown that reducing the dFLC below 10 mg/L correlates with better organ responses than 20 mg/L [17]. It is becoming more evident that even patients in CR have a better organ response when they have their plasma cells eliminated from the bone marrow to a point of less than 1:10,000, designated as $< 10^{-5}$ cells minimal residual disease (MRD) measurement [18]. Subsequently, the goal of treatment is to achieve a deep response [19, 20].
10. Organ responses (Table 4) are assessed utilizing the cardiac biomarkers proBNP and BNP. The classical binary system (response = reduction of more than 300 ng/ml or > 30%) was utilized to assess cardiac prognosis. Recently, a graded cardiac response criterion which correlates better with survival was suggested (i.e. proBNP and BNP reduction: 30–60% reduction is CarPR; > 60% is CarVGPR and normalization of proBNP or BNP is CarCR) [21].

Table 3 Hematological response criteria

Response criteria	Definition
MRD negative status	Plasma cells eliminated from the bone marrow to a point of less than 1:10,000, designated as < 10^{-5} cells
CR	Negative serum and urine immunofixation and normal FLC ratio
VGPR	dFLC < 40 mg/L
PR	dFLC decrease > 50%
NR	Less than 50% dFLC decrease

Abbreviations: *MRD* minimal residual disease; *CR* complete response; *FLC* free light chain; *VGPR* very good partial response; *dFLC* difference between involved and uninvolved free light chain; *PR* partial response; *NR* no response

Table 4 Cardiac organ response criteria

	Response criteria
Classical binary response criteria [2, 5]	Heart (BNP based) = reduction of BNP of 30% and > 50 ng/L over the starting value Heart (NT-proBNP based) = reduction of NT-proBNP of 30% and > 300 ng/L over the starting value
Graded cardiac response criteria [6, 7]	CarCR = nadir NT-proBNP ≤ 350 pg/mL or BNP ≤ 80 pg/mL CarVGPR > 60% reduction in NT-proBNP/BNP CarPR = 31–60% reduction in NT-proBNP CarNR ≤ 30% reduction in NT-proBNP

Abbreviations: *CarCR* cardiac complete response; CarVGPR, cardiac very good partial response; *CarPR* cardiac partial response; *CarNR* cardiac no response; *NT-proBNP* N-terminal prohormone brian natriuretic peptide; *BNP* brian natriuretic peptide

11. Unlike MM, clinical trials, particularly phase 3 clinical trials, are scanty in AL. Until recently, there were no official approved therapies for AL, and all data regarding the ability of anti-PC MM-derived therapies to rectify AL was based on the agents approved for MM, subsequently reported in large AL case series and small prospective trials. The reasons for this, are: (a) the rarity of AL (generally, and compared to MM), and (b) the frailty of patients, as most have cardiac involvement, with moderate to severe heart failure.
12. Nevertheless, the tumor load in AL is minimal as compared with MM, allowing deep and sustained responses, once achieved.
13. Although this approach is directed towards the root (the PCs secreting the LC), and not the stem (the amyloid formation in the organs) of this disease, it is the only established therapy allowing subsequent organ restoration. Therapy to prevent amyloid sedimentation or clearance from the organs is not yet available, but is being investigated extensively.

Prognosis of AL Amyloidosis

The extent of heart involvement is the major determinant of survival in AL [22, 23]. While clinical parameters and cardiac imaging studies can be utilized to assess the extent of heart involvement, cardiac biomarkers (troponin and proBNP) levels in the blood are the mainstay of prognostication. Cardiac biomarker levels are not only the simplest way of cardiac assessment, but also are reliable and validated reflectors of the severity of heart disease and predictors of patients' outcome [13, 14].

The t(11:14) was correlated with reduced response rates with bortezomib but favorable response rates following autologous stem cell transplant (ASCT) [24, 25]. Other factors which were found to be associated with poorer outcomes are multi-organ involvement [23], degree of marrow plasmacytosis [23], dFLC level > 50 mg/l [17], factor X deficiency [26] and high von-Willebrand factor levels [27].

Therapies for AL Amyloidosis

The various agents to target the amyloidogenic plasma cells are diagrammatically shown in Fig. 1.

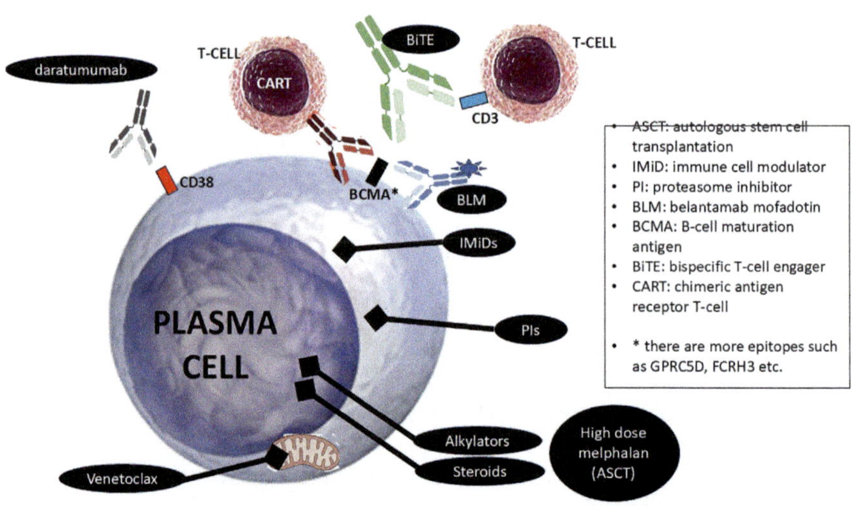

Fig. 1 Available agents for the treatments of AL amyloidosis

Conventional-Dose Therapy: Alkylating Agents and Steroids

Alkylating agents, particularly melphalan and cyclophosphamide, have been used to treat AL for many years, and were the standard of therapy until the advent of novel therapies for MM [28]. These agents cross-link DNA strands, causing DNA damage, disrupting DNA replication and transcription, and ultimately inducing apoptosis and cell death. The role of high-dose melphalan in the context of autologous stem cell transplantation (ASCT) is discussed further in a separate section.

Combined with other agents, cyclophosphamide, an alkylating agent prodrug, although administered at low doses to minimize hematological and cardiac toxicity, is widely used as part of standard frontline therapy together with dexamethasone and newer agents such as bortezomib and daratumumab (discussed below) [29].

Being the first anti-PC agent introduced, steroids (prednisone and dexamethasone) have long been a cornerstone in AL therapy [30]. Until the implementation of bortezomib (see below), oral melphalan combined with high dose dexamethasone has been a standard and mainstay initial treatment for AL [31], feasible even in the frailest patients.

This combination has demonstrated hematologic overall response rates (ORR) ranging from 45 to 75%, with a median overall survival (OS) of 7 years. Achievement of the above desired CR was not common, and the melphalan-dexamethasone regimen has not been able to overcome the poor OS in patients with severe cardiac involvement, and was poorly tolerated in this population, largely due to cytopenias, fluid retention and gastrointestinal adverse effects. Dexamethasone, still a part of standard treatment regimens, should be used cautiously in cardiac patients, as it causes fluid retention and extreme cardiac overload. Patients with advanced heart involvement did not tolerate high-dose dexamethasone, but lowering the dose from 40 to 20 mg on days 1–4 was associated with significantly lower CR rates [32], arguing for the dire need for more efficient yet less toxic therapies [29].

High-Dose Therapy and Autologous Stem Cell Transplantation (ASCT)

ASCT was first reported in 1998 as a major breakthrough in the treatment of AL amyloidosis [33], following its prior use in MM. Melphalan 200 mg/m^2 was reported to induce hematologic ORR of 76%, and a CR in 33% of patients, while transplant related mortality (TRM) was 12–13% [34–36], but reported to be as high as 40% [37]. Reduction of the melphalan dose may be suitable for patients with moderate cardiac dysfunction, but results in some lower hematologic response rates, and varying TRM rates, which may still be high [34, 36–40]. The procedure is suitable for only about 20–25% of AL patients, with cardiac dysfunction being the significant factor for ineligibility. Another major difficulty limiting ASCT use is the high initial mortality rate before ASCT—during induction chemotherapy and during the period of stem cell mobilization. Moreover, a head-to-head randomized controlled trial failed to demonstrate an advantage for ASCT over melphalan and prednisone, possibly due to high TRM (24%) obscuring the beneficial effects of ASCT, and a higher risk patient population [36]. Albeit the high TRM which precludes ASCT from many AL patients, patients who eventually tolerate ASCT and achieve CR were reported to have an excellent prognosis [39]. Interestingly, AL patients selected for ASCT were found to have a significantly better prognosis than parallel MM patients receiving ASCT [40]. Hence, accurate patient selection for this rigorous procedure based on cardiac risk assessment is crucial. Left ventricular ejection fraction < 40% is considered a contraindication, and cardiac biomarkers (troponin and proBNP levels) are essential for eligibility assessment [41]. ProBNP level of above 5000 ng/L was shown to be associated with very high mortality rates, and was set as an acceptable threshold. Even when a patient is deemed eligible, the procedure carries significant risks, though with careful patient selection and vigorous supportive care before and during ASCT, mortality and morbidity can be reduced. Until the introduction of novel effective PC-targeted therapies, ASCT following high-dose melphalan was the standard treatment for patients who could tolerate this rigorous procedure [34]. Due to the availability of other treatment options, ASCT utilization has been reduced over the last few years.

Proteasome Inhibitors (PIs)

Proteasome inhibitors, bortezomib being the first-in-class, are an attractive treatment strategy, as amyloidogenic PC relies on the proteasome to manage the proteotoxic stress caused by amyloidogenic LC [42]. Since 2009, bortezomib has been administered in combination with dexamethasone and alkylating agents as the frontline treatment, demonstrating rapid and deep hematologic responses with a favorable safety profile, making it suitable even for patients with end-stage renal disease [43, 44]. Multiple large case series supporting bortezomib use in AL have been reported to date. The combination of melphalan and dexamethasone was compared to the addition of bortezomib, in one of the only randomized controlled clinical trials in AL, the latter showing superiority and establishing triad-therapy as standard. Non-randomized historical comparisons have found cyclophosphamide to be an effective combo [45, 46]. CyBorD is now the accepted frontline regimen for newly diagnosed patients (combined with daratumumab, as will be discussed further on).

Its notable side effect is peripheral neuropathy, which typically improves or resolves with dose reductions or discontinuation of the treatment, yet limits this therapy for patients with baseline neuropathy related to AL. The presence of 11:14 chromosomal translocation, in about a half of AL patients, has been identified as a predictive factor for suboptimal response to bortezomib-based regimens in AL, with chromosome 11-located cyclin D1 overexpression being associated with this resistance to bortezomib [24].

Carfilzomib, a second-generation PI with a higher potency and lower neuropathy rates is generally avoided in AL due to its potential cardiac and renal toxicities [42].

On the other hand, ixazomib has proven effective in inducing both hematologic and organ responses in relapsed/refractory AL, both as a single agent and in combinations [47]. A large prospective randomized clinical trial comparing ixazomib and dexamethasone with standard of care for relapsed AL revealed the safety and efficacy of ixazomib based therapy [48]. However, the trial failed to show superiority of ixazomib and dexamethasone over other regimens, and daratumumab, which has become the agent of choice (see below), was not a comparator.

Immunomodulatory Drugs (IMiDs)

Immunomodulatory drugs are an important class of drugs with various mechanisms of action, including direct effects on the abnormal PC, but mainly the enhancement of NK and T-cells anti-tumoral effects. However, they also carry significant risks, including an increased likelihood of venous and arterial thromboembolism, rash, GI side effects and cytopenias. Thalidomide tolerability may be limited in AL due to neuropathy and GI effects, and lenalidomide may be challenging in patients with cardiac and/or renal disease [23]. IMiDs are also associated with a significant rise in proBNP levels measurements [49]. The latter phenomenon is not entirely understood and is not necessarily associated with cardiac exacerbations. Yet, caution is advised at treatment initiation in cardiac patients. In addition, lenalidomide has been linked to an increased risk of secondary malignancies (solid and myeloid) especially when used in combination with melphalan [50]. Pomalidomide, a third generation IMiD, is the most potent of the three and also the most tolerable, however, it may also be associated with worsening of heart failure symptoms [23]. It has shown high efficacy in combination with dexamethasone, inducing frequent hematologic remissions in heavily pre-treated refractory AL [51]. Emerging evidence indicates that lower dosing and careful monitoring may reduce these risks, making IMiDs, and mostly pomalidomide, a viable option for selected patients [23].

Anti CD38 Antibodies

Two anti-CD38 antibodies, daratumumab and isatuximab, have been approved by the Food and Drug Administration (FDA) for the treatment of MM, and the former was subsequently incorporated into standard first-line therapy in AL following the results of the ANDROMEDA trial in 2021. In this trial, 388 patients with newly-diagnosed AL were randomized to receive treatment with a standard induction regimen of bortezomib, cyclophosphamide and dexamethasone, either alone (CyBorD) or with daratumumab (D-CyBorD) [29]. The addition of daratumumab resulted in a nearly three-fold increase in the rate of hematologic CR (53% vs. 18%), and the rate of target organ response (cardiac/renal) was approximately doubled with the addition of daratumumab. The trial also highlighted a relatively favorable safety profile for

D-CyBorD, with only a slight increase in hematologic and infectious adverse events when compared to CyBorD, and a nearly identical rate of treatment discontinuation due to adverse events. Patients with severe cardiovascular disease (including a proBNP level of more than 8500 ng/L, a systolic blood pressure of less than 90 mmHg, or a stage IIIB disease by Mayo 2004) were excluded from the trial, but daratumumab is being investigated in this population. Treatment with single agent daratumumab for stage 3b cardiac patients has shown a favorable safety profile and relatively high efficacy, yet the prognosis remained poor [52]. The duration of treatment with first line daratumumab is controversial and the effect of daratumumab maintenance therapy following successful induction with D-CyBorD is being studied in a phase 2 trial (NCT05898646). The success of the D-CyBorD combination has made it the first registered treatment for AL amyloidosis, and the standard of care in first line.

Although daratumumab is currently part of the standard of care at first-line, many patients with relapsed/refractory (r/r) disease were not previously exposed to this agent. A large number of retrospective studies have reported on the use of daratumumab in the r/r setting [53, 54], and daratumumab as monotherapy in previously treated disease was prospectively evaluated in two phase 2 clinical trials, with relatively high rates (55–86%) of rapid and deep responses [55, 56]. Various combination treatments with daratumumab are currently being tested, including daratumumab with pomalidomide (NCT04270175, NCT04895917), ixazomib (NCT03283917), or venetoclax (NCT05486481) in patients with the 11:14 translocation. The high efficacy achieved with daratumumab, albeit the lack of a phase 3 study, has made daratumumab based combinations the first choice for r/r AL patients.

Several trials of isatuximab in AL amyloidosis are ongoing. In the upfront setting, isatuximab is being evaluated in combination with bortezomib, cyclophosphamide, and dexamethasone in patients with high-risk disease (NCT04754945). This study includes patients with advanced cardiac disease, including Mayo stages 3 and 4, and utilizes what has been termed a “slow-go” approach, comprising the sequential addition of therapies and gradual dose escalations to limit treatment-related toxicity and early mortality. In the r/r setting, trials are evaluating both isatuximab monotherapy (NCT03499808) and the combination of isatuximab, pomalidomide, and dexamethasone (NCT05066607).

Venetoclax

Given the encouraging results in t(11:14) multiple myeloma [57] and the high prevalence of t(11:14) in AL amyloidosis in over 50% of patients, venetoclax is an attractive treatment option in this setting. However, it is not a registered therapy even in MM, and as such, is still considered an experimental therapy.

Few retrospective cohorts reported encouraging efficacy with this agent at variable doses, with the largest two studies (43/26 patients) reporting an overall hematologic response rate of 72/88% with event-free survival of more than 2 years [58, 59]. The treatment was relatively safe, with low rates of cytopenias, low rate of severe infections and no cases of tumor lysis syndrome (TLS). Dose reductions were frequent, but did not affect the efficacy. These promising results led to studies testing now venetoclax in AL prospectively (NCT05996406, NCT03000660, NCT05451771, NCT04847453, NCT06629818, NCT0548648).

Belantamab Mafodotin

Belantamab mafodotin (BLM) is an antibody–drug conjugate (ADC) consisted of the anti-BCMA monoclonal antibody belantamab conjugated to monomethyl auristatin F (MMAF), a tubulin inhibitor. This agent is approved for MM as a single agent in advanced lines, and recently regained attention following very supportive data in combination with dexamethasone and pomalidomide/bortezomib [60, 61]. Few retrospective studies in r/r AL showed great efficacy, with response rates as a single agent that were twice than seen in MM—60–80% versus 30–45% [62–65]. Similar to MM, keratopathy was the most frequent adverse event, manageable with appropriate dose interruptions and reductions. Besides the apparently greater efficacy, the data suggests lower rates of hematological toxicity in AL compared to MM, likely related to reduced marrow involvement and better marrow reserve in AL patients. Preliminary results of a prospective study with BLM in AL are supportive of the data above [66].

Bispecific Antibodies (BSA)

BSAs are antibodies recognizing two different epitopes, most commonly CD3 and a tumor epitope, to facilitate T-cell redirection and activation ultimately resulting in T-cell-mediated target cell killing [67]. BSAs have shown impressive results in r/r MM, although high rates of infectious complications remain a concern. Teclistamab is a BCMA-CD3 BSA and was the first BSA approved by the FDA for the treatment of r/r MM [68]. Few retrospective series with teclistamab in AL were published, and reported a very high response rates of 88–100% [68–70]. Importantly, responses were deep (most patients had a decrease in the serum level of the involved light chain to below the normal range) and rapid (a median time to best hematologic response of one month), with some early cardiac responses documented. Cytokine release syndrome (CRS), a potentially fatal side effect with high body temperatures, severe hypotension and pulmonary infiltrates causing respiratory failure is the most worrisome side effect of BSAs, and may be lethal in frail cardiac AL patients. CRS was reported in more than half of the patients in different series, but generally of the lowest grade (fever only, without other detrimental effects) and was very manageable. Although one case of infectious death and one case of severe immune cell associated neurotoxicity syndrome (ICANS) were reported, overall, the rate of adverse events was consistent with what was seen in MM, and no additional signals relating to cardiac or kidney toxicity specific to AL patients were observed. Thus, although limited in extent, these reports provide reassurance to safety concerns which are specific to AL in general and cardiac disease in particular, while also showing high efficacy as expected from previous experience in r/r MM. These deep responses show great promise in achieving the goals of therapy in advanced patients. The role of other BSAs in AL, such as talquetamab, elranaramab and cevostamab has yet to be proved.

Chimeric Antigen Receptor T-Cell Therapy (CART)

CART has revolutionized the treatment of r/r MM, with two anti-BCMA CART products, ciltacabtagene autoleucel (cilta-cel) and idecabtagene vicleucel (ide-cel) now approved by the Federal Drub Agency (FDA) and European Medicines Agency (EMA) for the treatment of r/r MM as early as second line (cilta-cel) or third line (ide-cel) [71, 72]. This unique modality involves the collection of autologous T-lymphocytes from the patient and the manipulation of these cells to enable the recognition of a tumor antigen and the consequent activation of the T-cells, resulting in the elimination of the tumor cells. While BCMA is the main target antigen in MM tested to date, encouraging data on other targets and approaches are gradually accumulating [73, 74]. Several drawbacks remain, including limited availability due to the complexity of the manufacturing process and unique adverse events mentioned above-CRS and ICANS, at higher rates than seen with BSAs [75].

Trepidation with exposure of already frail AL amyloidosis patients to these adverse events, along with the relative rarity of this disease, probably underlie the fact that commercial CART products have not been tested in AL amyloidosis thus far. Few reports of successful administration of CART to MM patients who also had AL were reported [76–78].

The first prospective experience of CART in AL was reported with the academic anti-BCMA CART HBI0101, showing both preclinical and clinical evidence for a proof-of-concept of utilizing this therapy in Al [79]. The phase 1a-b study with this product, which showed promising efficacy and manageable toxicity in MM patients [79], enrolled also AL patients. Sixteen AL patients with relapsed/refractory disease were included and reported to date-14 were treated within the study and 2 on a compassionate basis [80]. The AL patients were treated within the following cohorts: 1 received 150×10^6 CART cells, 2 received 450×10^6 CART cells and 13 received 800×10^6 CART cells. The patients were heavily pretreated, and most (13/16, 81%) had cardiac involvement, including 5 with MAYO-stage 3a/3b at study entry.

Hematologic adverse events were milder and resolved quicker compared to MM, probably due to the better marrow reserve in AL. There were 9 occurrences of AL-related organ deterioration (heart/kidney/liver) in a total of 7/16 patients, all of which resolved to baseline function with supportive care. CRS was observed in 14/16 (grade 1–2:11 patients; grade 3:3 patients; no grade 4 or 5 CRS), and was manageable with frequent use of tocilizumab (12/14). None of the patients developed ICANS or other neurotoxicity. There were no treatment-related deaths.

The overall hematological response rate was 15/16 (94%) and the CR rate was 12/16 (75%). Minimal residual disease (MRD) negativity based on flow cytometry 10^{-5} was achieved in 9/14 evaluable patients. The median time to response was 17 days. Eight of thirteen evaluable patients had organ responses (heart/kidney/liver/autonomic dysfunction). Seven patients died during follow-up, of whom 3 while in hematologic response.

In summary, in this largest cohort of AL patients treated with CART reported to date acceptable toxicity was demonstrated in this frail population, with a remarkable hematologic efficacy, leading to organ responses in many patients. Among patients with baseline advanced cardiac disease, deaths in the first year were frequent, suggesting that this effective therapy should be considered earlier, before end-stage heart disease is established. Overall, this data suggests that anti-BCMA CART modality may become a powerful clinical tool to improve organ function and survival in AL.

Stabilization of Amyloid Fibrils

Unlike WT-TTR amyloidosis, stabilization of LC fibrils was not proven effective. While initial non-randomized historically controlled reports suggested that the addition of doxycycline to the bortezomib based therapy may prolong survival [81], a randomized trial in combination with CyBorD failed to show and survival advantage or cardiac advantage [82].

Antibodies Promoting Fibril Clearance

As mentioned, the treatment for AL nowadays is based on anti-PC therapy and there are no approved therapies promoting the clearance of amyloid fibrils from damaged organs. However, there is growing interest in such treatment and relevant studies are ongoing, with birtamimab and anselamimab being the agents in the most advanced development stage.

NEOD001 (birtamimab) is an antibody that specifically binds AL amyloid (both κ and λ isotype) and promotes Fc-receptor-mediated phagocytosis of amyloid fibrils. Though early results with this agent were promising [83], a phase 3 clinical trial (VITAL study) assessing this agent added to frontline therapy failed to show benefit in survival of the patients or enhanced cardiac responses. The post-hoc analysis of VITAL study showed a potential survival benefit for the subgroup of Mayo Stage IV patients with birtamimab, without additional toxicity [84], leading to a phase 3 randomized placebo-controlled study of birtamimab in selected patients with newly diagnosed Mayo stage IV AL that is ongoing (NCT04973137).

CAEL-101 (anselamimab) is a different antibody designed to bind the misfolded LCs and promote their clearance. In a phase 1a/b clinical trial of CAEL-101, 17 of 27 patients (63%) achieved organ responses [85]. The preliminary results of the phase 2 study of CAEL-101 combined with CyBorD ± daratumumab showed promising organ responses, paving the route to two randomized, double-blind phase 3 studies of CAEL-101 combined with CyBorD ± daratumumab for the treatment of newly diagnosed AL with stage IIIa/IIIb (NCT04512235, NCT04504825) that are ongoing.

Other approaches preventing the accumulation or promoting the clearance of amyloid fibrils are being investigated [86].

Summary

AL amyloidosis has turned in the last two decades from a progressive disease with dismal outcomes to most patients with cardiac involvement, to a disease with a variety of effective therapies enabling the eradication of abnormal PC secreting the toxic LC, and ultimately improvement in the function of involved organs. This subsequently led to improved survival and quality of life for the majority of these patients. Promising data is emerging regarding newer anti-PC therapies, as well as therapies targeting the clearance of amyloid fibrils. Together with effective agents targeting the root of this disease, a multidisciplinary approach with supportive care for these patients, especially for heart failure, is crucial for the treatment of these patients.

References

1. Palladini G, Milani P, Merlini G. Management of AL amyloidosis in 2020. Blood. 2020;136(23):2620–7.
2. Palladini G, Merlini G. How I treat AL amyloidosis. Blood. 2022;139(19):2918–30.
3. Bou Zerdan M, Nasr L, Khalid F, Allam S, Bouferraa Y, Batool S, et al. Systemic AL amyloidosis: current approach and future direction. Oncotarget. 2023;14(1):384–94.
4. Puertas B, González-Calle V, Sobejano-Fuertes E, Escalante F, Queizán JA, Bárez A, et al. Novel agents as main drivers for continued improvement in survival in multiple myeloma. Cancers (Basel). 2023;15(5):1558.
5. Moore KLF, Turesson I, Genell A, Klausen TW, Knut-Bojanowska D, Redder L, et al. Improved survival in myeloma patients–a nationwide registry study of 4,647 patients ≥75 years treated in Denmark and Sweden. Haematologica. 2022;108(6):1640–51.
6. Eisfeld C, Kajüter H, Möller L, Wellmann I, Shumilov E, Stang A. Time trends in survival and causes of death in multiple myeloma: a population-based study from Germany. BMC Cancer. 2023;23(1):317.
7. Muchtar E, Gertz MA, Kumar SK, Lacy MQ, Dingli D, Buadi FK, et al. Improved outcomes for newly diagnosed AL amyloidosis between 2000 and 2014: cracking the glass ceiling of early death. Blood. 2017;129(15):2111–9.
8. Staron A, Zheng L, Doros G, Connors LH, Mendelson LM, Joshi T, et al. Marked progress in AL amyloidosis survival: a 40-year longitudinal natural history study. Blood Cancer J. 2021;11(8):139.

9. Kaufman GP, Dispenzieri A, Gertz MA, Lacy MQ, Buadi FK, Hayman SR, et al. Kinetics of organ response and survival following normalization of the serum free light chain ratio in AL amyloidosis. Am J Hematol. 2015;90(3):181–6.
10. Kumar SK, Gertz MA, Lacy MQ, Dingli D, Hayman SR, Buadi FK, et al. Recent improvements in survival in primary systemic amyloidosis and the importance of an early mortality risk score. Mayo Clin Proc. 2011;86(1):12–8.
11. Chee CE, Rajkumar V, Gertz M, Lacy M, Zeldenrust S, Kumar S, et al. Unraveling early mortality in patients with AL amyloidosis. Blood. 2010;116(21):4990–4990.
12. Wechalekar AD, Schonland SO, Kastritis E, Gillmore JD, Dimopoulos MA, Lane T, et al. A European collaborative study of treatment outcomes in 346 patients with cardiac stage III AL amyloidosis. Blood. 2013;121(17):3420–7.
13. Dispenzieri A, Gertz MA, Kyle RA, Lacy MQ, Burritt MF, Therneau TM, et al. Serum cardiac troponins and N-terminal pro-brain natriuretic peptide: a staging system for primary systemic amyloidosis. J Clin Oncol. 2004;22(18):3751–7.
14. Kumar S, Dispenzieri A, Lacy MQ, Hayman SR, Buadi FK, Colby C, et al. Revised prognostic staging system for light chain amyloidosis incorporating cardiac biomarkers and serum free light chain measurements. J Clin Oncol. 2012;30(9):989–95.
15. Imperlini E, Gnecchi M, Rognoni P, Sabidò E, Ciuffreda MC, Palladini G, et al. Proteotoxicity in cardiac amyloidosis: amyloidogenic light chains affect the levels of intracellular proteins in human heart cells. Sci Rep. 2017;7(1):15661.
16. Maritan M, Romeo M, Oberti L, Sormanni P, Tasaki M, Russo R, et al. Inherent biophysical properties modulate the toxicity of soluble amyloidogenic light chains. J Mol Biol. 2020;432(4):845–60.
17. Milani P, Basset M, Russo F, Foli A, Merlini G, Palladini G. Patients with light-chain amyloidosis and low free light-chain burden have distinct clinical features and outcome. Blood. 2017;130(5):625–31.
18. Kastritis E, Kostopoulos IV, Theodorakakou F, Fotiou D, Gavriatopoulou M, Migkou M, et al. Next generation flow cytometry for MRD detection in patients with AL amyloidosis. Amyloid. 2021;28(1):19–23.
19. Muchtar E, Dispenzieri A, Leung N, Lacy MQ, Buadi FK, Dingli D, et al. Depth of organ response in AL amyloidosis is associated with improved survival: grading the organ response criteria. Leukemia. 2018;32(10):2240–9.
20. Palladini G, Schönland SO, Sanchorawala V, Kumar S, Wechalekar A, Hegenbart U, et al. Clarification on the definition of complete haematologic response in light-chain (AL) amyloidosis. Amyloid. 2021;28(1):1–2.
21. Muchtar E, Dispenzieri A, Wisniowski B, Palladini G, Milani P, Merlini G, et al. Graded cardiac response criteria for patients with systemic light chain amyloidosis. J Clin Oncol. 2023;41(7):1393–403.
22. Gertz MA, Dispenzieri A. Systemic amyloidosis recognition, prognosis, and therapy. JAMA. 2020;324(1):79.
23. Gertz MA. Immunoglobulin light chain amyloidosis: 2018 Update on diagnosis, prognosis, and treatment. Am J Hematol. 2018;93(9):1169–80.
24. Bochtler T, Hegenbart U, Kunz C, Granzow M, Benner A, Seckinger A, et al. Translocation t(11;14) is associated with adverse outcome in patients with newly diagnosed AL amyloidosis when treated with bortezomib-based regimens. J Clin Oncol. 2015;33(12):1371–8.
25. Bochtler T, Hegenbart U, Kunz C, Benner A, Kimmich C, Seckinger A, et al. Prognostic impact of cytogenetic aberrations in AL amyloidosis patients after high-dose melphalan: a long-term follow-up study. Blood. 2016;128(4):594–602.
26. Patel G, Hari P, Szabo A, Rein L, Kreuziger LB, Chhabra S, et al. Acquired factor X deficiency in light-chain (AL) amyloidosis is rare and associated with advanced disease. Hematol Oncol Stem Cell Ther. 2019;12(1):10–4.
27. Kastritis E, Papassotiriou I, Terpos E, Roussou M, Gavriatopoulou M, Komitopoulou A, et al. Clinical and prognostic significance of serum levels of von Willebrand factor and ADAMTS-13 antigens in AL amyloidosis. Blood. 2016;128(3):405–9.

28. Merlini G, Dispenzieri A, Sanchorawala V, Schönland SO, Palladini G, Hawkins PN, et al. Systemic immunoglobulin light chain amyloidosis. Nat Rev Dis Primers. 2018;4(1):38.
29. Kastritis E, Palladini G, Minnema MC, Wechalekar AD, Jaccard A, Lee HC, et al. Daratumumab-based treatment for immunoglobulin light-chain amyloidosis. N Engl J Med. 2021;385(1):46–58.
30. Palladini G, Anesi E, Perfetti V, Obici L, Invernizzi R, Balduini C, et al. A modified high-dose dexamethasone regimen for primary systemic (AL) amyloidosis. Br J Haematol. 2001;113(4):1044–6.
31. Palladini G, Perfetti V, Obici L, Caccialanza R, Semino A, Adami F, et al. Association of melphalan and high-dose dexamethasone is effective and well tolerated in patients with AL (primary) amyloidosis who are ineligible for stem cell transplantation. Blood. 2004;103(8):2936–8.
32. Palladini G, Milani P, Foli A, Obici L, Lavatelli F, Nuvolone M, et al. Oral melphalan and dexamethasone grants extended survival with minimal toxicity in AL amyloidosis: long-term results of a risk-adapted approach. Haematologica. 2014;99(4):743–50.
33. Comenzo RL, Vosburgh E, Falk RH, Sanchorawala V, Reisinger J, Dubrey S, et al. Dose-intensive melphalan with blood stem-cell support for the treatment of AL (amyloid light-chain) amyloidosis: survival and responses in 25 patients. Blood. 1998;91(10):3662–70.
34. Sanchorawala V, Skinner M, Quillen K, Finn KT, Doros G, Seldin DC. Long-term outcome of patients with AL amyloidosis treated with high-dose melphalan and stem-cell transplantation. Blood. 2007;110(10):3561–3.
35. Skinner M, Sanchorawala V, Seldin DC, Dember LM, Falk RH, Berk JL, et al. High-dose melphalan and autologous stem-cell transplantation in patients with AL amyloidosis: an 8-year study. Ann Intern Med. 2004;140(2):85.
36. Gertz MA, Lacy MQ, Dispenzieri A, Ansell SM, Elliott MA, Gastineau DA, et al. Risk-adjusted manipulation of melphalan dose before stem cell transplantation in patients with amyloidosis is associated with a lower response rate. Bone Marrow Transplant. 2004;34(12):1025–31.
37. Moreau P. Autologous stem cell transplantation for AL amyloidosis: a standard therapy? Leukemia. 1999;13(12):1929–31.
38. Sanchorawala V, Hoering A, Seldin DC, Finn KT, Fennessey SA, Sexton R, et al. Modified high-dose melphalan and autologous SCT for AL amyloidosis or high-risk myeloma: analysis of SWOG trial S0115. Bone Marrow Transplant. 2013;48(12):1537–42.
39. Cibeira MT, Sanchorawala V, Seldin DC, Quillen K, Berk JL, Dember LM, et al. Outcome of AL amyloidosis after high-dose melphalan and autologous stem cell transplantation: long-term results in a series of 421 patients. Blood. 2011;118(16):4346–52.
40. Dispenzieri A, Seenithamby K, Lacy MQ, Kumar SK, Buadi FK, Hayman SR, et al. Patients with immunoglobulin light chain amyloidosis undergoing autologous stem cell transplantation have superior outcomes compared with patients with multiple myeloma: a retrospective review from a tertiary referral center. Bone Marrow Transplant. 2013;48(10):1302–7.
41. Sanchorawala V, Boccadoro M, Gertz M, Hegenbart U, Kastritis E, Landau H, et al. Guidelines for high dose chemotherapy and stem cell transplantation for systemic AL amyloidosis: EHA-ISA working group guidelines. Amyloid. 2022;29(1):1–7.
42. Jelinek T, Kryukova E, Kufova Z, Kryukov F, Hajek R. Proteasome inhibitors in AL amyloidosis: focus on mechanism of action and clinical activity. Hematol Oncol. 2017;35(4):408–19.
43. Palladini G, Sachchithanantham S, Milani P, Gillmore J, Foli A, Lachmann H, et al. A European collaborative study of cyclophosphamide, bortezomib, and dexamethasone in upfront treatment of systemic AL amyloidosis. Blood. 2015;126(5):612–5.
44. Kastritis E, Leleu X, Arnulf B, Zamagni E, Cibeira MT, Kwok F, et al. Bortezomib, melphalan, and dexamethasone for light-chain amyloidosis. J Clin Oncol. 2020;38(28):3252–60.
45. Venner CP, Lane T, Foard D, Rannigan L, Gibbs SDJ, Pinney JH, et al. Cyclophosphamide, bortezomib, and dexamethasone therapy in AL amyloidosis is associated with high clonal response rates and prolonged progression-free survival. Blood. 2012;119(19):4387–90.
46. Mikhael JR, Schuster SR, Jimenez-Zepeda VH, Bello N, Spong J, Reeder CB, et al. Cyclophosphamide-bortezomib-dexamethasone (CyBorD) produces rapid and complete hematologic response in patients with AL amyloidosis. Blood. 2012;119(19):4391–4.

47. Cohen OC, Sharpley F, Gillmore JD, Lachmann HJ, Sachchithanantham S, Mahmood S, et al. Use of ixazomib, lenalidomide and dexamethasone in patients with relapsed amyloid light-chain amyloidosis. Br J Haematol. 2020;189(4):643–9.
48. Dispenzieri A, Kastritis E, Wechalekar AD, Schönland SO, Kim K, Sanchorawala V, et al. A randomized phase 3 study of ixazomib–dexamethasone versus physician's choice in relapsed or refractory AL amyloidosis. Leukemia. 2022;36(1):225–35.
49. Dispenzieri A, Dingli D, Kumar SK, Rajkumar SV, Lacy MQ, Hayman S, et al. Discordance between serum cardiac biomarker and immunoglobulin-free light-chain response in patients with immunoglobulin light-chain amyloidosis treated with immune modulatory drugs. Am J Hematol. 2010;85(10):757–9.
50. Palumbo A, Bringhen S, Kumar SK, Lupparelli G, Usmani S, Waage A, et al. Second primary malignancies with lenalidomide therapy for newly diagnosed myeloma: a meta-analysis of individual patient data. Lancet Oncol. 2014;15(3):333–42.
51. Palladini G, Milani P, Foli A, Basset M, Russo F, Perlini S, et al. A phase 2 trial of pomalidomide and dexamethasone rescue treatment in patients with AL amyloidosis. Blood. 2017;129(15):2120–3.
52. Theodorakakou F, Briasoulis A, Fotiou D, Petropoulos I, Georgiopoulos G, Lama N, et al. Outcomes for patients with systemic light chain amyloidosis and Mayo stage 3B disease. Hematol Oncol. 2023;41(4):725–32.
53. Shragai T, Gatt M, Lavie N, Vaxman I, Tadmor T, Rouvio O, et al. Daratumumab for relapsed AL amyloidosis—when cumulative real-world data precedes clinical trials: a multisite study and systematic literature review. Eur J Haematol. 2021;106(2):184–95.
54. Wechalekar AD, Sanchorawala V. Daratumumab in AL amyloidosis. Blood. 2022;140(22):2317–22.
55. Roussel M, Merlini G, Chevret S, Arnulf B, Stoppa AM, Perrot A, et al. A prospective phase 2 trial of daratumumab in patients with previously treated systemic light-chain amyloidosis. Blood. 2020;135(18):1531–40.
56. Sanchorawala V, Sarosiek S, Schulman A, Mistark M, Migre ME, Cruz R, et al. Safety, tolerability, and response rates of daratumumab in relapsed AL amyloidosis: results of a phase 2 study. Blood. 2020;135(18):1541–7.
57. Kumar S, Kaufman JL, Gasparetto C, Mikhael J, Vij R, Pegourie B, et al. Efficacy of venetoclax as targeted therapy for relapsed/refractory t(11;14) multiple myeloma. Blood. 2017;130(22):2401–9.
58. Premkumar VJ, Lentzsch S, Pan S, Bhutani D, Richter J, Jagannath S, et al. Venetoclax induces deep hematologic remissions in t(11;14) relapsed/refractory AL amyloidosis. Blood Cancer J. 2021;11(1):10.
59. Lebel E, Kastritis E, Palladini G, Milani P, Theodorakakou F, Aumann S, et al. Venetoclax in relapse/refractory AL amyloidosis—a multicenter international retrospective real-world study. Cancers (Basel). 2023;15(6):1710.
60. Hungria V, Robak P, Hus M, Zherebtsova V, Ward C, Ho PJ, et al. Belantamab mafodotin, bortezomib, and dexamethasone for multiple myeloma. N Engl J Med. 2024;391(5):393–407.
61. Dimopoulos MA, Beksac M, Pour L, Delimpasi S, Vorobyev V, Quach H, et al. Belantamab mafodotin, pomalidomide, and dexamethasone in multiple myeloma. N Engl J Med. 2024;391(5):408–21.
62. Shragai T, Magen H, Lavi N, Gatt M, Trestman S, Zektser M, et al. Real-world experience with belantamab mafodotin therapy for relapsed/refractory multiple myeloma: a multicentre retrospective study. Br J Haematol. 2023;200(1):45–53.
63. Lonial S, Lee HC, Badros A, Trudel S, Nooka AK, Chari A, et al. Belantamab mafodotin for relapsed or refractory multiple myeloma (DREAMM-2): a two-arm, randomised, open-label, phase 2 study. Lancet Oncol. 2020;21(2):207–21.
64. Zhang Y, Godara A, Pan S, Toskic D, Mann H, Sborov D, et al. Belantamab mafodotin in patients with relapsed/refractory AL amyloidosis with myeloma. Ann Hematol. 2022;101(9):2119–21.
65. Khwaja J, Bomsztyk J, Atta M, Bygrave C, Forbes A, Durairaj S, et al. Real-world efficacy of single-agent belantamab mafodotin in relapsed systemic AL amyloidosis. Br J Haematol. 2024;204(5):1811–5.

66. Kastritis E, Palladini G, Dimopoulos MA, Jaccard A, Merlini G, Theodorakakou F, et al. S198: efficacy and safety of belantamab mafodotin monotherapy in patients with relapsed or refractory light chain amyloidosis: a phase 2 study by the European myeloma network. Hemasphere. 2023;7(S3): e2301416.
67. Labrijn AF, Janmaat ML, Reichert JM, Parren PWHI. Bispecific antibodies: a mechanistic review of the pipeline. Nat Rev Drug Discov. 2019;18(8):585–608.
68. Moreau P, Garfall AL, van de Donk NWCJ, Nahi H, San-Miguel JF, Oriol A, et al. Teclistamab in relapsed or refractory multiple myeloma. N Engl J Med. 2022;387(6):495–505.
69. Forgeard N, Elessa D, Carpinteiro A, Belhadj K, Minnema M, Roussel M, et al. Teclistamab in relapsed or refractory AL amyloidosis: a multinational retrospective case series. Blood. 2024;143(8):734–7.
70. Chakraborty R, Bhutani D, Maurer MS, Mohan M, Lentzsch S, D'Souza A. Safety and efficacy of teclistamab in systemic immunoglobulin light chain amyloidosis. Blood Cancer J. 2023;13(1):172.
71. Rodriguez-Otero P, Ailawadhi S, Arnulf B, Patel K, Cavo M, Nooka AK, et al. Ide-cel or standard regimens in relapsed and refractory multiple myeloma. N Engl J Med. 2023;388(11):1002–14.
72. San-Miguel J, Dhakal B, Yong K, Spencer A, Anguille S, Mateos MV, et al. Cilta-cel or standard care in lenalidomide-refractory multiple myeloma. N Engl J Med. 2023;389(4):335–47.
73. Zhang M, Wei G, Zhou L, Zhou J, Chen S, Zhang W, et al. GPRC5D CAR T cells (OriCAR-017) in patients with relapsed or refractory multiple myeloma (POLARIS): a first-in-human, single-centre, single-arm, phase 1 trial. Lancet Haematol. 2023;10(2):e107–16.
74. Li C, Xu J, Luo W, Liao D, Xie W, Wei Q, et al. Bispecific CS1-BCMA CAR-T cells are clinically active in relapsed or refractory multiple myeloma. Leukemia. 2024;38(1):149–59.
75. Martino M, Canale FA, Alati C, Vincelli ID, Moscato T, Porto G, et al. CART-Cell therapy: recent advances and new evidence in multiple myeloma. Cancers (Basel). 2021;13(11):2639.
76. Oliver-Caldes A, Jiménez R, Español-Rego M, Cibeira MT, Ortiz-Maldonado V, Quintana LF, et al. First report of CART treatment in AL amyloidosis and relapsed/refractory multiple myeloma. J Immunother Cancer. 2021;9(12): e003783.
77. Das S, Ailawadhi S, Sher T, Roy V, Fernandez A, Parrondo RD. Anti-B cell maturation antigen chimeric antigen receptor T cell therapy for the treatment of AL amyloidosis and concurrent relapsed/refractory multiple myeloma: preliminary efficacy and safety. Curr Oncol. 2023;30(11):9627–33.
78. Goel U, Dima D, Davis J, Ahmed N, Shaikh H, Lochner J, et al. Safety and efficacy of B cell maturation antigen-directed CAR T-cell therapy in patients with relapsed/refractory multiple myeloma and concurrent light chain amyloidosis. Eur J Haematol. 2024;113(6):817–23.
79. Kfir-Erenfeld S, Asherie N, Grisariu S, Avni B, Zimran E, Assayag M, et al. Feasibility of a novel academic BCMA-CART (HBI0101) for the treatment of relapsed and refractory AL amyloidosis. Clin Cancer Res. 2022;28(23):5156–66.
80. Lebel E, Asherie N, Kfir-Erenfeld S, Grisariu S, Avni B, Elias S, et al. Efficacy and safety of anti–B-cell maturation antigen chimeric antigen receptor T-cell for the treatment of relapsed and refractory AL amyloidosis. J Clin Oncol. 2024.
81. Wechalekar AD, Whelan C. Encouraging impact of doxycycline on early mortality in cardiac light chain (AL) amyloidosis. Blood Cancer J. 2017;7(3):e546–e546.
82. Shen K-n, Fu W-j, Wu Y, Dong Y-j, Huang Z-x, Wei Y-q, et al. Doxycycline combined with bortezomib-cyclophosphamide-dexamethasone chemotherapy for newly diagnosed cardiac light-chain amyloidosis: a multicenter randomized controlled trial. Circulation. 2022;145(1):8–17.
83. Gertz MA, Landau H, Comenzo RL, Seldin D, Weiss B, Zonder J, et al. First-in-human phase I/II study of NEOD001 in patients with light chain amyloidosis and persistent organ dysfunction. J Clin Oncol. 2016;34(10):1097–103.
84. Gertz MA, Cohen AD, Comenzo RL, Kastritis E, Landau HJ, Libby EN, et al. Birtamimab plus standard of care in light-chain amyloidosis: the phase 3 randomized placebo-controlled VITAL trial. Blood. 2023;142(14):1208–18.

85. Edwards CV, Rao N, Bhutani D, Mapara M, Radhakrishnan J, Shames S, et al. Phase 1a/b study of monoclonal antibody CAEL-101 (11–1F4) in patients with AL amyloidosis. Blood. 2021;138(25):2632–41.
86. Wang J, Li J, Zhong L. Current status and prospect of anti-amyloid fibril therapy in AL amyloidosis. Blood Rev. 2024;66: 101207.

New Frontiers and Evolving Therapies in ATTR Cardiac Amyloidosis

Abdirahman Wardhere, Dimitrios Bampatsias, and Mathew S. Maurer

Abstract In the past decade, treatment of transthyretin cardiomyopathy (ATTR-CM) has been revolutionized mainly due to the deepened understanding of the cellular biology of the disease. Intervening in TTR synthesis, by gene editing or RNA silencing, TTR tetramer stabilization and TTR amyloid removal from tissues could all serve as therapeutic targets. There are now three FDA approved disease modifying therapies for ATTR-CM. These therapies targeting different mechanisms in the pathophysiology of ATTR-CM provide new alternatives for treating the disease. This chapter will discuss available and investigational therapies, their mechanism of action, indications, evidence for their efficacy, and safety profile. Finally, this chapter will summarize all major completed and ongoing trials for the treatment of ATTR-CM.

Keywords Transthyretin cardiomyopathy · Disease modifying therapies · Indications · Safety profile

Background

The treatment landscape for transthyretin cardiac amyloidosis (ATTR-CM) has undergone a remarkable transformation over the past decade [1]. This triumph in the management of ATTR-CM stems from a deepened biological understanding of the disease's underlying pathophysiology. This newfound knowledge has paved the way for the development of various disease-modifying therapies aimed at targeting various pathophysiologic pathways of ATTR amyloidosis [2]. The emerging therapies have not only expanded the treatment armamentarium but have also demonstrated meaningful effects on both the quality and quantity of affected individuals' lives [1].

A. Wardhere · D. Bampatsias · M. S. Maurer (✉)
Cardiac Amyloidosis Program, Department of Cardiology, Columbia University Irving Medical Center, New York Presbyterian Hospital, New York, NY, USA
e-mail: msm10@cumc.columbia.edu

E. Herzog (ed.), *Cardiac Amyloidosis*, https://doi.org/10.1007/978-3-031-88342-2_15

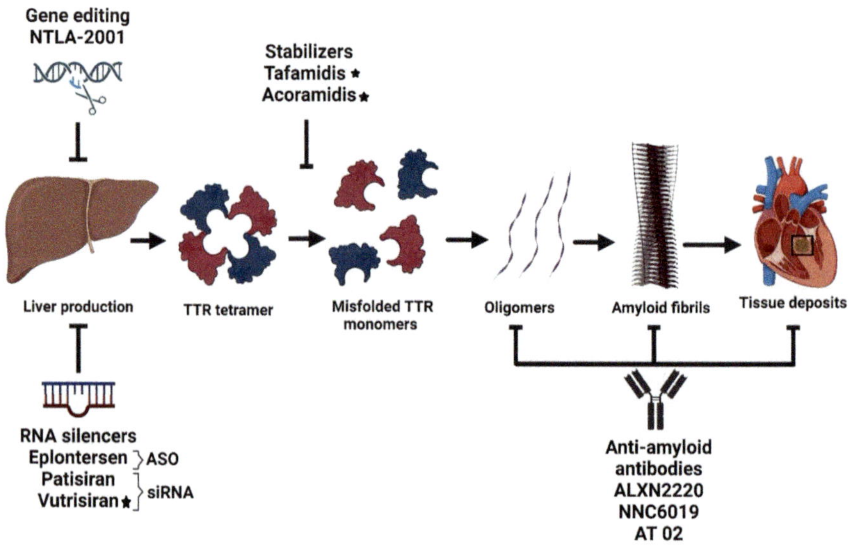

Fig. 1 An illustration of different targets of TTR amyloidosis approved and investigational therapies. Adapted from a review article on ATTR-CM treatment [5]

Therapeutics Targets

Clinical and investigational therapies for ATTR amyloidosis target one of three pathways in the pathophysiology including (1) silencing/knocking down production of the ATTR protein, (2) stabilization of the TTR tetramer, or (3) disruption or extraction of the ATTR amyloid fibrils, termed anti-fibrillar or anti-amyloid therapies [3] (Fig. 1). Approved therapies have different indications based on the specific phenotype and genotype of ATTR amyloidosis [4] (Fig. 2). There are currently three FDA-approved therapies for the treatment of ATTR-CM: 2 stablizers (tafamidis and acoramidis) and a silencer (vutrisiran).

ATTR Tetramer Stabilizers

Tafamidis. Tafamidis is a TTR tetramer stabilizing compound that binds with high affinity to the thyroxine binding site of TTR, raising the threshold for kinetic destabilization into monomers and oligomers that ultimately form amyloid fibrils [2]. Tafamidis is commercially available as tafamidis meglumine (20 mg) [Vyndaqel], and as tafamidis free salt (61 mg) [Vyndamax].

In the 2018 randomized controlled ATTR-ACT trial assessing patients with wild-type (ATTRwt) and variant (ATTRv) transthyretin amyloid cardiomyopathy, tafamidis meglumine (administered at doses of 20 mg or 80 mg) was compared

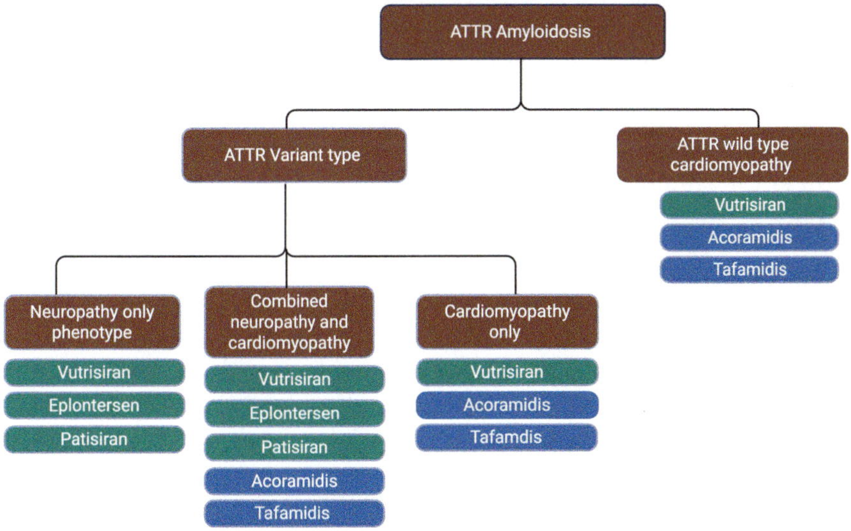

Fig. 2 A flow chart demonstrating indications of different disease modifying therapies for ATTR-CM. Brown color are the stabilizers, and green colors represent the silencers

against a placebo control [6]. The primary hierarchical endpoint, comprising first all-cause mortality and subsequently rates of cardiovascular hospitalizations, was evaluated utilizing the Finkelstein–Schoenfeld method. Results demonstrated a statistically significant "win ratio" favoring tafamidis over placebo, with a ratio of 1.70 (P = 0.0006). More traditional analysis using Kaplan–Meier time-to-event analysis revealed a 30% reduction in the hazard for all-cause mortality and a 32% reduction in the hazard for cardiovascular hospitalization among patients randomized to tafamidis (both 20 mg and 80 mg doses were pooled for the primary analysis) compared to those receiving placebo. Furthermore, tafamidis resulted in a slowing of the decline in 6-min walk test (6-MWT) distances and Kansas City Cardiomyopathy Questionnaire (KCCQ) scores compared to placebo. The benefits of tafamidis were particularly pronounced in early-stage disease, as evidenced by a higher rate of CV hospitalizations among patients with NYHA class III symptoms on placebo [4]. This was thought to be due to the longer survival in patients with more advanced disease who were then more susceptible to CV hospitalizations. A survival benefit in NYHA Class III participants was confirmed by results from the long-term extension of ATTR-ACT trial [7]. Furthermore, tafamidis demonstrated a favorable safety profile, with adverse effects such as diarrhea and constipation being predominantly mild to moderate in severity [8–10]. The high cost of tafamidis remains a significant barrier to widespread access, both domestically and globally, notwithstanding assistance programs aimed at mitigating this limitation [8, 9, 11].

Acoramidis. Acoramidis is another TTR stabilizer which binds to a different site on TTR compared to tafamidis. It mimics the TTR stabilization achieved by the Thr119Met mutation leading to stabilization of the TTR tetramer in the context of a destabilizing variant, such as Val30Met[10]. Experimental evidence suggests that acoramidis exhibits greater TTR stabilization in vitro compared to tafamidis [12, 13]. Administered at a dose of 712 mg twice daily for 30 months, acoramidis demonstrated superiority over placebo in ATTRibute-CM trial by reducing the combined hierarchical endpoint of mortality, CV hospitalizations, NT-proBNP change, and 6-MWT distance, with a win ratio of (1.8 95% CI: 1.4–2.2) [14]. Moreover, acoramidis significantly slowed the decline in quality of life, as evidenced by a mean difference of 9.94 points in the KCCQ score compared to placebo at 30 months. However, the reduction in all-cause mortality did not reach statistical significance, with an absolute reduction of 6.4% compared to placebo. Acoramidis demonstrated a 50% reduction in CV hospitalizations, from 42.6% to 26.7%. The survival rates in the placebo group of ATTRibute-CM trial were higher (74.3%) than those in the active treatment arm of the ATTR-ACT trial (70.5%), which reflected a shift toward early-stage disease [15, 16]. The differences in the participants in the two trials likely account for the differences in survival and CV hospitalizations, as early-stage patients are less likely to suffer a morbid event and are at greater risk for CV hospitalization. Acoramidis and placebo had a similar safety profile and favored acoramidis with respect to serious adverse events (54.6% and 64.9%, respectively). Despite experimental evidence suggesting greater ATTR stabilization by acoramidis compared to tafamidis, there is currently no randomized head-to-head trial available comparing the efficacy of tafamidis versus acoramidis. Acoramidis was FDA-approved for the treatment of ATTR-CM and is now commercially available as Attruby 356 mg tablets.

Silencers of the TTR Gene

Patisiran. Patisiran is a small double-stranded siRNA encapsulated within a lipid nanoparticle and serves as a potent agent for targeting the 3′ untranslated region of TTR messenger RNA (mRNA). This targeted approach promotes the cleavage of TTR mRNA, effectively reducing the production of amyloidogenic TTR protein [17, 18]. The APOLLO-A trial showed the efficacy of patisiran in patients with polyneuropathy due to transthyretin variant type (ATTRv-PN), regardless of concomitant cardiomyopathy [19]. In this trial, patisiran demonstrated significant benefits over placebo, as evidenced by an 18-month difference in modified Neurological Impairment Score plus 7 (mNIS + 7) of $-$ 6.0 $\pm$ 1.7 versus 28.0 $\pm$ 2.6 for placebo ($p < 0.001$). Post-hoc analyses within the cardiac subpopulation revealed additional benefits, including stable global longitudinal strain (GLS), reduced left ventricular (LV) wall thickness, and a notable reduction in NT-proBNP levels [20]. Moreover, pressure–volume loop analysis indicated sustained stroke volume attributed to preserved LV capacitance [21].

In the APOLLO-B trial, which enrolled 360 patients with ATTR-CM, patisiran demonstrated efficacy in maintaining functional capacity and improving quality of life [22]. Although the composite endpoint was not met due to the short-term nature of the study and the early stage of disease, patients treated with patisiran maintained their 6-MWT distance and had stable KCCQ score compared to placebo. Despite meeting the primary and secondary endpoints, patisiran did not receive FDA approval due to perceived lack of clinical meaningfulness in primary and secondary outcomes. Specifically, the reported changes in 6-MWT distance (14.69 m) and KCCQ) score (3.7 points) did not meet the minimal clinically important difference thresholds of approximately 33 m and 5 points, respectively [23]. However, long-term extension of the APOLLO-B trial has shown promising trends in slowing disease progression and preserving functional capacity [24]. These findings demonstrate that what patients with amyloidosis lose, they do not recover, emphasizing the importance of early recognition and institution of disease modifying therapy. Drug-related adverse events with patisiran include infusion-related reactions, arthralgia, and muscle spasm. The promising results of the APOLLO-B study which occurred over only 12 months, provided hope that that a larger and longer-term study of TTR silencing therapy is likely to be beneficial.

Vutrisiran. Vutrisiran is another siRNA therapy which targets hepatic production of ATTR mRNA by leveraging a unique biochemical design. It is conjugated to N-acetylgalactosamine (GalNAc) ligand, enhancing its hepatic-specific uptake, and thereby facilitating potent suppression of ATTR expression [17, 25]. This targeted approach ensures increased potency and metabolic stability, enabling a dosing interval of 25 mg administered subcutaneously every three months. The HELIOS-A trial demonstrated the efficacy of vutrisiran in treating ATTRv-PN [26]. In that study, vutrisiran showed a statistically significant reduction in mNIS + 7 at month 9 compared to a historical placebo group derived from the APOLLO-A trial. Furthermore, an exploratory sub-analysis highlighted vutrisiran's favorable impact on cardiac parameters, including NT-proBNP levels, cardiac output, and left ventricular (LV) stroke volume [27]. Notably, vutrisiran also demonstrated a reduction in cardiac technetium-99m-pyrophosphate (99mTc-PYP) uptake.

The HELIOS-B trial [28] evaluated the cardiac efficacy and safety of vutrisiran in patients with ATTR-CM. A total of 655 patients were randomized in a 1:1 ratio to receive either vutrisiran or placebo, with follow-up over 42 months. At baseline, 40% of the cohort was also receiving tafamidis. The primary outcome, which included all-cause death or recurrent cardiovascular events, demonstrated that vutrisiran significantly reduced the risk of these outcomes compared to placebo (HR = 0.72; 95% CI, 0.56–0.93; P = 0.01). Additionally, patients treated with vutrisiran experienced less decline in their 6-min walk test performance, with a least-squares mean difference of 26.5 m (95% CI, 13.4–39.6; P < 0.001), and showed a smaller reduction in their Kansas City Cardiomyopathy Questionnaire Overall Summary (KCCQ-OS) score, with a least-squares mean difference of 5.8 points (95% CI, 2.4–9.2; P < 0.001). Adverse events were similar between the vutrisiran and placebo groups, and there was no significant difference in serious adverse events. In the context of this study, vutrisiran provides another alternative in the treatment of ATTR-CM and might offer clinical benefits specially for patients with mixed phenotype who have both ATTR-CM and ATTR-PN. Based on the results of the Helios-B trial, vutrisiran got FDA approval for the treatment of ATTR-CM and is now commercially available as Amvuttra, 25 mcg subcutaneous injections.

Eplontersen. Eplontersen is an antisense oligonucleotide (ASO), which has a similar design and sequence to inotersen but is conjugated to a GalNAc ligand to enhance liver uptake [25]. This conjugation allows for subcutaneous administration at a dose of 45 mg, administered less frequently compared to inotersen, with dosing intervals extended to once every month. In the NEURO-TTRansform study, eplontersen demonstrated significant efficacy in reducing serum transthyretin concentration, mitigating neuropathy impairment, and improving quality of life [29]. Notably, in a post-hoc analysis focusing on the cardiac subpopulation, eplontersen treatment was associated with improvements in left ventricular ejection fraction (LVEF) and stroke volume compared to historical placebo group [30]. Other markers of cardiac structure and function, including NT-proBNP, remained stable, suggesting potential benefits in cardiac function. Further evidence from a study including patients with cardiac involvement from the NEURO-TTRansform study revealed that eplontersen treatment was associated with reduced uptake in 99mTc-PYP scan after a median follow-up of 544 days [31].

The ongoing CARDIO-TTRansform trial will evaluate the efficacy and safety of eplontersen in a larger cohort of > 1400 participants [32]. Participants receive eplontersen or placebo in a 1:1 ratio every 4 weeks for up to 140 weeks (about 2 and a half years), with the primary endpoint being a composite of cardiovascular mortality and recurrent cardiovascular clinical events. Anticipated to report results in 2026, this trial holds promise in further elucidating the therapeutic potential of eplontersen in managing ATTR-CM and for elucidating if combination therapy with a silencer and a stabilizer is beneficial on hard outcomes.

Gene Editing with CRISPR/Cas9

NTLA-2001 represents a potential alternative to traditional TTR mRNA silencing therapies, utilizing clustered regularly interspaced short palindromic repeats and associated Cas9 endonuclease (CRISPR-Cas9) technology for in vivo gene editing. Administered via a single-dose intravenous infusion, NTLA-2001 targets the TTR gene in hepatocytes, resulting in reduced production of both wild-type and mutant TTR [33]. A recently published phase 1 trial showed that a single infusion of Nexiguran Ziclumeran (Nex-Z) resulted in an 89% reduction in serum TTR at 28 days (95% CI, −92 to −87) and 90% at 12 months (95% CI, −93 to −87). Adverse events occurred in 94% of participants (34/36), including 14 serious events and 5 infusion-related reactions; one patient died from ischemic heart disease, unrelated to treatment. Secondary outcomes showed a geometric mean NT-proBNP change of 1.02 (95% CI, 0.88 to 1.17), troponin T change of 0.95 (95% CI, 0.89 to 1.01), median 5 m increase in 6MWD, and 61% had ≥ 5-point KCCQ improvement; 92% had stable or improved NYHA class [34]. The MAGNITUDE trial, is an ongoing Phase 3 study of NTLA-2001 in patients with ATTR-CM, which aims to enroll 765 participants and randomize them in a 2:1 ratio to receive NTLA-2001 or placebo

[35]. The primary endpoint is a composite of cardiovascular mortality and cardiovascular events, with secondary endpoints including changes in ATTR levels and KCCQ score at 18 months. Notably, patients who are already treated with silencers will be excluded from the study.

Anti-amyloid Therapy

Two monoclonal antibodies, NNC6019 (formerly PRX004) and ALXN2220 (formerly NI006), have shown promise in phase 1 clinical trials and are currently in phase 2 and 3 trials, respectively. ALXN2220, a recombinant human anti-ATTR monoclonal IgG1 antibody, selectively binds to ATTR amyloid deposits, demonstrating safety and efficacy in reducing cardiac scintigraphy tracer uptake and extracellular volume on cardiac MRI in patients with ATTR-CM [36]. The ongoing phase 3 trial, DepleTTR-CM, will evaluate its efficacy and safety in a larger cohort of 1000 patients with ATTR-CM. NNC6019 (Coramitug), designed to clear existing deposits and prevent new fibril formation, is undergoing evaluation in a placebo-controlled double-blind Phase 2 trial in patients with ATTR-CM. The primary outcomes include changes from baseline in 6-MWT and NT-proBNP levels at 52 weeks [37, 38].

AT-02, a fusion of an amyloid-targeting peptide called pan-amyloid removal (PAR) peptide with an IgG1 antibody, is being evaluated in a phase 2 trial in patients with systemic amyloidosis of any type [39]. The trial aims to assess the long-term safety and efficacy of AT-02 for up to 120 weeks.

Conclusion

The therapeutic landscape for ATTR-CM is undergoing rapid evolution, with a high likelihood of additional treatment options emerging soon, offering patients multiple effective choices. Ongoing and future studies need to address existing knowledge gaps, and proactive advocacy from clinicians across all levels can help bridge the disparity between optimal medical therapies for ATTR-CM and patients' ability to access them affordably (Tables 1, 2 and 3).

Table 1 Results of phase 3 landmark studies for stabilizers

Drug Study Year	Study design	Sample size	Randomization assignment	Follow up (months)	Primary endpoints	Dosing	Side-effects	Pre-treatment	Concomitant treatment	Cost
Tafamidis ATTR-ACT 2018 [5]	Randomized, Double-blind, Placebo-controlled Phase 3	441 patients with ATTR-CM	2:2:1 ratio for 80 mg, 20 mg tafamidis meglumine and placebo	30 months	Reduced mortality risk compared to placebo (HR = 0.7) Reduced hospitalization risk (RR = 0.68) compared to placebo	Vyndamax 61 mg orally once daily Vyndaqel 80 mg orally once daily	No significant difference compared to placebo	None	None	$268,000/y
Acoramidis ATTRibute-CM 2023 [13]	Randomized, Double-blind, Placebo-controlled Phase 3	632 patients with ATTR-CM	2:1 ratio to acoramidis or placebo	30 months	Acoramidis treatment was superior to placebo (Win ratio = 1.8, 95%CI: 1.4–2.2) in a hierarchical endpoint of death, CVRH, NT-proBNP and 6-MWT change	800 mg orally twice daily	No significant difference compared to placebo	None	None	$244,000/y

Abbreviations: *ATTR-CM* transthyretin amyloidosis cardiomyopathy, *ATTRv* variant ATTR, *HR* hazard ratio, *RR* relative risk, *CVRH* cardiovascular related hospitalizations, *NT-proBNP* N-terminal pro B natriuretic peptide, *6-MWT* Six minute walk test, *IV* intravenous, *GLS* global longitudinal strain, *LVWT* left ventricle wall thickness, *LVEDV* left ventricle end-diastolic volume, *KCCQ-OS* Kansas City Cardiomyopathy Questionnaire Overall Score, *AEs* adverse events, *N/A* non-available, *LVEF* left ventricle ejection fraction, *CV* cardiovascular, *OLE* open label extension, *ECV* extracellular volume, *NIS* neuropathy impairment score, *KCCQ-CSS* Kansas City Cardiomyopathy Questionnaire-Clinical Summary Score, *CRISPR-Cas-9* clustered regularly interspaced short palindromic repeats and associated Cas9 endonuclease

Table 2 Completed and ongoing trials of silencers

Drug Study name Year published	Study design	Sample size	Randomization assignment	Follow up (months)	Primary endpoints	Dosing	Side-effects	Pre-treatment	Concomitant treatment	Cost
Patisiran APOLLO-A 2018 [19]	Randomized, Double-blind, Placebo-controlled Phase 3	126 ATTRv with cardiac involvement patients	90 on patisiran 36 on placebo	18 months	Improved GLS (Mean difference 1.4%) Reduced LVWT (Mean difference − 0.9 mm) Increased LVEDV (Mean difference 8.3 mL)	IV administration every 3 weeks 0.3 mg/kg, up to 30 mg	Mild or moderate in severity, including peripheral edema and infusion-related reactions	Premedication: IV corticosteroid (dexamethasone, 10 mg, or equivalent) Oral acetaminophen IV or oral H1 blocker IV or oral H2 blocker Daily	Daily Vitamin A supplement	$450,000/y
Patisiran APOLLO-B 2023 [22]	Randomized, Double-blind, Placebo-controlled Phase 3	360 patients with ATTR-CM	181 on patisiran 179 on placebo	12 months	Preserved functional capacity and quality of life (median difference of 14.47 m in 6MWT and 3.7 points in KCCQ-OS) compared to placebo at 12 months	IV administration every 3 weeks 0.3 mg/kg, up to 30 mg	Mild or moderate in severity, including infusion-related reactions, [(19%), 5% led to infusion interruption] arthralgia, and muscle spasms	Premedication: IV corticosteroid (dexamethasone, 10 mg, or equivalent) Oral acetaminophen IV or oral H1 blocker IV or oral H2 blocker	Daily Vitamin A supplement	$450,000/y for ATTRv with or without cardiomyopathy Not approved for ATTR-CM

(continued)

Table 2 (continued)

Drug Study name Year published	Study design	Sample size	Randomization assignment	Follow up (months)	Primary endpoints	Dosing	Side-effects	Pre-treatment	Concomitant treatment	Cost
Vutisiran HELIOS-A 2018 [26]	Open label, Phase 3	122 patients with ATTRv-PN received vutrisiran and were compared to 77 external placebo controls from APOLLO study and 42 controls on patisiran	3:1 ratio to vutrisiran or external placebo controls from APOLLO-A study	18 months	Vutrisiran treatment reduced the progression of neurologic impairment (modified NIS + 7 difference: 17 points), preserved quality of life (16.2-point difference in Norfolk QOL-DN score) at 9 months	25 mg subcutaneous every 3 months	Mild Adverse events include nasopharyngitis, headache, arthralgias, and injection-site reaction	None	Daily Vitamin A supplement	$572,884/y

(continued)

Table 2 (continued)

Drug Study name Year published	Study design	Sample size	Randomization assignment	Follow up (months)	Primary endpoints	Dosing	Side-effects	Pre-treatment	Concomitant treatment	Cost
Eplontersen NEURO-TTRansform 2023 [29]	Open label Phase 3	79 ATTRv with cardiac involvement patients	49 on eplontersen to 30 from historical placebo arm from a prior NEURO-TTR trial	65 weeks	At week 65, eplontersan caused significant reduction in serum transthyretin, difference: 70% eplontersen reduced neurological progression modified NIS + 7 difference: 24.8) and preserved quality of life, 20 points differences for Norfolk QoL-DN score Post-hoc analysis: 4.9% change in LVEF 10.64 mL change in stroke volume	45 mg subcutaneous injection every 4 weeks	Mild or moderate in severity including diarrhea, urinary tract infection, vitamin A deficiency, and nausea	None	Daily Vitamin A supplement	$525,564/y

(continued)

Table 2 (continued)

Drug Study name Year published	Study design	Sample size	Randomization assignment	Follow up (months)	Primary endpoints	Dosing	Side-effects	Pre-treatment	Concomitant treatment	Cost
Vutisiran HELIOS-B 2024 [28]	Randomized, Double-blind, Placebo-controlled Phase 3	655 patients with ATTR-CM	1:1 ratio to vutrisiran or placebo	36 months	At 42 weeks, Vutrisiran led to 28% reduction in the risk of developing composite endpoint including all-cause mortality or recurrent cardiovascular events. Vutrisiran also led to less decline in the 6-MWT and KCCQ-OS	25 mg subcutaneous every 3 months	Mild Adverse events include nasopharyngitis, headache, arthralgias, and injection-site reaction	None	Daily Vitamin A supplement	$477,404/y
Eplontersen CARDIO-TTRansform [32]*	Randomized, Double-blind, Placebo-controlled Phase 3	>1400 patients with ATTR-CM	1:1 ratio to eplontersen or placebo	140 weeks	Primary endpoint: Composite outcome of CV Mortality and frequency of CV clinical events at Week 120 Secondary endpoint: Change from Baseline on the 6-MWT at Week 61	45 mg subcutaneous injection every 4 weeks	N/A	None	Daily Vitamin A supplement	Unknown

Abbreviations: *ATTR-CM* transthyretin amyloidosis cardiomyopathy, *ATTRv* variant ATTR, *HR* hazard ratio, *RR* relative risk, *CVRH* cardiovascular related hospitalizations, *Nt-proBNP* N-terminal pro B natriuretic peptide, *6-MWT* Six minute walk test, *IV* intravenous, *GLS* global longitudinal strain, *LVWT* left ventricle wall thickness, *LVEDV* left ventricle end-diastolic volume, *KCCQ-OS* Kansas City Cardiomyopathy Questionnaire Overall Score, *AEs* adverse events, *N/A* non-available, *LVEF* left ventricle ejection fraction, *CV* cardiovascular, *OLE* open label extension, *ECV* extracellular volume, *NIS* neuropathy impairment score, *KCCQ-CSS* Kansas City Cardiomyopathy Questionnaire-Clinical Summary Score. * Indicates the ongoing trials

Table 3 Ongoing gene editing and anti-amyloid trials

Drug	Study design	Sample size	Randomization assignment	Follow up (months)	Dosing	Primary endpoints	Side-effects	Pre-treatment	Concomitant treatment
Anti-fibrillar/anti-amyloid therapies									
ALXN2220/NI006 [40]	Randomized, Double-blind, Placebo-controlled, Phase 3	1000 patients with ATTR-CM	2:1 ratio to NI006 versus placebo	4 months placebo controlled followed by 8 months of open label extension	Intravenous every 4 weeks	Primary endpoint: Composite endpoint of all-cause mortality and CV-event frequency	Mild arthralgias and arthritis, transient decrease in platelet count. Two cases of cytokine release syndrome of mile severity were reported in the treatment group	Corticosteroids, Antihistamine, Acetaminophen may be administered in subjects with infusion related reactions, based on institutional protocols	N/A

(continued)

Table 3 (continued)

Drug	Study design	Sample size	Randomization assignment	Follow up (months)	Dosing	Primary endpoints	Side-effects	Pre-treatment	Concomitant treatment
NNC6019-0001 (Coramitug) [38]	Phase 2, randomized, double-blind, placebo controlled	99 patients with ATTR-CM	2:1 ratio to NNC6019-0001 versus placebo	Up to 64 weeks	N/A	Primary: Change in 6-MWT and NT-proBNP Secondary: Changes in ECV, KCCQ-CSS, NIS, GLS, Troponin I, safety, mortality, CV events	N/A	N/A	N/A
AT-02 [39]	Open-label extension study, Phase 2		120 patients with any type of systemic amyloidosis	120 weeks	Dose not determined yet	Primary outcome: Incidence, frequency, and severity of adverse event, safety, and tolerability of AT-02	N/A	Corticosteroids	N/A

(continued)

Table 3 (continued)

Drug	Study design	Sample size	Randomization assignment	Follow up (months)	Dosing	Primary endpoints	Side-effects	Pre-treatment	Concomitant treatment
Gene editing by CRISPR-Cas-9 technology									
NTLA-2001 or Nexiguran Ziclumeran (Nex-Z) [34]	Phase 1 open label trial	36 patients	N/A	At least 12 months	A single intravenous infusion of Nex-Z	Primary outcome: 89% reduction in serum TTR at 28 days and 90% at 12 months. Secondary outcomes: At 12 months, no significant changes of NT-proBNP and hs-cTnT levels were noted. Median 6-MWT increased by 5 meters, and 92% of patients had stable or improved NYHA class.	Mild transient infusion-related reactions, and transient liver-enzyme elevations.	Oral dexamethasone 8 mg or equivalent administered between 8 and 24 hours before the infusion of Nex-Z and one dose each of a glucocorticoid, an H1 receptor antagonist, and an H2 receptor antagonist administered approximately 1 hour before the infusion	Daily Vitamin A supplement
NTLA-2001 [35] MAGNITUDE	Phase 3 Randomized	765 patients with ATTR (36 ATTR-PN, 29 ATTR-CM)	NA	28 days	Single IV dose 0.1 mg/kg	Primary outcome: Composite endpoint of death and CV events Secondary: Change in serum TTR and KCCQ-OS score at 18 months	Mild severity infusion related reactions. Transient increase in d-dimers and liver enzymes	Oral dexamethasone 8 to 24 h before administration of study intervention Dexamethasone, antihistamines, and acetaminophen 1 to 2 h before the infusion	Daily Vitamin A supplement

Abbreviations: *ATTR-CM* transthyretin amyloidosis cardiomyopathy, *NT-proBNP* N-terminal pro B natriuretic peptide, *CRISPR-Cas-9* clustered regularly interspaced short palindromic repeats and associated Cas9 endonuclease

References

1. Griffin JM, Rosenthal JL, Grodin JL, et al. ATTR amyloidosis: current and emerging management strategies. JACC CardioOncol. 2021;3(4):488–505.
2. Maurer MS, Mann DL. The tafamidis drug development program: a translational triumph. JACC Basic Transl Sci. 2018;3(6):871–3.
3. Maurer MS. Overview of current and emerging therapies for amyloid transthyretin cardiomyopathy. Am J Cardiol. 2022;185(Suppl 1):S23-s34.
4. Addison D, Slivnick JA, Campbell CM, et al. Recent advances and current dilemmas in the diagnosis and management of transthyretin cardiac amyloidosis. J Am Heart Assoc. 2021;10(9): e019840.
5. Bampatsias D, Wardhere A, Maurer MS. Treatment of transthyretin cardiac amyloidosis. Curr Opin Cardiol. 2024 Apr 22.
6. Maurer MS, Schwartz JH, Gundapaneni B, et al. Tafamidis treatment for patients with transthyretin amyloid cardiomyopathy. N Engl J Med. 2018;379(11):1007–16.
7. Elliott P, Gundapaneni B, Sultan MB, et al. Improved long-term survival with tafamidis treatment in patients with transthyretin amyloid cardiomyopathy and severe heart failure symptoms. Eur J Heart Fail. 2023;25(11):2060–4.
8. Kazi DS, Bellows BK, Baron SJ, et al. Cost-effectiveness of tafamidis therapy for transthyretin amyloid cardiomyopathy. Circulation. 2020;141(15):1214–24.
9. Gurwitz JH, Maurer MS. Tafamidis-A pricey therapy for a not-so-rare condition. JAMA Cardiol. 2020;5(3):247–8.
10. Wardhere A, Bampatsias D, Fine N, et al. Heterogeneous worldwide access and pricing of Tafamidis. Amyloid. 2024;31(1):73–5.
11. Hammarström P, Schneider F, Kelly JW. Trans-suppression of misfolding in an amyloid disease. Science. 2001;293(5539):2459–62.
12. Miller M, Pal A, Albusairi W, et al. Enthalpy-driven stabilization of transthyretin by AG10 mimics a naturally occurring genetic variant that protects from transthyretin amyloidosis. J Med Chem. 2018;61(17):7862–76.
13. Zhou S, Ge S, Zhang W, et al. Conventional molecular dynamics and metadynamics simulation studies of the binding and unbinding mechanism of TTR stabilizers AG10 and tafamidis. ACS Chem Neurosci. 2020;11(19):3025–35.
14. Gillmore JD, Judge DP, Cappelli F, et al. Efficacy and safety of acoramidis in transthyretin amyloid cardiomyopathy. N Engl J Med. 2024;390(2):132–42.
15. Ioannou A, Patel RK, Razvi Y, et al. Impact of earlier diagnosis in cardiac ATTR amyloidosis over the course of 20 years. Circulation. 2022;146(22):1657–70.
16. Chan N, Teruya S, Mirabal A, et al. Temporal outcomes of patients diagnosed with transthyretin cardiac amyloidosis. J Card Fail. 2024.
17. Aimo A, Castiglione V, Rapezzi C, et al. RNA-targeting and gene editing therapies for transthyretin amyloidosis. Nat Rev Cardiol. 2022;19(10):655–67.
18. Ioannou A, Fontana M, Gillmore JD. RNA targeting and gene editing strategies for transthyretin amyloidosis. BioDrugs. 2023;37(2):127–42.
19. Adams D, Gonzalez-Duarte A, O'Riordan WD, et al. Patisiran, an RNAi therapeutic, for hereditary transthyretin amyloidosis. N Engl J Med. 2018;379(1):11–21.
20. Solomon SD, Adams D, Kristen A, et al. Effects of Patisiran, an RNA interference therapeutic, on cardiac parameters in patients with hereditary transthyretin-mediated amyloidosis. Circulation. 2019;139(4):431–43.
21. Rosenblum HR, Griffin JM, Minamisawa M, et al. Effect of patisiran on stroke volume in hereditary transthyretin-mediated amyloidosis: insights from pressure-volume analysis of the APOLLO study. Eur J Heart Fail. 2023;25(5):727–36.
22. Maurer MS, Kale P, Fontana M, et al. Patisiran treatment in patients with transthyretin cardiac amyloidosis. N Engl J Med. 2023;389(17):1553–65.
23. Maurer MS, Gillmore JD. Patisiran in patients with transthyretin cardiac amyloidosis. Reply N Engl J Med. 2024;390(3):286–7.

24. Maurer MS, Berk JL, Hanna MA, et al. Primary results from APOLLO-B open-label extension study of Patisiran in patients with transthyretin cardiac amyloidosis. J Cardiac Failure. 2024;30(1):130–131.
25. Kim Y, Jo M, Schmidt J, et al. Enhanced potency of GalNAc-conjugated antisense oligonucleotides in hepatocellular cancer models. Mol Ther. 2019;27(9):1547–57.
26. Adams D, Tournev IL, Taylor MS, et al. Efficacy and safety of vutrisiran for patients with hereditary transthyretin-mediated amyloidosis with polyneuropathy: a randomized clinical trial. Amyloid. 2023;30(1):1–9.
27. Garcia-Pavia P, Grogan M, Kale P, et al. Impact of vutrisiran on exploratory cardiac parameters in hereditary transthyretin-mediated amyloidosis with polyneuropathy. Eur J Heart Fail. 2024;26(2):397–410.
28. Fontana M, Berk JL, Gillmore JD, et al. Vutrisiran in patients with transthyretin amyloidosis with cardiomyopathy. N Engl J Med. 2024;NEJMoa2409134.
29. Coelho T, Marques W Jr, Dasgupta NR, et al. Eplontersen for hereditary transthyretin amyloidosis with polyneuropathy. JAMA. 2023;330(15):1448–58.
30. Masri A, Maurer MS, Claggett BL, et al. Effect of eplontersen on cardiac structure and function in patients with hereditary transthyretin amyloidosis. J Card Fail. 2023.
31. Yu AL, Chen YC, Tsai CH, et al. Use of technetium-99m-pyrophosphate single-photon emission computed tomography/computed tomography in monitoring therapeutic changes of eplontersen in patients with hereditary transthyretin amyloid cardiomyopathy. J Am Heart Assoc. 2024;13(2): e030512.
32. CARDIO-TTRansform: a study to evaluate the efficacy and safety of eplontersen (formerly known as ION-682884, IONIS-TTR-LRx and AKCEA-TTR-LRx) in participants with transthyretin-mediated amyloid cardiomyopathy (ATTR CM)—full text view—ClinicalTrials.gov [Internet]. clinicaltrials.gov. Available from: https://classic.clinicaltrials.gov/ct2/show/NCT04136171.
33. Gillmore JD, Gane E, Taubel J, et al. CRISPR-Cas9 in vivo gene editing for transthyretin amyloidosis. N Engl J Med. 2021;385(6):493–502.
34. Fontana M, Solomon SD, Kachadourian J, et al. CRISPR-Cas9 gene editing with nexiguran ziclumeran for ATTR cardiomyopathy. N Engl J Med. 2024 Dec 12;391(23):2231–2241. https://doi.org/10.1056/NEJMoa2412309.
35. MAGNITUDE: a phase 3 study of NTLA-2001 in participants with transthyretin amyloidosis with cardiomyopathy (ATTR-CM)—full text view—ClinicalTrials.gov [Internet]. clinicaltrials.gov. Available from: https://classic.clinicaltrials.gov/ct2/show/NCT06128629.
36. Garcia-Pavia P, Aus dem Siepen F, Donal E, et al. Phase 1 Trial of antibody NI006 for depletion of cardiac transthyretin amyloid. N Engl J Med. 2023;389(3):239–250.
37. Galant NJ, Bugyei-Twum A, Rakhit R, et al. Substoichiometric inhibition of transthyretin misfolding by immune-targeting sparsely populated misfolding intermediates: a potential diagnostic and therapeutic for TTR amyloidoses. Sci Rep. 2016;28(6):25080.
38. Fontana M, Buchholtz K, Engelmann M, et al. NNC6019-0001, a humanized monoclonal antibody, in patients with transthyretin amyloid cardiomyopathy (ATTR-CM): rationale and study design of a phase 2, randomized, placebo-controlled trial [Internet]. Available from: https://academic.oup.com/eurheartj/article/43/Supplement_2/ehac544.1767/6745267.
39. Attralus, Inc., Novotech (Australia) Pty Limited. A Phase 2, open-label extension study to evaluate the long-term safety and tolerability of AT-02 [Internet]. clinicaltrials.gov. 2024. Available from: https://classic.clinicaltrials.gov/ct2/show/NCT05951049.
40. Alexion Pharmaceuticals, Inc. A Phase 3, randomized, double-blind, placebo-controlled, multicenter study to evaluate the efficacy and safety of amyloid depleter ALXN2220 in adult participants with transthyretin amyloid cardiomyopathy (ATTR-CM) [Internet]. clinicaltrials.gov. 2024. Available from: https://classic.clinicaltrials.gov/ct2/show/NCT06183931.

Treatment of Cardiac Amyloidosis—Disease Modifying Therapies in ATTR: Pharmacological Point of View

Bruria Hirsh-Raccah

Abstract Transthyretin amyloidosis (ATTR amyloidosis) is a progressive disease, ATTR amyloidosis can be treated specifically in three different mechanisms. The first mechanism stops of amyloidogenic TTR synthesis through various methods. Inotersen and Eplontersen are antisense oligonucleotide, which "silence" or block TTR protein synthesis, results in a decrease in TTR expression. Patisiran and Vutrisiran are RNA interference therapies targeting the gene encoding transthyretin (TTR) resulting in reduction the amount of mutant transthyretin that is synthesized by the liver. Clustered regularly interspaced short palindromic repeats (CRISPR or CRISPR-associated protein 9 (CRISPR Cas9) is technology of a gene editing that enable to modifies the genome sequence by produce base substitutions, insertion, or deletions in the genome. The second mechanism include medication that stabilized the TTR tetramer by binding to the T4-binding site on the TTR to prevent misfolding and deposition of monomers and oligomers. In phase III clinical trials, Tafamidis and Acoramidis have been shown to reduce cardiovascular-related hospitalizations. TTR stabilizers and silencers can prevent disease deterioration but do not improve advanced staged of ATTR CMs. Indeed, the third newly mechanism enhance protein misfolding removal. NI301A and PRX004 bind to specific epitope, located in misfolding monomers and oligomers but unexposed in TTR's naturally folded conformation, this enhance amyloid deposit removal through phagocytic cells specific monoclonal antibodies that directly enhance the clearance of toxic amyloid by stimulating their removal through phagocytic cells to improve organ function.

Keywords Antisense oligonucleotide · RNA interference therapies · Tetramer stabilizer · Gene editing · Protein misfolding removal

---

B. Hirsh-Raccah (✉)
Division of Clinical Pharmacy, Faculty of Medicine, School of Pharmacy, Institute for Drug Research, Hebrew University of Jerusalem, Jerusalem, Israel
e-mail: bruria.hirsh@mail.huji.ac.il

Department of Cardiology, Hadassah University Hospital, Jerusalem, Israel

E. Herzog (ed.), *Cardiac Amyloidosis*, https://doi.org/10.1007/978-3-031-88342-2_16

Transthyretin amyloidosis (ATTR amyloidosis) is a progressive disease characterized by the formation of fibrils composed of misfolded transthyretin (TTR) resulting from either dissociation of wild-type ATTR (ATTRwt) or mutations in the TTR gene called Hereditary or variant amyloidosis (ATTRv) [1].

ATTR amyloidosis can be treated specifically in three different mechanisms [2]:

1. stopping of amyloidogenic TTR synthesis
2. stabilizing the TTR tetramer
3. Protein misfolding removal.

According to a disease simulation model, early treatment extends mean life expectancy by 5.46 and 7.76 years, for ATTRwt and ATTRv respectively. Early treatment were also associated with improve quality of life (QoL) [3].

Stopping of Amyloidogenic TTR Synthesis

The use of those agents, which "silence" or block TTR protein synthesis, results in a decrease in TTR expression. ATTR-silencer approved for the treatment of patients with polyneuropathy involved ATTRv, either with or without cardiac disease. However, recently, the FDA approved Vutrisiran as the first ATTR-silencer specifically indicated for the treatment of ATTR cardiomyopathy.

Antisense Oligonucleotide (ASO)

Inotersen

Inotersen is a type of antisense oligonucleotide (ASO)-single-stranded deoxyribonucleotide strands that binds specifically to the target mRNA and block TTR protein production. Inotersen is weekly subcutaneous injections [4].

In phase-3 randomized, double-blind, placebo-controlled, inotersen was administered in adults with hereditary transthyretin amyloidosis with polyneuropathy. Although 63% of the patients had cardiomyopathy, patients with heart failure of New York Heart Association class III or higher were excluded. In the intervention period, neither tafamidis nor diflunisal were allowed. In this study, the primary endpoint was the change in the modified Neuropathy Impairment Score, and cardiac outcomes were not included [5].

To ensure adequate delivery of dietary vitamin A to tissues in the context of low transthyretin levels, all the patients received vitamin A supplements at the recommended daily allowance (approximately 3000 IU).

Inotersen treatment was associated with a 79% reduction in median serum transthyretin levels.

Change in Neuropathy Impairment Score were favor the inotersen group. However, after 15 months, echocardiographic variables such as global longitudinal strain did not differ significantly between the inotersen group and the placebo group.

All five deaths during the trial were occurred in the inotersen group include fatal intracranial hemorrhage in association with a platelet count of less than 10,000 cubic millimeters. The most common serious adverse events in the inotersen group were thrombocytopenia and glomerulonephritis, both occurring in 3% of patients. Nausea, pyrexia, chills, vomiting, anemia and lowered platelet counts were at least twice as high in the inotersen group as in the placebo group. In an open-label extension trial at 36 months patients treated with Inotersen maintained their quality of life (Tables 1 and 2) [6].

Eplontersen

Eplontersen is an investigational ligand-conjugated antisense oligonucleotide being investigated for patients with ATTRv polyneuropathy in the NEURO-TTRansform study.

The Eplontersen trial had similar design, demographic variables, and outcomes as the Inotersen trial. For this trial, the placebo group consists of patients treated with placebo in the inotersen trial with similar eligibility criteria and endpoints. Eplontersen was administered subcutaneously every 4 weeks at a dose of 45 mg to 144 patients. At baseline cardiomyopathy were diagnosed by echocardiography in 34% of the treatment group and 50% of the placebo group. However, patients with heart failure of New York Heart Association class III or higher were excluded. Patients used any approved drug for hereditary TTR amyloidosis were also exclude.

Eplontersen treatment was associated was associated with a significant reduction in serum transthyretin concentration (81.7% vs. 11.2%), less neuropathy impairment, and better quality of life in comparison to the historical placebo group.

Among eplontersen patients, 2 deaths were reported that were consistent with known disease-related sequelae (cardiac arrhythmia; intracerebral hemorrhage); none occurred among placebo recipients (Tables 1 and 2) [7].

The CARDIO-TTRansform is an ongoing study design to evaluate the efficacy and safety of eplontersen in about 1400 patients with transthyretin-mediated amyloid cardiomyopathy [8].

siRNA, Small Interfering RNA Therapies and Gene Editing

Patisiran

Patisiran is RNA interference therapies targeting the gene encoding transthyretin (TTR) resulting in reduction the amount of mutant transthyretin that is synthesized by the liver [9]. Patisiran trial was similar in design, demographic variables, and

Table 1 Clinical trials on therapies for amyloid transthyretin (ATTR):

	Study name	Study design	Population	Inclusion criteria	Primary outcomes	Secondary outcomes	Duration	Main results:
Antisense oligonucleotide (ASO)								
Inotersen		Phase 3 RCT	112 In the inotersen group and 60 in the placebo group	Adults with ATTRv amyloidosis with polyneuropathy	Change in the modified mNIS+7 and the change in the score on the patient-reported QOL-DN questionnaire		66 weeks	Inotersen improved the Norfolk QOL-DN score, glomerulonephritis and severe thrombocytopenia were observed in the inotersen group
Eplontersen	NEURO-TTRansform	Open-label, single-group, phase 3 trial	144 In the Eplontersen group and 60 in the historical placebo group	Adults with ATTRv amyloidosis with polyneuropathy	Changes from baseline in serum transthyretin concentration, mNIS+7 composite score, and Norfolk QoL-DN total score	Changes from baseline in neuropathy symptom and change total score3 at weeks 35 and 66, 36-Item Short Form Survey physical component summary score29 at week 65, PND score10 at week 65, and modified BMI 30 at week 65	65/66 weeks	Eplontersen reduce TTR, improved mNISþ7 score, mNIS+7 composite score and for Norfolk QoL-DN. overall incidence and types of adverse events were similar in the placebo and treatment groups execpt high frequency of vitamin D deficiency.
siRNA								
Patisiran	APOLLO study	Phase 3 RCT	148 To the patisiran group and 77 to the placebo group	Adults with ATTRv amyloidosis with polyneuropathy	Change from baseline in the mNIS+7 score	The Norfolk QOL-DN questionnaire, 10-m walk test, modified BMI	18 months	Patisiran improved the mean (±SD) baseline Norfolk QOL-DN score, gait speed and modified BMI, the overall incidence and types of adverse events were similar in the placebo and treatment groups.

(continued)

Table 1 (continued)

	Study name	Study design	Population	Inclusion criteria	Primary outcomes	Secondary outcomes	Duration	Main results:
	APOLLO - B study	Phase 3 RCT	181 to the patisiran group and 179 to the placebo group	Adults with ATTRv-or ATTRwt cardiac amyloidosis	Change from baseline in the distance covered on the 6-minute walk test at 12 months	KCCQ-OS scores composite of death from any cause, cardiovascular events, and change from baseline in the 6-minute walk test distance at 12 months	12 months	Patisiran had a lower decline in the 6-minute walk distance than placebo, no diffrence were observed for secondary composite end point
Vutrisiran	HELIOS-A	Phase 3, global, open-label study	164 in the Vutrisiran group and external placebo group (APOLLO study)	Adults with ATTRv amyloidosis with polyneuropathy	Change in mNIS+7	Change from baseline in QOL (total score on the Norfolk Quality of Life-Diabetic Neuropathy questionnaire [Norfolk QOL-DN]) at Month 9; gait speed (10-meter walk test [10-MWT]) at Month 9; mNISþ7 at Month 18; Norfolk QOL-DN total score at Month 18; 10-MWT at Month 18;nutritional status (modified body mass index [mBMI]) at Month 18; and disability (Rasch-built Overall Disability Scale [R-ODS] score) at Month 18. In addition, non-inferiority in serum TTR level percent reduction through Month 18 in the vutrisiran group compared with the within-study patisiran group	18 months	Vutrisiran reduce TTR, improved the mNISþ7 score , Norfolk Quality of Life-Diabetic Neuropathy, 10-meter walk test, modified BMI, and Rasch-built Overall Disability Scale.

(continued)

Table 1 (continued)

	Study name	Study design	Population	Inclusion criteria	Primary outcomes	Secondary outcomes	Duration	Main results:
	HELIOS-B	Phase 3, randomized, double-blind, placebo-controlled study	326 patients were assigned to receive vutrisiran and 329 to receive placebo	Patients with cardiomyopathy and ATTRv or ATTRwt amyloidosis	Composite of death from any cause and recurrent cardiovascular events	Death from any cause, change from baseline in the KCCQ-OS score and the change from baseline in the distance covered on the 6-minute walk test	11 months	Compare to placebo Vutrisiran significantly decreased mortality, cardiovascular events, markers of disease progression, decline in the KCCQ-OS score and in the distance covered on the 6-minute. The incidence of adverse events was similar in the two groups
CRISPR Cas9								
NTLA-2001		Phase1 clinical study	Six patients receive single dose of NTLA-2001	Adults with diagnosis of polyneuropathy due to ATTRv amyloidosis (with or without CM), without current treatments for ATTR amyloidosis.	Serum TTR concentration		24 months	NTLA-2001 was associated with durable knockout of TTR and dose depended reduction in serum TTR protein concentration
Nexiguran ziclumeran		Phase1 clinical study	36 Patients receive single dose	Patients with cardiomyopathy and ATTRv or ATTRwt amyloidosis	Serum TTR level and adverse drug reaction.	Changes in NT-proBNP, troponin T levels, the 6-minute walk distance, and the NYHA class	12 months	90% Reduction from baseline in serum transthyretin (TTR) levels. 92% of patients showed either improvement or no change in their NYHA class Adverse events included infusion-related reactions and transient elevations in AST levels.

(continued)

Table 1 (continued)

	Study name	Study design	Population	Inclusion criteria	Primary outcomes	Secondary outcomes	Duration	Main results:
ATTR stabilizers								
Diflunisal		Single-arm, open-label study	13 patients	Adults with ATTRv amyloidosis or ATTRwt-CM	Diabetic polyneuropathy metric and mNIS+7 score		11 months	There was no significant mean change in cardiac structure, function, or biomarkers during the study period. Glomerular filtration rate were decline by 6%.
		Single-arm, open-label study	40 patients	Adults with ATTRv amyloidosis	Ulnar and tibial nerve conduction velocities and compound muscle action potential amplitudes, clinical FAP score (Kumamoto score) serum TTR concentration, modified BMI, plasma BNP and echocardiographic parameters, including intraventricular septum thickness, left ventricular posterior wall thickness, and EF.		38 months	Diflunisal stabilized TTR tetramer structure. after 24 months of treatment, ulnar compound muscle action potential amplitude, cardiac wall thickness, and ejection fraction were not deteriorated. Deterioration of renal function and thrombocytopeniawedrded observed in three patients.

(continued)

Table 1 (continued)

	Study name	Study design	Population	Inclusion criteria	Primary outcomes	Secondary outcomes	Duration	Main results:
Tafamidis	ATTR-ACT Study	phase 3 RCT	264 Patients in the tafamidis group ,177 patients received placebo	Adults with ATTRv amyloidosis or ATTRwt-CM	Al-cause mortality, followed by frequency of cardiovascular-related hospitalizations	Change from baseline to month 30 for the 6-minute walk test and the score on the Kansas City Cardiomyopathy Questionnaire–Overall Summary (KCCQ-OS)	30 months	Tafamidis was associated with reductions in all-cause mortality and cardiovascular-related hospitalizations and improve 6-minute walk test and the score as compared with placebo. The incidence and types of adverse events were similar in the two groups.
Acoramidis	ATTRibute-CM	Phase 3 RCT	421 to the acoramidis group and 211 to the placebo group	Adults with diagnosis of ATTRv-CM or ATTRwt-CM	The four-step primary hierarchical analysis included death from any cause, cardiovascular-related hospitalization, the change from baseline in the NT-proBNP, level, and the change from baseline in the 6-minute walk distance	Death from any cause, the 6-minute walk distance, the score on the Kansas City Cardiomyopathy Questionnaire–Overall Summary, and the serum TTR level	30 months	Acoramidis was assosiated with improve in the four-step primary hierarchical analysis. Adverse events were similar in the two groups
Tolcapone		Phase IIa trial single arm	Seventeen patients	Adults with diagnosis of ATTRwt or ATTRv	TTR stabilization measured in plasma samples		24 hours	All participants in this study experienced TTR stabilization

(continued)

Table 1 (continued)

	Study name	Study design	Population	Inclusion criteria	Primary outcomes	Secondary outcomes	Duration	Main results:
Protein misfolding removal								
Doxycyclin + TUDCA		Phase II, open-label study	Seventeen patients	Adults with diagnosis of ATTRv-CM or ATTRwt-CM	Response rate: nonprogression of the cardiomyopathy and of the neuropathy score	Neuropathy score, quality of life (QoL), echocardiography and saftey parameters	12 months	No clinical progression of the cardiac status and the neuropathy score remained substantially stable over 1 year
		phase II	Twenty-eight patients	Adults with diagnosis of ATTRv-CM or ATTRwt-CM	Changes in s-pro-BNP and neuropathy score from baseline		18-months	There were no changes in pro-BNP and neuropathy score after 6 months of treatment but after 12 months it had increased significantly. High dropout rate from the study
NI006	NCT04360434.	Phase 1, double-blind trial	40 patients were randomized to receive either NI006 or placebo	Adults with diagnosis of ATTRv-CM or ATTRwt-CM	Saftey parametres, changes in ECGs, echocardiograms, cardiac telemetry, vital signs, and laboratory evaluations	Pharmacokinetic parameters	12 months	Improve surrogate markers of cardiac amyloid load (e.g. extracellular volume on cardiac magnetic resonance imaging and cardiac tracer uptake on scintigraphy) were observed. Troponin T and pro-B-type natriuretic peptide levels also appeared to have declined.
PRX004	NCT03336580	Phase 1 , open-label study	Seven patients	Adults with diagnosis of ATTRv-CM	Saftey parametres, changes in ECGs, echocardiograms, cardiac telemetry, vital signs, and laboratory evaluations	Pharmacokinetic parameters and immunogenicity indicators	9 mounths	All patients showed improvement in global longitudinal strains. Three of seven patients showed improvement in the mNIS+7 score from baseline. The study was terminated early because of the impact of COVID-19 pandemic

ATTRwt: Wild-type amyloidosis, ATTRv: Hereditary amyloidosis, mNIS+7: modified Neuropathy Impairment Score+7, QOL-DN: Norfolk Quality of Life–Diabetic Neuropathy, KCCQ-OS: Kansas City Cardiomyopathy Questionnaire–Overall Summary TTR: transthyretin, BMI: body mass index, Norfolk QOL-DN: Norfolk Quality of Life–Diabetic Neuropathy, PND: polyneuropathy disability, NT-proBNP: N-terminal pro–B-type natriuretic peptide, BNP: B-type natriuretic peptide, EF: ejection fraction

Table 2 Pharmacokinetic and pharmacodynamic characteristics of therapies for amyloid transthyretin (ATTR) amyloidosis

	Inotersen	Eplontersen	Patisiran	Vutrisiran	Diflunisal	Tafamidis
Indication	ATTRv	ATTRv	ATTRv, ATTRwt,	ATTRv	ATTRwt, ATTRv	ATTRwt, ATTRv
Mechanism of action	Antisense oligonucleotide (ASO)	Antisense oligonucleotide (ASO)	siRNA	siRNA	ATTR stabilizers	ATTR stabilizers
Route of administration	S.C	S.C	IV	S.C	P.O	P.O
Dosage	Three dose of 300 mg during the first week, followed by a once-weekly injection	45 mg every 4 weeks	0.3 mg per kilogram of body weight every 3 weeks over 80 min	25 mg every 3 months (Q3M)	250 BID or 500 OD	80 mg*1day
Serious adverse events	Thrombocytopenia and glomerulonephritis	Atrioventricular block	NR		Like other adverse effects reported with other non-steroidal anti-inflammatory agents: cardiovascular thrombotic events, renal failure, serious gastrointestinal adverse events including bleeding, ulceration, and perforation	NR
Other adverse events	Nausea, pyrexia, chills, vomiting, anemia and lowered platelet counts	Diarrhea, urinary tract infection, vitamin A deficiency, and nausea	Upper respiratory infection, peripheral edema, Infusion-related reaction	Dyspnoea, Arthralgia, Pain in extremity, Injection site reaction, An investigation into an increase in blood alkaline phosphatase is conducted	Like other adverse effects reported with other non-steroidal anti-inflammatory agents included: nausea, vomiting, dyspepsia, gastrointestinal pain, diarrhea, constipation, and flatulence	Diarrhea, rash, pruritus

(continued)

Table 2 (continued)

	Inotersen	Eplontersen	Patisiran	Vutrisiran	Diflunisal	Tafamidis
Drug interaction	Anti platelets, NSAIDs, anticoagulants: increased risk of bleeding	NR	NR	Vutrisiran is not expected to cause interactions or to be affected by inhibitors or inducers of cytochrome P450 enzymes	Diminish the antihypertensive effect of ACE-inhibitors and angiotensin II antagonists, antacids may reduce plasma levels of Diflunisal, increase in cyclosporine-induced toxicity, reduce the natriuretic effect of furosemide and thiazides, elevation of lithium and methotrexate plasma levels, prolongation of prothrombin time with vitamin K antagonist, anti platelets, increased risk of bleeding with NSAIDs, anticoagulants	May increased BCRP and UGT1A1 substrate exposure and an increased risk of the substrate-related toxicities (do not exceed a dose of rosuvastatin 20 mg once daily, Caution is needed when combining Tafmidiis and BCRP ubstrate such as: Imatinib, Irinotecan, Methotrexate, Ozanimod, Sulfasalazine, Tenofovir Alafenamide Tenofovir Alafenamide, Ubrogepant)
Renal impairment	Inotersen has not been studied in patients with CKD-EPI formula < 60 mL/min/1.73 m^2 at Screening	Severe renal impairment or end-stage renal disease: No specific recommendations for dosage adjustment are available	Patisiran has not been studied in patients with severe renal impairment or end-stage renal disease	Vutrisiran has not been studied in patients with severe renal impairment or end-stage renal disease	Diflunisal should not be used in patients with renal failure	Dosage adjustment in patients with renal impairment is considered not necessary

(continued)

Table 2 (continued)

	Acoramidis	Tolcapone	Doxycyclin + T/UDCA	NI006	PRX004
Indication	Acoramidis has not been studied in patients with end-stage renal disease (eGFR < 15 mL/min/1.73 m^2)	ATTRwt, ATTRv	ATTRwt, ATTRv	ATTRwt, ATTRv	ATTRv
Mechanism of action	ATTR stabilizers	ATTR stabilizers	Protein misfolding removal	Recombinant human anti-ATTR antibody	Recombinant human anti-ATTR antibody
Route of administration	P.O	P.O	P.O	IV	IV
Dosage	800 mg*2/day	200 mg*1/day or 100 mg*3/day	100 mg BID + 250 mg TID	10 mg/kg every 4 weeks	3 mg/kg once every 28 days
Serious adverse events	NR	Liver failure, Rhabdomyolysis	Stevens Johnson syndrome, hepatotoxicity, pseudotumor cerebri, esophagitis	Cytokine release syndrome, thrombocytopenia	NR
Other adverse events	Diarrhea, abdominal pain	Fatigue, Myalgia, Peripheral edema, Vertigo, Gastric disorder	Diarrhea, nausea	Arthralgias and arthritis	Fall, anaemia, upper respiratory tract infection, back pain, constipation, diarrhea, and insomnia
Drug interaction	May increased CYP2C9 substrate exposure (warfarin), Concomitant use of UGT inducers can potentially decrease acoramidis exposure (such as: rifampin, carbamazepine, Ritonavir, Phenytoin, Testosterone, Ethinylestradiol and Desogestrel,	CYP 2C9 inhibitor	Aluminum-based antacids, vitamin A, isotretinoin or tretinion	NR	NR
Renal impairment	Acoramidis has not been studied in patients with end-stage renal disease (eGFR < 15 mL/min/1.73 m^2)	Patients with severe renal impairment should be treated with caution	Dosage adjustment in patients with renal impairment is considered not necessary	NI006 has not been studied in patients with severe renal impairment or end-stage renal disease	PRX004 has not been studied in patients with estimated glomerular filtration rate (eGFR) below 45 mL/min/1.73 m^2

NR not reported, *NSAID's* non-steroidal anti-inflammatory agents, *TUDCA* tauroursodeoxycholic acid, *eGFR* estimated glomerular filtration rate outcome measures to Inotersen trial. However, there were differences in mode of administration (subcutaneous or intravenous) and treatment duration [9].

In phase-3 randomized, double-blind, placebo-controlled, Patisiran was administered in adults with hereditary transthyretin amyloidosis with polyneuropathy [10]. New York Heart Association class II were presented in 50% of the patients, patients with heart failure of New York Heart Association class III or higher were excluded [10]. Patients with previous liver transplantation or who were candidate to undergo liver transplantation during the trial period were also excluded. Among these patients, 53% had previously been treated with transthyretin tetramer stabilizers (tafamidis or diflunisal). There was an 81% reduction in median serum transthyretin levels after the Parisian treatment [10].

Parisian reduced neuropathy clinical manifestations measured by the modified Neuropathy Impairment Score + 7.Parisian improve quality of life and show better 10-m walk test compare to placebo [10].

The rate of severe and serious adverse events was similar in the two groups. Patients with patisiran experienced peripheral edema (30% vs. 22%) and reactions related to the infusion (19% vs. 9%) more often than those treated with placebo [10].

In open label extension study, at 12 months, patisiran treatment improved or sustained stability for patients in measures of quality of life, polyneuropathy, disability, autonomic function, and nutritional status compared with their treatment baseline values, while keeping an acceptable safety profile [11].

An assessment of patisiran's effects on cardiac structure and function was conducted in a subgroup of 126 patients (56% of total population) with evidence of cardiac amyloid involvement. At month 18, patisiran decreased mean left ventricular wall thickness (least-squares mean difference ± SEM: − 0.9 ± 0.4 mm, P = 0.017), global longitudinal strain (− 1.4 ± 0.6%, P = 0.015) and N-terminal prohormone of brain natriuretic peptide compared with placebo. Patisiran also increased cardiac output (0.38 ± 0.19 L/min, P = 0.044) and end-diastolic volume (8.3 ± 3.9 mL, P = 0.036) compared with placebo [12].

Parisian treatment related to approximates a reduction in event rate of ≈50% for all-cause hospitalization and mortality and ≈45% for cardiac hospitalization and all-cause mortality. The proportion of patients with cardiac adverse events was similar between the groups. The proportion of patients with cardiac arrhythmia was lower in the patisiran group (18.9%) than the placebo group (30.6%) [12].

Patisiran's effectiveness in the treatment of Transthyretin Cardiac Amyloidosis was evaluated in a phase 3 randomized, double-blind, placebo-controlled trial. 360 patients with ATTRv or ATTRwt were randomized to receive patisiran (0.3 mg per kilogram of body weight every 3 weeks) or placebo for 12 months. All patients have echocardiography evidence of cardiac involvement. At baseline, Tafamidis was administered to approximately 25% of patients. Patients with ATTR amyloidosis stage of 3, New York Heart Association class of III or IV, a 6-min walk distance of less than 150 m and a polyneuropathy disability score greater than II were excluded. In the patisiran group, serum transthyretin levels dropped rapidly and sustainably and had a significantly lower 6-min walk distance at 12 months compared with the placebo group (median difference of 14.69 m). A subgroup analysis including variant and wild-type ATTR amyloidosis produced the same results. The patisiran group had a significantly higher KCCQ-OS score (mean change, − 3.4 points). Mean NT-proBNP and troponin were also lower in the patisiran group. However, the composite end point of death from any cause, cardiovascular events, and change from baseline in the distance covered on the 6-min walk test was not significant (Tables 1 and 2) [13].

Vutrisiran

Vutrisiran was approved in June 2022 by The United States Food and Drug Administration (FDA) for the treatment of the polyneuropathy in adults with ATTRv polyneuropathy. The HELIOS-A—study was an open-label, phase 3 study. Efficacy and safety of 122 patients treated with Vutrisiran were compared to 42 patients treated with patisiran and 77 patients served as an external placebo group from the APOLLO study. Patients with previous use of TTR stabilizer must have completed a wash-out period before enrolled in the study. The study excluded patients with New York Heart Association heart failure class > II. A comparison of HELIOS-A and APOLLO placebo did not reveal any significant differences in baseline characteristics.

At 9 months, Vutrisiran significantly improved quality of life and neuropathy scores compare to external placebo. Similar to patisiran group, over 18 months, TTR levels were reduced rapidly and sustainably following vutrisiran treatment. There were no discontinuations or deaths associated with the drug [14]. Multiple measures of quality of life and 10-m walk test improved from baseline with vutrisiran group, In contrast, all measures in the external placebo group declined from baseline. Treatment was most effective in patients with earlier stages of disease, illustrating the importance of treating patients as early as possible [15].

Cardiac amyloid involvement was detected in around 30% of the HALLOS A population [14]. The cardiac subpopulation were defined as baseline left ventricular wall thickness $\geq$ 1.3 cm and no medical history of hypertension or aortic valve disease. At 18 months NT-ProBNP and cardiac output were significantly improved in the vutrisiran group compare to the external placebo group [16].

The HELIOS-B was a global, Phase 3, randomized, double-blind, placebo-controlled study that evaluated the efficacy and safety of vutrisiran in adult patients with cardiomyopathy and ATTRv or ATTRwt amyloidosis. 326 patients were assigned to receive vutrisiran (25 mg) and 329 to receive placebo every 12 weeks for up to 36 months. At basline, 60% of the patients were not taking tafamidis. 78% of the patients had NYHA class II heart failure. The primary end point was a composite of death from any cause and recurrent cardiovascular events. Secondary end points included death from any cause, the change from baseline in the KCCQ-OS score and the change from baseline in the distance covered on the 6-min walk test. The primary and secondary endpoints were assessed in the overall population and in patients taking vutrisiran monotherapy (i.e. those not taking tafamidis at baseline).

Vutrisiran significantly decreased mortality, cardiovascular events and markers of disease progression in the overall population and in the monotherapy population.

Treatment with vutrisiran resulted in less of a decline in the KCCQ-OS score and in the distance covered on the 6-min walk test than placebo. The incidence of adverse events was similar in the two groups (Tables 1 and 2) [17]. Recently, the FDA approved Vutrisiran as the first ATTR-silencer specifically indicated for treating ATTR cardiomyopathy.

Other therapies

Revusiran is a GalNAc conjugated siRNA that was investigated in the phase III trial. In The ENDEAVOUR trial, Patients with ATTRv amyloidosis with cardiomyopathy were randomized to revusiran or placebo. The study was stopped early due to "mortality imbalance between treatment arms", 12.9% patients on revusiran group were dies compare to 3.0% on the placebo group. In accordance with the disease's natural history, most deaths were due to heart failure in both groups. A post hoc safety analysis found that the majority of those who died were over 75 years old and had clinical signs of more advanced heart failure [18].

Gene Editing

CRISPR Cas9

Clustered regularly interspaced short palindromic repeats (CRISPR or CRISPR-associated protein 9 (CRISPR Cas9) is technology of a gene editing that enable to modifies the genome sequence by produce base substitutions, insertion or deletions in the genome. This technology use naturally system of bacteria and archaea to protect themselves against phage infection and plasmid transfer. In a variety of fields, such as cardiovascular disease, cancer, and neurodegenerative disease, the technology is used to modify undesirable DNA in living organisms [19]. NTLA-2001 is a lipid nanoparticle served as delivery system to CRISPR—Cas9 to produced human TTR gene knockout [20]. In phase1 clinical study administration of NTLA-2001 to six patients with hereditary ATTR amyloidosis with polyneuropathy was associated with durable knockout of TTR after a single dose and dose depended reduction in serum TTR protein concentration (52% and 87% reduction in the groups that received dose of 0.1 and 0.3 mg per kilogram respectively) [21]. Adverse events were in mild grade and included nausea, infusion-related reaction, thyroxine decreased and rhinorrhea. D-dimer levels increased in five of six patients 4 to 24 h after infusion, In day 7 the values returned to baseline in all six patients [21].

MAGNITUDE is an ongoing phase 3 study of NTLA-2001 in participants with transthyretin amyloidosis with cardiomyopathy. The study will complete on 2028 [20].

Nexiguran ziclumeran (Nex-Z) is an investigational CRISPR-Cas9-based therapy currently being evaluated. In a Phase 1, open-label trial, a single intravenous infusion of Nex-Z was administered to 36 patients with ATTR-CM. Of these, 25 patients had wild-type ATTR, and 50% were in NYHA class III at baseline.

Adverse events were reported in 34 patients. Five patients experienced infusion-related reactions, one of which was classified as serious. Two patients had transient elevations in AST levels.

After 12 months of follow-up, the mean percent reduction from baseline in serum transthyretin (TTR) levels was 90%. Furthermore, 92% of patients showed either improvement or no change in their NYHA class. Levels of NT-proBNP and high-sensitivity cardiac troponin T did not show significant changes [22].

Stabilizing the TTR Tetramer

A tetramer stabilizer binds to the T4-binding site on the TTR in order to prevent misfolding and deposition of monomers and oligomers [1].

Diflunisal

Diflunisal is a non-steroidal anti-inflammatory (NSAID) drug with non-selective ATTR stabilizing properties. In a single-arm, open-label study, 13 patients with ATTRwt- or ATTRv receive Diflunisal. The study has shown no significant mean change in cardiac structure, function, or biomarkers during the course of 0.9 ± 0.3 years [23].

An additional study including 40 Japanese with ATTRv amyloidosis found that diflunisal stabilized TTR tetramers structure. In addition, ejection fraction and cardiac wall thickness were not deteriorated over a mean follow-up of 38.0 ± 31.2 months.

Long term adverse events of NSAID were observed in the study as three patients discontinued the drug as a result of adverse events related to diflunisal, including deterioration of renal function and thrombocytopenia (Tables 1 and 2) [24].

Tafamidis

By binding to transthyretin, Tafamidis serves as a tetramer stabilizer, preventing the dissociation of tetramers and the formation of amyloids. In a phase III, multi-center, double blind, placebo controlled trial, 441 patients with ATTRwt or ATTRv cardiomyopathy were randomized in 2:1:2 ratio to receive oral tafamidis 80 mg daily, tafamidis 20 mg daily, or placebo for 30 months. Compare to placebo, Tafamidis was associated with lower all-cause mortality (29.5% vs. 42.9%, hazard ratio, 0.70; (95% confidence interval [CI], 0.51 to 0.96). reduce cardiovascular related hospitalizations, risk ratio of 0.68 (0.48 per year vs. 0.70 per year; 95% CI, 0.56 to 0.81). At month 30, tafamidis was also associated with benefit in the KCCQ-OS score and the distance for the 6-min walk test, The overall incidence of adverse events or serious adverse events during treatment period was similar in the tafamidis group and the placebo group [25].

The study found an interaction between treatment and NYHA baseline classification, indicating that the benefits of tafamidis regarding all-cause mortality and cardiovascular-related hospitalization were not observed in patients with NYHA class III disease at baseline. An interaction between treatment and TTR status (ATTRwt or ATTRv) were not observed (Tables 1 and 2) [25].

Acoramidis

Acoramidis mimic a rare protective T119M mutation cause unique hydrogen bonding resulting in better stabilization of the tetramer than wild-type TTR. Acoramidis has shown improved potency, binding-site occupancy, binding affinity, and TTR stabilization compare to diflunisal, and tolcapone. Although Acoramidis and Tafamidis have similar binding affinities (Kd) to TTR ($Kd = 4.8 \pm 1.9$ and 4.4 ± 1.3 nM, respectively), Acoramidis is more selective for binding and stabilizing TTR in human serum and was more potent in stabilizing TTR in buffer [26].

In a phase III, multicenter, double blind, placebo controlled trial, 632 patients with ATTRwt or ATTRv cardiomyopathy were randomized in a 2:1 ratio to receive acoramidis hydrochloride or matching placebo for 30 months. Patients with an eGFR of less than 15 ml per minute per 1.73 m^2 were excluded from the study. Patients with stage 4 chronic kidney disease (an eGFR of less than 30 ml per minute per 1.73 m^2) included in an the safety analysis but were excluded from the primary efficacy analysis [27].

Acoramidis was associated with improve in the four-step primary hierarchical analysis included: death from any cause, cardiovascular-related hospitalization, NT-proBNP, and 6-min walk distance. For the 6-min walk distance, KCCQOS score, and TTR serum level, there were significant between-group differences, but not for death from any cause. This can be attributed to the trial's lower death rate.

The overall incidence of adverse events or serious adverse events during treatment period was similar in the acoramidis group and the placebo group [27].

In an open-label extension study, 263 patients who received continuous acoramidis and 126 patients who switched from placebo to acoramidis were followed for 12 months. The hazard ratio for all-cause mortality or first cardiovascular-related hospitalization was 43% lower in patients treated early with acoramidis compared to those who switched from placebo. Additionally, improvements were seen in NT-proBNP levels, quality of life as assessed by KCCQ-OS, and 6-min walk distance, all favoring continuous acoramidis. No new clinically significant safety issues were identified during this long-term evaluation. These findings emphasize the importance of early diagnosis and the initiation of disease-modifying therapy (Tables 1 and 2) [28].

Tolcapone

Tolcapone is a catechol-O-methyltransferase (COMT) inhibitor indicated for the treatment of Parkinson's disease. Concurrent administration of COMT inhibitors with levodopa and peripheral AADC inhibitor such as carbidopa or benserazide increase the amount of levodopa brain penetration, levodopa bioavailability and increase the elimination half-life of levodopa [29].

Molecular studies have shown that tolcapone also binds strongly to thyroxine binding sites of TTR, preventing it from dissociating into monomers [30]. In a phase IIa trial, seventeen patients with ATTRwt or ATTRv receive single 200 mg dose of tolcapone in phase A and three 100 mg doses taken at 4 h intervals in phase B. All participants in this study experienced TTR stabilization [30]. However, Clinical outcomes from large RCTs are lacking. Tolcapone also carries a black box warning about the risk of acute fulminant liver failure, which can be fatal (Tables 1 and 2) [31].

Protein Misfolding Removal

TTR stabilizers and silencers can prevent disease deterioration but do not improve advanced staged of ATTR CMs. Indeed, most studies excluded patients with end stage heart failure.

Doxycyclin + T/UDCA

In mouse models, high doses of doxycyclin have been shown to remove TTR amyloid deposit. Tauroursodeoxycholic acid (TUDCA), a biliary acid, reduces non-fibrillar TTR deposits, with evidence of synergistic effects when combined with doxycycline [32].

In an open label phase II study, doxycycline (100 mg BID) and TUDCA (250 mg three times/day) were administered to twenty patients. During the 12 months, both the cardiac status and the neuropathy score remained relatively stable. Only seven of the 20 patients enrolled completed 12-month treatment [33].

In another phase 2 study, doxycycline and ursodeoxycholic acid (UDCA) were administered to twenty-eight patients for 18 months. After six months of treatment, there was no change in pro-BNP and neuropathy scores, but after 12 months, the levels had increased significantly. Only four patients had completed the whole study (Tables 1 and 2) [34].

Monoclonal Antibodies (mAb)

Specific monoclonal antibodies (mAbs) are therapies that directly enhance the clearance of toxic amyloid by stimulating their removal through phagocytic cells to improve organ function [35].

PRX004

The antibodies are targeting epitopes that are exposed in the misfolding monomers and oligomers. As a result, it can target amyloidogenic TTR deposits while maintaining the native TTR protein's functions. In preclinical studies, PRX004 reduced insoluble amyloid fibrils through phagocytosis, and inhibited amyloid fibril formation [35].

In phase 1 dose-escalation study, I.V. PRX004 was administered to twenty-one ATTRv patients. The dose-escalation phase included three infusions at doses of between 0.1 and 30 mg/kg (every 28-day) with long-term extension phase for up to 15 infusions. Neither serious adverse events nor deaths related to the drug have been reported. The most frequent adverse events (more than 10%) were constipation, diarrhea, anemia, upper respiratory tract infection, insomnia, back pain, and fall. Based on pharmacokinetic/pharmacodynamic models, dose levels of 3 mg/kg were predicted to facilitate clearance of > 90% of amyloid deposits. Data reports from seven patients enrolled in the long-term extension phase indicate slower progression vs natural history and an improvement in global longitudinal strains. Three of seven patients showed improvement in the Neuropathy Impairment Scale (NIS) from baseline [36]. The study was terminated early due to COVID-19 pandemic. Patients with New York Heart Association (NYHA) Functional Class III-IV or LVEF $\leq$ 45% were excluded from the study [37]. Phase 2 study (NCT05442047) will evaluate the efficacy and safety of PRX004 in adult patients with cardiomyopathy and ATTRv or ATTRwt amyloidosis. The study is expected to be completed in 2025 (Tables 1 and 2) [38].

NI006

NI006 is the drug name of the human monoclonal antibodies NI301A. The development of NI301A was based on high-throughput screening of human memory B-cell libraries, which generated a library of ATTR-binding antibodies. NI301A bind to specific epitope WEPFA, located in misfolding monomers and oligomers but unexposed in TTR's naturally folded conformation, this enhance amyloid deposite removal through phagocytic cells [35].

In phase 1 double-blind trial, dose-escalation study, 40 patients with ATTRwt or ATTRv cardiomyopathy and chronic heart failure were randomized in a 2:1 ratio to receive either NI006 at doses of between 0.3 to 60 mg/kg or placebo every 4 weeks for

4 months. In the open-label extension phase, patients received eight NI006 infusions with stepwise dose increases after four infusions. The study included patients with heart failure corresponding to NYHA class I-III.

Neither serious adverse events nor deaths related to the drug have been reported. The most frequent adverse events were arthralgia's and arthritis, in the high dose group, three patients from the high dose group developed cytokine release syndrome at grade 1 or 2, and one patient was withdrawn from the study due to thrombocytopenia.

At 12 months, doses of at least 10 mg per kilogram were predicted to improve surrogate markers of cardiac amyloid load (e.g. extracellular volume on cardiac magnetic resonance imaging and cardiac tracer uptake on scintigraphy). Troponin T and pro-B-type natriuretic peptide levels also appeared to have declined [39].

Phase 3 randomized, double-blind, placebo-controlled study (NCT06183931) will evaluate the efficacy and safety ALXN2220 (formerly NI006) in adult patients with cardiomyopathy and ATTRv or ATTRwt amyloidosis. The study is expected to be completed in 2028 (Tables 1 and 2) [40].

Conclusion

There have been significant advances in the treatment of ATTR-CM in recent years. Current therapies for ATTR amyloidosis focus on reducing TTR protein production, stabilizing its structure, or eliminating its source.

As amyloidogenic TTR deposits can continue to cause progressive organ damage, particularly to the heart, leading to early mortality, it is essential to evaluate the outcomes of combination therapies and to emphasize treatments targeting the depletion or removal of already amyloidogenic TTR deposits.

Promising studies are currently exploring amyloid deposits depletion, which could expand the available treatment options and help determine whether removing preexisting deposits improves survival and quality of life for patients.

References

1. Quarta CC, Fontana M, Damy T, et al. Changing paradigm in the treatment of amyloidosis: from disease-modifying drugs to anti-fibril therapy. Front Cardiovasc Med. 2022;9. https://doi.org/10.3389/fcvm.2022.1073503.
2. Ando Y, Adams D, Benson MD, et al. Guidelines and new directions in the therapy and monitoring of ATTRv amyloidosis. Amyloid. 2022;29(3):143–55. https://doi.org/10.1080/13506129.2022.2052838.
3. Rozenbaum MH, Large S, Bhambri R, et al. Estimating the health benefits of timely diagnosis and treatment of transthyretin amyloid cardiomyopathy. J Comp Eff Res. 2021;10(11):927–38. https://doi.org/10.2217/cer-2021-0071.

4. Dhuri K, Bechtold C, Quijano E, et al. Antisense oligonucleotides: an emerging area in drug discovery and development. J Clin Med. 2020;9(6):1–24. https://doi.org/10.3390/JCM9062004.
5. Benson MD, Waddington-Cruz M, Berk JL, et al. Inotersen treatment for patients with hereditary transthyretin amyloidosis. N Engl J Med. 2018;379(1):22–31. https://doi.org/10.1056/nejmoa1716793.
6. Karam C, Brown D, Yang M, et al. Long-term treatment effects of inotersen on health-related quality of life in patients with hATTR amyloidosis with polyneuropathy: analysis of the open-label extension of the NEURO-TTR trial. Muscle Nerve. 2021;2022:438–46. https://doi.org/10.1002/mus.27675.
7. Coelho T, Marques W, Dasgupta NR, et al. Eplontersen for hereditary transthyretin amyloidosis with polyneuropathy. JAMA. 2023;330(15):1448–58. https://doi.org/10.1001/jama.2023.18688.
8. CARDIO-TTRansform: a study to evaluate the efficacy and safety of AKCEA-TTR-LRx in participants with transthyretin-mediated amyloid cardiomyopathy (ATTR CM). Case Medical Research. https://doi.org/10.31525/ct1-nct04136171.
9. Buxbaum JN. Oligonucleotide drugs for transthyretin amyloidosis. N Engl J Med. 2018;379(1):82–5.
10. Adams D, Gonzalez-Duarte A, O'Riordan WD, et al. Patisiran, an RNAi therapeutic, for hereditary transthyretin amyloidosis. N Engl J Med. 2018;379(1):11–21. https://doi.org/10.1056/nejmoa1716153.
11. Adams D, Polydefkis M, González-Duarte A, et al. Long-term safety and efficacy of patisiran for hereditary transthyretin-mediated amyloidosis with polyneuropathy: 12-month results of an open-label extension study. Lancet Neurol. 2021;20(1):49–59. https://doi.org/10.1016/S1474-4422(20)30368-9.
12. Solomon SD, Adams D, Kristen A, et al. Effects of Patisiran, an RNA interference therapeutic, on cardiac parameters in patients with hereditary transthyretin-mediated amyloidosis: analysis of the APOLLO study. Circulation. 2019;139(4):431–43. https://doi.org/10.1161/CIRCULATIONAHA.118.035831.
13. Maurer MS, Kale P, Fontana M, et al. Patisiran treatment in patients with transthyretin cardiac amyloidosis. N Engl J Med. 2023;389(17):1553–65. https://doi.org/10.1056/nejmoa2300757.
14. Adams D, Tournev IL, Taylor MS, et al. Efficacy and safety of vutrisiran for patients with hereditary transthyretin-mediated amyloidosis with polyneuropathy: a randomized clinical trial. Amyloid. 2023;30(1):18–26. https://doi.org/10.1080/13506129.2022.2091985.
15. Obici L, Ajroud-Driss S, Lin KP, et al. Impact of vutrisiran on quality of life and physical function in patients with hereditary transthyretin-mediated amyloidosis with polyneuropathy. Neurol Ther. 2023;12(5):1759–75. https://doi.org/10.1007/s40120-023-00522-4.
16. Mussinelli R, Garcia-Pavia P, Gillmore JD, Kale P, Berk JL, Maurer MS, Conceição I, Dicarli M, Solomon S, Chen C, Arum S, Vest J, Grogan M. Helios-A: 18-month exploratory cardiac results from the phase 3 study of vutrisiran in patients with hereditary transthyretin-mediated amyloidosis. Eur Heart J. 2022;24(Supplement_K):K232. https://doi.org/10.1093/eurheartjsupp/suac121.654.
17. Fontana M, Berk JL, Gillmore JD, et al. Vutrisiran in patients with transthyretin amyloidosis with cardiomyopathy. N Engl J Med. Published online 2024:1–12. https://doi.org/10.1056/NEJMoa2409134
18. Judge DP, Kristen A V., Grogan M, et al. Phase 3 multicenter study of revusiran in patients with hereditary transthyretin-mediated (hATTR) amyloidosis with cardiomyopathy (ENDEAVOUR). Cardiovasc Drugs Ther. 2020;34(3):357–70. https://doi.org/10.1007/s10557-019-06919-4. Cardiovasc Drugs Ther. 2020;34(6):889. https://doi.org/10.1007/s10557-020-07023-8.
19. Li T, Yang Y, Qi H, et al. CRISPR/Cas9 therapeutics: progress and prospects. Signal Transduct Target Ther. 2023;8(1). https://doi.org/10.1038/s41392-023-01309-7.
20. Finn JD, Smith AR, Patel MC, et al. A single administration of CRISPR/Cas9 lipid nanoparticles achieves robust and persistent in vivo genome editing. Cell Rep. 2018;22(9):2227–35. https://doi.org/10.1016/j.celrep.2018.02.014.

21. Gillmore JD, Gane E, Taubel J, et al. CRISPR-Cas9 in vivo gene editing for transthyretin amyloidosis. N Engl J Med. 2021;385(6):493–502. https://doi.org/10.1056/nejmoa2107454.
22. Kachadourian J, Pharm D, Walsh L, et al. CRISPR-Cas9 gene editing with Nexiguran Ziclumeran for ATTR cardiomyopathy. N Engl J Med. Published online 2024:1–10. https://doi.org/10.1056/NEJMoa2412309.
23. Castaño A, Helmke S, Alvarez J, Delisle S, Maurer MS. Diflunisal for ATTR cardiac amyloidosis. Congest Hear Fail. 2012;18(6):315–9. https://doi.org/10.1111/j.1751-7133.2012.00303.x.
24. Sekijima Y, Tojo K, Morita H, Koyama J, Ikeda SI. Safety and efficacy of long-term diflunisal administration in hereditary transthyretin (ATTR) amyloidosis. Amyloid. 2015;22(2):79–83. https://doi.org/10.3109/13506129.2014.997872.
25. Maurer MS, Schwartz JH, Gundapaneni B, et al. Tafamidis treatment for patients with transthyretin amyloid cardiomyopathy. N Engl J Med. 2018;379(11):1007–16. https://doi.org/10.1056/nejmoa1805689.
26. Penchala SC, Connelly S, Wang Y, et al. AG10 inhibits amyloidogenesis and cellular toxicity of the familial amyloid cardiomyopathy-associated V122I transthyretin. Proc Natl Acad Sci USA. 2013;110(24):9992–7. https://doi.org/10.1073/pnas.1300761110.
27. Gillmore JD, Judge DP, Cappelli F, et al. Efficacy and safety of acoramidis in transthyretin amyloid cardiomyopathy. N Engl J Med. 2024;390(2):132–42. https://doi.org/10.1056/nejmoa2305434.
28. Judge DP, Gillmore JD, Alexander KM, et al. Long-term efficacy and safety of acoramidis in ATTR-CM: initial report from the open-label extension of the ATTRibute-CM trial. Circulation. Published online 2024. https://doi.org/10.1161/CIRCULATIONAHA.124.072771.
29. Fabbri M, Ferreira JJ, Rascol O. COMT inhibitors in the management of Parkinson's disease. CNS Drugs. 2022;36(3):261–82. https://doi.org/10.1007/s40263-021-00888-9.
30. Gamez J, Salvadó M, Reig N, et al. Transthyretin stabilization activity of the catechol-O-methyltransferase inhibitor tolcapone (SOM0226) in hereditary ATTR amyloidosis patients and asymptomatic carriers: proof-of-concept study#. Amyloid. 2019;26(2):74–84. https://doi.org/10.1080/13506129.2019.1597702.
31. Discussion C, The OF, Patient THE, Provided HAS. Tasmar (tolcapone) interview form. In Vitro. 2005;5:1–17.
32. Cardoso I, Martins D, Ribeiro T, Merlini G, Saraiva MJ. Synergy of combined Doxycycline/TUDCA treatment in lowering Transthyretin deposition and associated biomarkers: studies in FAP mouse models. J Transl Med. 2010;8:1–11. https://doi.org/10.1186/1479-5876-8-74.
33. Obici L, Cortese A, Lozza A, et al. Doxycycline plus tauroursodeoxycholic acid for transthyretin amyloidosis: a phase II study. Amyloid. 2012;19(SUPPL. 1):34–6. https://doi.org/10.3109/13506129.2012.678508.
34. Wixner J, Pilebro B, Lundgren HE, Olsson M, Anan I. Effect of doxycycline and ursodeoxycholic acid on transthyretin amyloidosis. Amyloid. 2017;24:78–9. https://doi.org/10.1080/13506129.2016.1269739.
35. Nuvolone M, Nevone A, Merlini G. Targeting amyloid fibrils by passive immunotherapy in systemic amyloidosis. BioDrugs. 2022;36(5):591–608. https://doi.org/10.1007/s40259-022-00550-w.
36. Committee TS, Academy A. Neurological and cardiac improvements with PRX004 in amyloidosis patients: results of a phase 1 study, 2021 Emerging Science Abstracts. 2021 AAN Annual meeting abstracts. Neurology. 2021;96(22):2783–8. https://doi.org/10.1212/wnl.0000000000012044.
37. NCT03336580. A study of PRX004 in subjects with amyloid transthyretin (ATTR) amyloidosis. Published 2020. https://clinicaltrials.gov/ct2/show/NCT03336580.
38. EUCTR2021-006226-49-DE. A research study to look at how a new medicine called NNC6019-0001 works and how safe it is for people who have heart disease due to TTR amyloidosis. https://trialsearch.who.int/Trial2.aspx?TrialID=EUCTR2021-006226-49-DE. Published 2022. https://doi.org/10.1002/central/CN-02513038/full.

39. Garcia-Pavia P, aus dem Siepen F, Donal E, et al. Phase 1 Trial of antibody NI006 for depletion of cardiac transthyretin amyloid. N Engl J Med. 2023;389(3):239–50. https://doi.org/10.1056/nejmoa2303765.
40. Study of ALXN2220 versus placebo in adults with ATTR-CM—full text view—ClinicalTrials.gov. https://classic.clinicaltrials.gov/ct2/show/NCT06183931.

Neurology in Cardiac Amyloidosis

Marc Gotkine and Roy Dayan

Abstract The neurological manifestations associated with cardiac amyloidosis are often overlooked, as they overlap with a wide variety of other conditions. Involvement of the nervous system is generally restricted to the peripheral nervous system and includes length-dependent neuropathy, autonomic neuropathy, carpal tunnel syndrome, and lumbosacral radiculopathy due to spinal stenosis. Though many of these syndromes are common, their appearance together or in certain contexts should alert the clinician to the possibility of amyloidosis. Early recognition of these manifestations is critical, as they may precede the diagnosis of cardiac amyloidosis or prompt initiation of specific targeted therapies.

Keywords Neuropathy · Autonomic neuropathy · Amyloidosis · Carpal tunnel syndrome

Introduction

Recognizing the neurological manifestation of systemic amyloidosis is essential for any clinician seeing patients with cardiological manifestations that could be due to amyloidosis, since they are common manifestations of the disease and are often the initial presentation. Some complaints, particularly symptoms that are caused by involvement of the autonomic nervous system, may be wrongly attributed to the cardiological disease of the patient. Other complaints, such as carpal tunnel syndrome, which is a common neurological manifestation of amyloidosis, [1] may be overlooked due to the condition's high prevalence. Therefore, it is essential to be aware of the neurological symptoms of amyloidosis, the diagnostic approaches, and the treatment of this aspect of the disease.

In this chapter, we briefly present the basic pathophysiology of neurological amyloidosis, the common presenting symptoms, and the diagnostic methods. We

M. Gotkine (✉) · R. Dayan
Department of Neurology, Hadassah Medical Organization and Faculty of Medicine, Hebrew University of Jerusalem, Jerusalem, Israel
e-mail: marc@gotkine.com

E. Herzog (ed.), *Cardiac Amyloidosis*, https://doi.org/10.1007/978-3-031-88342-2_17

also summarize the staging systems for neurological manifestations of amyloidosis and the current treatment options. The focus will be on AL and TTR amyloidosis, with different approaches to each disease type.

It is important to note that other types of amyloidosis play an important role in several diseases of the central nervous system, such as Alzheimer's disease and cerebral amyloid angiopathy. However, these are generally unrelated to cardiac amyloidosis—which is primarily due to AL and TTR amyloidosis. These amyloidoses, when they affect the nervous system, almost exclusively affect the peripheral, rather than central nervous system, causing amyloid neuropathy.

Pathophysiology of Amyloid Neuropathy: Different Causes, Common Pathway

While many different proteins tend to form amyloids, they all share a common pathway in which the backbone of a part of the protein is exposed and forms hydrogen bonds with similar proteins by forming β-sheets [3]. Several conditions are required for the creation of amyloids, including a high concentration of the soluble protein, caused either by insufficient degradation or increased synthesis, and the forming of a nucleus as a template that initiates the abnormal bonding [3].

AL amyloidosis is derived from plasma cells in the bone marrow generating monoclonal antibodies and free light chains [2]. The specific sequence of the free light chains, in addition to external factors such as the presence of serum amyloid P component, are responsible for protein aggregation [2, 4]. In this process, the free light chains are misfolded, forming oligomers and later cross-β amyloid fibrils deposited next to the involved tissue [2].

Conversely, TTR amyloidosis is either a hereditary disease—due to mutated TTR—or a disease of the elderly, where the wild-type TTR amyloid accumulates. TTR, formerly known as prealbumin, is a tetrameric transport protein synthesized in the liver, choroid plexus and the retinal epithelium [5]. Many cases of hereditary TTR amyloidosis are caused by a Val30Met substitution in the TTR gene, which is endemic in several regions (i.e., Portugal, Sweden, Japan) and is referred to as the amyloidosis TTR variant (ATTRv). The pathophysiology involves the dissociation of the TTR tetramers and the misfolding of the monomers, followed by the aggregation of oligomers and later of fibrils. However, abnormal cleavage is also suspected as an alternative mechanism. In addition to the hereditary form, amyloidosis also similarly occurs with wild-type TTR proteins [5].

In both AL and TTR amyloidosis, the amyloids tend to aggregate in the endoneurium of the dorsal root ganglia and the sympathetic ganglia, causing damage to the Schwann cells of the small fibers [1]. It has been suggested that, at least in TTR, the mechanism involves a vascular component with disruption of the blood nerve barrier [6]. TTR amyloids have a high affinity for Schwann cell membranes, resulting in cell stress that affects mainly the small fiber axons while the large myelinated fibers are relatively protected [5].

To conclude, amyloid neuropathy may be caused either by the formation of monoclonal free light chains or the misfolding of mutated or wild-type TTR. This results in the protein aggregating in β-sheets form and deposition into the Schwann cell membranes, affecting predominantly the small nerve fibers but also the large fibers.

Clinical Manifestations of Amyloid Neuropathy: Sensory Neuropathy, Carpal Tunnel Syndrome and Autonomic Manifestations

The peripheral somatic and autonomic nerves are often affected in both AL and ATTRv amyloidosis [1]. The neurological symptoms relating to dysfunction of these systems often constitute the initial presentation of the disease [1].

In AL amyloidosis, the presentation of axonal polyneuropathy is more common than small-fiber polyneuropathy, although both manifestations are prevalent. Patients may commonly present with sensory neuropathy, orthostatic hypotension, complaints of gastrointestinal motility, early satiety, neurogenic bladder, and erectile dysfunction. In the clinic, patients with sensory neuropathy often complain of numbness that is length-dependent and frequently begins at the feet, distally (Fig. 1). On neurological examination, these patients demonstrate reduced deep-tendon reflexes, reduced pinprick and temperature sensation, impaired sense of vibration (tested with a 128 Hz tuning fork) and proprioception (the patient is asked to tell the position of the distal joints in the hands and feet while eyes are closed).

It is worth noting that the only abnormality that can be attributed to small fiber neuropathy is the reduced pinprick and temperature sensation, whilst the other findings require the involvement of large fibers. Large fibers are amenable to assessment by nerve conduction studies, while small fibers are not; the corollary is that nerve conduction studies only become abnormal when large fibers are involved.

Autonomic symptoms are numerous and varied. Features of orthostatic hypotension include lightheadedness and transient loss of vision on standing or could be vaguer and described as extreme fatigue. Symptoms related to dysfunction of involuntary sphincter control often relate to insufficient emptying of the bladder, leading to frequency, urgency, and nocturia. Erectile dysfunction is also common. Patients may also present with symptoms of small fiber neuropathy, such as distal burning pain. Additional features such as macroglossia and renal failure may also occur [1].

ATTR amyloidosis can be separated into two different entities (Table 1): an acquired "wild-type" form that develops with age (ATTRwt), and a hereditary form that is caused by a pathogenic variant (ATTRv), the latter being more intensely studied. Compared to the genetic ATTRv type, patients with ATTRwt have older age of onset, higher prevalence of males and more comorbidities, perhaps due to the

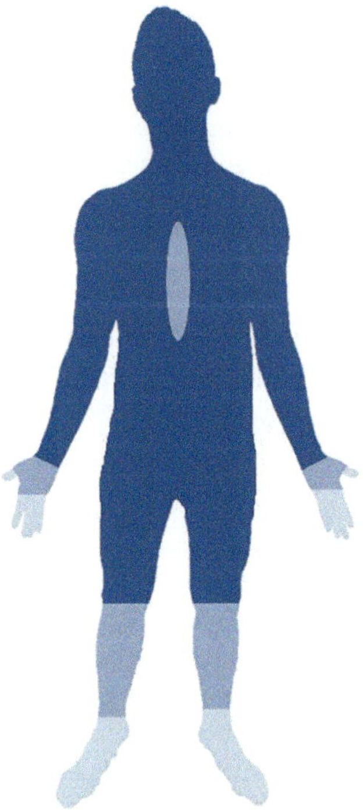

Fig. 1 Distribution of sensory symptoms and signs in length-dependent neuropathy. Lighter shade of blue represents more numbness and less sensation on examination

older age [7]. Patients with ATTRwt often have a predominantly cardiac presentation with dyspnea and arrhythmia, while ATTRv patients are more likely to present with neurological manifestations such as paresthesia. ATTRwt patients, however, had higher prevalence of carpal tunnel syndrome, but dysautonomia occurs at a similar frequency in the two groups [7].

A large prospective multicenter study of patients with ATTRv has shown that the manifestations may differ according to the genetic etiology. While the most common presenting syndrome for all patients with the Val30Met mutation was sensory neuropathy, GI and other autonomic symptoms were also common. In

Table 1 Clinical differences between ATTRv and ATTRwt, adapted from Fernandes et al. [7]

	ATTRv	ATTRwt
Age	Younger (median 54)	Older (median 78)
Males	~ 60%	~ 75%
Ethnicity	More in Africans	More in Caucasians
Carpal tunnel syndrome	~ 12%	~ 19%
Initial symptoms	Neuropathy: length-dependent sensory or diarrhea	Cardiac: dyspnea, arrhythmia
Phenotype	Mainly neurological	Mainly cardiologic

contrast, in patients with other mutations, the second most common presentation was cardiac involvement [8]. Even among the Val30Met mutation carriers, patients are divided into early onset (< 50 years) with more prominent autonomic neuropathy and progressive cardiac conduction disorders and late-onset with more prominent peripheral neuropathy and restrictive cardiomyopathy or cardiac insufficiency [9].

Within the neurological manifestations, one of the most common presentations, though non-specific, is carpal tunnel syndrome, which may present in two-thirds of patients, heralding the diagnosis of amyloidosis a decade before [10]. Carpal tunnel syndrome is a common neurological condition caused by compression of the median nerve at the wrist [11]. Patients commonly present with paresthesia, often upon awakening, in the distribution of the digital cutaneous branch of the median nerve, sparing the thenar eminence (Fig. 2). On neurological examination, eliciting the paresthesia with Phalen's sign (flexion of the wrist to 90° for 60s) or Tinel's sign (percussion on the carpal tunnel) may support the diagnosis [11]. Although CTS is very common, a high index of suspicion is important in order to alert the clinician that amyloidosis should be suspected. A clue towards the etiology of amyloidosis may be bilateral or severe non-dominant carpal tunnel syndrome, and it is more prevalent in ATTRv than AL amyloidosis [1]. In addition, the occurrence of CTS in atypical patient groups—i.e. those without risk factors for CTS (Table 2)—should prompt consideration of amyloidosis. Other mononeuropathies, predominantly in the upper limbs, may also occur [12].

Other red flags for considering amyloidosis are a rapidly progressive polyneuropathy unresponsive to immunotherapy, autonomic manifestations, weight loss, heart failure with preserved ejection fraction, and in ATTRv, spinal stenosis, and tendon rupture [1].

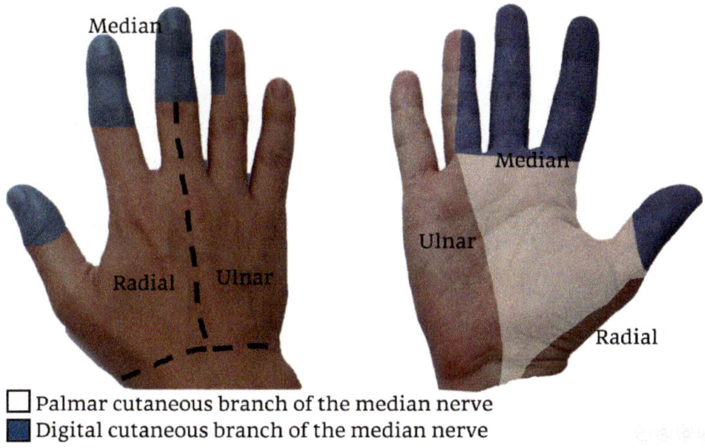

Fig. 2 Sensory territories of the median nerve in the hand. In carpal tunnel syndrome, the territory of the digital cutaneous branch of the median nerve is affected. In contrast, the palmar cutaneous branch, which divides from the median nerve proximal to the carpal tunnel, is spared

Table 2 Risk factors for carpal tunnel syndrome (adapted from Bland [11]; Kothari, uptodate, 2024)

Risk factors for carpal tunnel syndrome (besides amyloidosis)	
Age, sex and genetics	Advanced age, Female sex, genetic predisposition, Hereditary neuropathy with liability to pressure palsy
Medical conditions	Diabetes, arthritis, obesity, hypothyroidism, pregnancy
Environmental	Repetitive hand use

Rarely, ATTRv may involve the central nervous system. In these uncommon genetic variants, the clinical manifestations may include dementia, headache, and ataxia, with amyloid deposits in the leptomeningeal, subpial, and subependymal regions [13].

Clinical Case

Patient A, a 73-year-old woman of Yemenite-Jewish origin, presented with a complaint of fatigue, incontinence, and night sweats. The patient reported a history of right carpal tunnel syndrome that was treated surgically. She performed ECG, Holter-monitor, carotid US, brain, and cervical MRI with no specific results. At age 74, the patient started to suffer from pain in both hands. After being evaluated by specialists from various disciplines, she was treated for seronegative rheumatoid arthritis with no improvement and was later diagnosed with fibromyalgia.

After worsening of paresthesia in both upper limbs, the patient was reevaluated by a neurologist, finding prominently reduced proprioception and positive Romberg's sign (tendency to fall while standing with eyes closed, suggesting impaired proprioception) and was diagnosed with polyneuropathy.

At the age of 84, the patient performed sequencing of the *TTR* gene, which discovered a 290C > A mutation, causing a missense Ser97Tyr change previously reported as pathogenic. Following this finding, 11 years after the initial presentation, the neuromuscular team assessed the case, and it was concluded that the various neuropathic complaints were explained by sensory and autonomic polyneuropathy caused by ATTRv.

This case illustrates the non-specific symptoms commonly presented in patients with amyloid neuropathy, frequently leading to a long diagnostic.

Diagnosis of Amyloid Neuropathy

Due to the variability of presentation and similarities to other conditions, amyloid neuropathy is frequently misdiagnosed, particularly in cases with no family history [9]. The neurological manifestations are sometimes attributed to chronic inflammatory demyelinating polyradiculoneuropathy (CIDP), idiopathic axonal polyneuropathy, age-related spinal stenosis, or diabetic polyneuropathy [9]. In fact, spinal stenosis is in itself a feature of amyloidosis and can contribute to neurological impairment.

Nerve Conduction studies (NCS), often the first ancillary test, may typically demonstrate a length-dependent sensorimotor axonal neuropathy (Fig. 1) [14]. NCS may also support the diagnosis of carpal tunnel syndrome as a manifestation of amyloidosis (see clinical case 2 and Fig. 3). A study of 69 ATTRV30M asymptomatic carriers has found that sensory changes in NCS may predict the occurrence of symptoms by two years [14]. However, NCS in ATTRv patients may also demonstrate prolonged distal latency and abnormal temporal dispersion that may mimic a demyelinating disease and defer the correct diagnosis [15]. Patients with AL amyloidosis may also present with electrophysiological changes such as decreased motor conduction velocity (CV) and compound muscle action potential (CMAP) [16]. Notably, in cases of neuropathy affecting only the small fibers, which can be frequently seen in amyloidosis, the NCS may be completely normal despite considerable symptoms. Therefore, a normal NCS does not rule out neurological manifestations of amyloidosis.

Systemic amyloidosis is often confirmed by biopsy of the subcutaneous fat, which can be performed using fine-needle aspiration [2]. The tissue is stained with Congo red dye and is examined with polarized light microscopy, in which amyloid deposits appear with green birefringence. However, with neuropathy, a nerve biopsy, mostly from the sural nerve, may have higher sensitivity and specificity, particularly in ATTRv [1]. Nerve biopsy may also be falsely negative, as the amyloid deposition may be patchy or distal [1]. In selected cases with high suspicion and previous negative nerve biopsy, 18-F-florbetapir PET/MRI imaging may help to choose the right location for the procedure [17].

In AL amyloidosis, the diagnosis requires not only evidence of amyloidosis but also the presence of a hematological abnormality with production of monoclonal proteins (paraproteins) [2]. This condition can be detected by one of three tests: immunofixation electrophoresis (IEP) from serum or urine, immunoglobulin free light chain (FLC), or bone marrow biopsy demonstrating predominantly lambda or kappa plasma cells [2]. Even in the presence of monoclonal proteins, genetic testing for *TTR* mutations should still be considered, as there is a high prevalence of monoclonal gammopathy of undetermined significance in patients with ATTRv [18].

The genetic cause for TTR amyloidosis is confirmed by genetic testing, which usually includes sequencing of the *TTR* gene [1]. There are 146 known pathogenic mutations in the *TTR* gene registered in the amyloidosis mutations online registry

Nerve / Sites	Rec. Site	Onset Lat ms	Peak Lat ms	Amp µV	Segments	Distance mm	Peak Diff ms	Velocity m/s
L Median - Digit II (Antidromic)								
Wrist	Dig II	2.71	3.49	19.6	Wrist - Dig II	135		50
R Median - Digit II (Antidromic)								
Wrist	Dig II	2.97	3.65	21.6	Wrist - Dig II	140		47
L Ulnar - Digit V (Antidromic)								
Wrist	Dig V	1.67	2.66	11.5	Wrist - Dig V	114		68
R Ulnar - Digit V (Antidromic)								
Wrist	Dig V	1.98	2.76	19.1	Wrist - Dig V	123		62
R Sural - Ankle (Calf)								
Calf	Ankle	1.93	2.60	15.8	Calf - Ankle	105		54
L Sural - Ankle (Calf)								
Calf	Ankle	2.50	2.92	11.8	Calf - Ankle	125		50
L Superficial peroneal - Ankle								
Lat leg	Ankle	1.98	2.66	25.7	Lat leg - Ankle	100		51
R Superficial peroneal - Ankle								
Lat leg	Ankle	2.40	3.02	19.3	Lat leg - Ankle	115		48
L Median, Ulnar - Ring finger comparison								
Median Wrist	Ring finger	2.81	3.65	12.1	Median Wrist - Ring finger	140		50
Ulnar Wrist	Ring finger	2.66	3.28	3.8	Ulnar Wrist - Ring finger	140		53
					Median Wrist - Ulnar Wrist		0.36	
R Median, Ulnar - Ring finger comparison								
Median Wrist	Ring finger	3.13	3.85	6.5	Median Wrist - Ring finger	140		45
Ulnar Wrist	Ring finger	2.50	3.07	7.3	Ulnar Wrist - Ring finger	140		56
					Median Wrist - Ulnar Wrist		**0.78**	

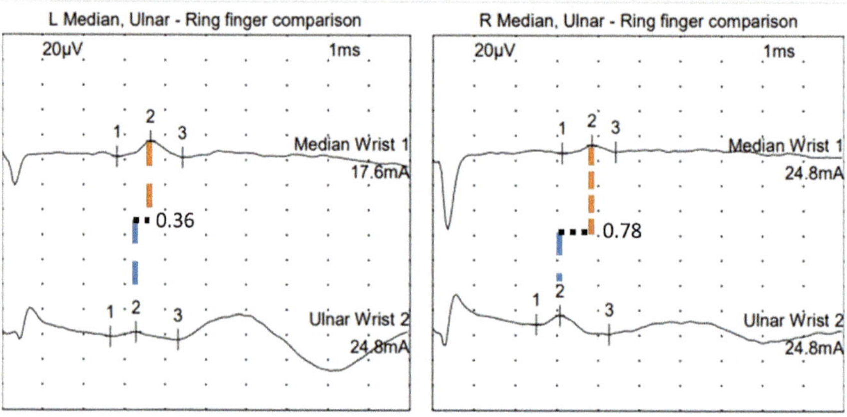

Fig. 3 Sensory nerve conduction studies (SNC) of the patient in clinical case 2. While most of the study is within the normal range, the difference in onset between the peak latency in the median (orange line) and ulnar (blue line) nerves at the right wrist is pathologically high, while normal in the left wrist. These findings are typical of early, mild carpal tunnel syndrome

[19]. The current approach prioritizes genetic testing over biopsy in patients with neurological symptoms raising suspicion for amyloidosis, [1] as the former is less invasive and has a relatively high yield in patients with polyneuropathy with unknown etiology [20].

Clinical Case—Continued

Patient B, the son of patient A, was a 52-year-old generally healthy male who presented with five years of paresthesia in all limbs. The patient performed nerve conduction studies (NCS), demonstrating mild right carpal tunnel syndrome with no other abnormalities (Fig. 3). Although these findings are non-specific, the patient completed genetic testing for the TTR gene due to the family history, discovering the pathogenic Ser97Tyr inherited from his mother. Cardiac workup, including ECG, Echo, NT-proBNP, and myocardial perfusion imaging, were completely normal. This case demonstrates how subtle neurological manifestations, particularly carpal tunnel syndrome, maybe the first manifestation of ATTRv.

Staging of Amyloid Neuropathy

Clinical trials investigating the therapy of neurological involvement of systemic amyloidosis have used grading scales that are based on the Neuropathy Impairment score, either the mNIS + 7-Alnylam scale used in the APOLLO trial or the mNIS + 7-Ionis scale used in the NEURO-TTR Trial [21]. Both scales include motor strength (192 points), reflexes (20 points), quantitative sensation testing (80 points), and nerve conduction studies, in addition to postural blood pressure in the mNIS + 7-Alnylam and sensation and heart rate with deep breathing in the mNIS + 7-Ionis [21].

The common staging systems for AL amyloidosis (Mayo 2004, Mayo 2012, European 2013, Boston 2019) do not include neurological parameters in the criteria, as they are focused on survival, which is mostly dependent on cardiac involvement [2]. However, since the neurological involvement in AL amyloidosis may cause substantial morbidity, it was suggested that the mNIS + 7 score, used in ATTRv, be adopted [22].

One biomarker that may indicate the severity of the neurological damage in systemic amyloidosis is the neurofilament light chain (Nfl). This cytoskeletal protein is increased in both plasma and CSF after neuronal injury [23]. Nfl levels increase in patients with polyneuropathy due to systemic amyloidosis, both in ATTRv and AL amyloidosis [23].

Treatment of Amyloid Neuropathy: Transplantation in AL Amyloidosis and New Disease-Modifying Drugs for ATTRv

Symptomatic drug treatment of neuropathic pain in amyloid neuropathy includes gabapentin, pregabalin, tricyclic antidepressants, and Serotonin-Norepinephrine reuptake inhibitors [2, 24]. In addition, orthostatic hypotension can be addressed with behavioral modifications, high stockings and pharmacological therapy [2, 25].

In AL amyloidosis, treatment with melphalan and autologous stem cell transplantation became the mainstay of treatment in eligible patients, with excellent long-term results [26]. Unlike severe cardiac and renal involvement, neurological manifestations are not considered as an exclusion criteria for this treatment [26]. Around 80% of patients are not eligible for stem cell transplantation and are commonly treated with a combination of cyclophosphamide, bortezomib, and dexamethasone [2]. Paradoxically, this regimen may cause worsening of the polyneuropathy since bortezomib may cause significant peripheral neuropathy [27].

The treatment of ATTRv was revolutionized by drugs that target the genetic pathophysiology of the disease and are currently indicated for treating patients with neurological manifestations.

Patisiran, an RNA interference drug, significantly improves the mNIS + 7 score compared to placebo, in addition to improvement in quality of life measures [28]. Inotersen is an antisense oligonucleotide drug that binds mutated TTR RNA and improves both neuropathy and quality of life measures [29]. Two other TTR silencing drugs, vutrisiran and eplontersen, are also promising [1].

Another therapeutic approach is based on the stabilization of the TTR tetramer to prevent its dissociation and thus suppresses the formation of the β-sheets. These drugs, such as diflunisal, have also proved to be effective in stopping the progression of neurological deterioration and improving quality of life [1, 30].

Prognosis of Amyloid Neuropathy

The Transthyretin amyloidosis Survey (THAOS), a multicenter study, demonstrated improved survival among TTR amyloidosis patients (both ATTRv and wild type) with neurological symptoms [31]. Conversely, another study on ATTRv patients did not find a difference in survival between patients with primary neurological manifestations, primary cardiac manifestations, or both [32]. As we enter the era of disease-modifying drugs and possibly higher awareness of ATTRv, prominent neurological manifestations may lead to earlier diagnosis and treatment, thus making possible better overall survival.

In AL amyloidosis, peripheral neuropathy detected on NCS—which only detects large fiber neuropathy—did not affect the overall prognosis of the hematological condition [33]. In contrast, small fiber neuropathy, detected by skin biopsy, was associated with poorer survival [34].

Conclusion

The current chapter provides a summary of the neurological aspects of cardiac amyloidosis. Both AL and ATTRv, which cause cardiac amyloidosis, tend to aggregate in the schwann cell membrane and to damage the smaller nerve fibers of the peripheral nervous system. The neurological manifestations commonly involve carpal tunnel syndrome, progressive polyneuropathy, and autonomic neuropathy. While nerve conduction studies may help the diagnosis, they should be verified by biopsy, proof for monoclonal antibodies in the case of AL amyloidosis, and genetic testing in the case of ATTRv. The mNIS + 7 is a conventional scoring system for staging neurological manifestations. Treatment is based on symptomatic therapy for all patients, autologous stem cell transplantation or chemotherapy for AL amyloidosis, and the novel TTR RNA silencing drugs or TTR tetramer stabilization for ATTRv.

References

1. Chompoopong P, Mauermann ML, Siddiqi H, Peltier A. Amyloid neuropathy: from pathophysiology to treatment in light-chain amyloidosis and hereditary transthyretin amyloidosis. Ann Neurol. 2024;ana.26965.
2. Sanchorawala V. Systemic light chain amyloidosis. N Engl J Med. 2024;390(24):2295–307.
3. Eisenberg D, Jucker M. The amyloid state of proteins in human diseases. Cell. 2012;148(6):1188–203.
4. Morgan GJ, Wall JS. The process of amyloid formation due to monoclonal immunoglobulins. Hematol Oncol Clin North Am. 2020;34(6):1041–54.
5. Adams D, Koike H, Slama M, Coelho T. Hereditary transthyretin amyloidosis: a model of medical progress for a fatal disease. Nat Rev Neurol. 2019;15(7):387–404.
6. Koike H, Ikeda S, Takahashi M, Kawagashira Y, Iijima M, Misumi Y, et al. Schwann cell and endothelial cell damage in transthyretin familial amyloid polyneuropathy. Neurology. 2016;87(21):2220–9.
7. Fernandes F, Luzuriaga GDCJ, Da Fonseca GWP, Correia EB, Carvalho AAS, Macedo AVS, et al. Clinical and genetic profiles of patients with hereditary and wild-type transthyretin amyloidosis: the Transthyretin Cardiac Amyloidosis Registry in the state of São Paulo, Brazil (REACT-SP). Orphanet J Rare Dis. 2024;19(1):273.
8. Coelho T, Conceição I, Waddington-Cruz M, Keohane D, Sultan MB, Chapman D, et al. A natural history analysis of asymptomatic *TTR* gene carriers as they develop symptomatic transthyretin amyloidosis in the Transthyretin Amyloidosis Outcomes Survey (THAOS). Amyloid. 2022;29(4):228–36.
9. Adams D, Ando Y, Beirão JM, Coelho T, Gertz MA, Gillmore JD, et al. Expert consensus recommendations to improve diagnosis of ATTR amyloidosis with polyneuropathy. J Neurol. 2021;268(6):2109–22.
10. Karam C, Dimitrova D, Christ M, Heitner SB. Carpal tunnel syndrome and associated symptoms as first manifestation of hATTR amyloidosis. Neur Clin Pract. 2019;9(4):309–13.
11. Bland JDP. Carpal tunnel syndrome. BMJ. 2007;335(7615):343–6.
12. Tracy JA, Dyck PJ, Dyck PJB. Primary amyloidosis presenting as upper limb multiple mononeuropathies. Muscle Nerve. 2010;41(5):710–5.
13. Ziskin JL, Greicius MD, Zhu W, Okumu AN, Adams CM, Plowey ED. Neuropathologic analysis of Tyr69His TTR variant meningovascular amyloidosis with dementia. Acta Neuropathol Commun. 2015 Dec;3(1):43.
14. Castro J, Miranda B, De Castro I, Conceição I. Changes in nerve conduction studies predate clinical symptoms onset in early onset Val30Met hereditary ATTR amyloidosis. Euro J Neurol. 2022;29(3):826–32.
15. Ohashi N, Kodaira M, Morita H, Sekijima Y. Electrophysiological demyelinating features in hereditary ATTR amyloidosis. Amyloid. 2019;26(1):15–23.

16. Matsuda M, Gono T, Morita H, Katoh N, Kodaira M, Ikeda S. Peripheral nerve involvement in primary systemic AL amyloidosis: a clinical and electrophysiological study: polyneuropathy in AL amyloidosis. Eur J Neurol. 2011;18(4):604–10.
17. Shouman K, Broski SM, Muchtar E, Pendleton CA, Johnson GB, Tracy J, et al. Novel imaging techniques using ^{18} F-florbetapir PET/MRI can guide fascicular nerve biopsy in amyloid multiple mononeuropathy. Muscle Nerve. 2021;63(1):104–8.
18. Phull P, Sanchorawala V, Connors LH, Doros G, Ruberg FL, Berk JL, et al. Monoclonal gammopathy of undetermined significance in systemic transthyretin amyloidosis (ATTR). Amyloid. 2018;25(1):62–7.
19. Rowczenio DM, Noor I, Gillmore JD, Lachmann HJ, Whelan C, Hawkins PN, et al. Online registry for mutations in hereditary amyloidosis including nomenclature recommendations. Hum Mutat. 2014;35(9):E2403–12.
20. Skrahina V, Grittner U, Beetz C, Skripuletz T, Juenemann M, Krämer HH, et al. Hereditary transthyretin-related amyloidosis is frequent in polyneuropathy and cardiomyopathy of no obvious aetiology. Ann Med. 2021;53(1):1787–96.
21. Dyck PJB, González-Duarte A, Obici L, Polydefkis M, Wiesman JF, Antonino I, et al. Development of measures of polyneuropathy impairment in hATTR amyloidosis: from NIS to mNIS + 7. J Neurol Sci. 2019;405: 116424.
22. Mauermann ML, Clarke JO, Litchy WJ, Obici L, Lousada I, Gertz MA, et al. Peripheral nervous, hepatic, and gastrointestinal endpoints for AL amyloidosis clinical trials: report from the amyloidosis forum multi-organ system working group. Adv Ther. 2023;40(11):4695–710.
23. Louwsma J, Brunger AF, Bijzet J, Kroesen BJ, Roeloffzen WWH, Bischof A, et al. Neurofilament light chain, a biomarker for polyneuropathy in systemic amyloidosis. Amyloid. 2021;28(1):50–5.
24. Rugnath R, Orzechowicz C, Newell C, Carullo V, Rugnath A. A literature review: the mechanisms and treatment of neuropathic pain—a brief discussion. Biomedicines. 2024;12(1):204.
25. Wieling W, Kaufmann H, Claydon VE, Van Wijnen VK, Harms MPM, Juraschek SP, et al. Diagnosis and treatment of orthostatic hypotension. The Lancet Neurol. 2022;21(8):735–46.
26. Gustine JN, Staron A, Szalat RE, Mendelson LM, Joshi T, Ruberg FL, et al. Predictors of hematologic response and survival with stem cell transplantation in AL amyloidosis: A 25-year longitudinal study. American J Hematol. 2022;97(9):1189–99.
27. Argyriou AA, Iconomou G, Kalofonos HP. Bortezomib-induced peripheral neuropathy in multiple myeloma: a comprehensive review of the literature. Blood. 2008;112(5):1593–9.
28. Adams D, Gonzalez-Duarte A, O'Riordan WD, Yang CC, Ueda M, Kristen AV, et al. Patisiran, an RNAi therapeutic, for hereditary transthyretin amyloidosis. N Engl J Med. 2018;379(1):11–21.
29. Benson MD, Waddington-Cruz M, Berk JL, Polydefkis M, Dyck PJ, Wang AK, et al. Inotersen treatment for patients with hereditary transthyretin amyloidosis. N Engl J Med. 2018;379(1):22–31.
30. Berk JL, Suhr OB, Obici L, Sekijima Y, Zeldenrust SR, Yamashita T, et al. Repurposing diflunisal for familial amyloid polyneuropathy: a randomized clinical trial. JAMA. 2013;310(24):2658.
31. Damy T, Kristen AV, Suhr OB, Maurer MS, Planté-Bordeneuve V, Yu CR, et al. Transthyretin cardiac amyloidosis in continental Western Europe: an insight through the Transthyretin Amyloidosis Outcomes Survey (THAOS). Eur Heart J. 2022;43(5):391–400.
32. Caponetti AG, Sguazzotti M, Accietto A, Saturi G, Ponziani A, Giovannetti A, et al. Characterization and natural history of different phenotypes in hereditary transthyretin amyloidosis: 40-year experience at a single Italian referral centre. Eur J Prev Cardiol. 2024;31(7):866–76.
33. Thimm A, Carpinteiro A, Oubari S, Papathanasiou M, Luedike P, Kessler L, et al. Prevalence and predictors of neurological manifestations in systemic AL amyloidosis. J Neurol Sci. 2022;440: 120341.
34. Kokotis P, Manios E, Schmelz M, Fotiou D, Dialoupi I, Gavriatopoulou M, et al. Involvement of small nerve fibres and autonomic nervous system in AL amyloidosis: comprehensive characteristics and clinical implications. Amyloid. 2020;27(2):103–10.

Orthopedic Manifestations of Cardiac Amyloidosis

Josh Schroeder

Abstract Amyloidosis is a heterogeneous acquired or hereditary disease, characterized by extracellular deposition of misfolded protein in the form of beta-pleated sheets (amyloid) fragments throughout the body. The amyloid can deposit in any tissue or organ in the body and can be localized (in one organ) or systemic (in multiple organs). The location and characteristics of the protein are related to the organ dysfunction. The systemic condition is relatively rare but can be life-threatening. The clinical manifestations of amyloidosis are varied and can affect multiple different organs and bodily functions. Musculoskeletal symptoms are common in the disease but are often overlooked and underdiagnosed. Orthopaedic manifestations are common in amyloidosis. Carpal tunnel syndrome (CTS) and spinal stenosis have been well described in association with amyloidosis and may proceed the diagnosis by many years. Other common orthopaedic symptoms include bone and join lesions. In this chapter, we review the incidence and presenting symptoms of common orthopedic manifestations associated with different subtypes of amyloidosis. We also outline the methods for diagnosing the disease and discuss current treatment strategies.

Keywords Amyloid · Carpal tunnel syndrome · Spinal stenosis

Introduction

Brief Overview of Amyloidosis: types, pathogenesis, and Systemic Involvement

Amyloidosis is a heterogeneous acquired or hereditary disease, characterized by extracellular deposition of misfolded protein in the form of beta-pleated sheets (amyloid) fragments throughout the body.

J. Schroeder (✉)
Department of Orthopedics, Hadassah Medical Center, Jerusalem, Israel
e-mail: jes@hadassah.org.il

Faculty of Medicine, Hebrew University, Jerusalem, Israel

E. Herzog (ed.), *Cardiac Amyloidosis*, https://doi.org/10.1007/978-3-031-88342-2_18

Amyloid proteins can accumulate in any tissue or organ. The type and characteristics of the protein determine the amyloid subtype and influence its specific tissue affinity, and is responsible for the corresponding organ dysfunction [1].

The disease can be localized or systemic. Systemic amyloidosis is relatively rare and classified as an orphan disease in Europe, however, is typically progressive and fatal. In contrast, localized site-specific forms of amyloid are very common. In both conditions, one of at least 15 plasma proteins forms amyloid fibrils distant from the site of protein synthesis. In systemic cases, amyloid deposits form in multiple organs and tissues, often leading to life-threatening conditions, whereas the localized cases, proteins are produced at the site of deposition. In both types, fibrils typically accumulate extracellularly, and can form noticeable conspicuous masses that distort tissues and disrupt normal functions [2].

The are multiple forms of amyloidosis, which can be grouped as primary (unknown cause), secondary (linked to other diseases like cancer), and familial (genetic). Common forms include AL amyloidosis (immunoglobulins), AA (inflammatory), and ATTR (transthyretin accumulation).

Cardiac amyloidosis occurs when amyloid deposits take the place of normal heart muscle. Cardiac amyloidosis is the most significant prognostic factor in AL amyloidosis, driving morbidity and mortality due to restrictive cardiomyopathy and subsequent heart failure. It is the leading cause of death in AL amyloidosis [3]. For patients with ATTR amyloidosis who have cardiac involvement, the median survival is generally under 60 months [3–6]. Once amyloid fibrils are deposited in the heart walls, the condition is irreversible [3–6].

Incidence

Amyloidosis is a rare condition and the exact incidence rates vary depending on the specific type of amyloidosis and geographic region.

Here are some general estimates:

- AL amyloidosis: This is a common type in Western countries.
- ATTR amyloidosis: This is more common in certain populations, particularly those of Scandinavian descent.
- AA amyloidosis: This is often associated with chronic inflammatory conditions and is more prevalent in developing countries.

It's important to note that these are general estimates, and actual incidence rates may vary depending on factors like age, gender, and geographic location.

Importance of Early Diagnosis and Management

Symptoms vary depending on the affected organs. The heterogenous, non-specific nature of amyloidosis as well as symptom overlap with other diseases poses significant diagnostic challenges and delays. Nonetheless, early diagnosis is a key determinant for improving patient outcomes, as advanced amyloid organ damage can limit the use of effective treatments [7]. Initiating early treatment with newly developed therapies can potentially change the disease course and extend survival. Since physiological mechanisms are ineffective at clearing amyloid deposits, early detection and prompt treatment are critical for patients with systemic amyloidosis [2, 7, 8].

Emphasis on the Underrecognized Nature of Orthopedic Manifestations

The clinical manifestations of amyloidosis are varied and can affect multiple different organs and bodily functions. Musculoskeletal symptoms are common in the disease but are often overlooked and underdiagnosed [9].

Common orthopaedic manifestations of amyloidosis include osteoarthritis with joint pain, bone lesions, and fractures, all of which are known disease targets [2, 10, 11]. Furthermore, carpal tunnel syndrome and spinal stenosis have been well-described clinical features across various amyloidosis subtypes and often precede a formal diagnosis by several years [10, 11].

Carpal Tunnel Syndrome

The biological link between deposition and accumulation of misfolded proteins known as amyloids and carpal tunnel syndrome has been well described, and often represents an early manifestation of systemic amyloidosis [2, 12].

For many years, hand surgeons observed the presence of amyloids in patients undergoing carpal tunnel release. However, the underlying correlation between amyloidosis and carpal tunnel syndrome (CTS) was never fully understood. This lack of clarity may be due to patients often presenting systemic symptoms of amyloidosis years after their initial encounter with the hand surgeon, or because diagnosing the condition was challenging and treatment options were limited [12].

In recent years and advances in treatment options the association has been observed across various amyloidosis subtypes and often indicates an early manifestation of systemic amyloidosis [9]. Initially, it was primarily linked to hemodialysis-associated β2-microglobulin systemic amyloidosis. However, recent findings indicate that it can precede both hereditary and wild-type ATTR amyloidosis, often by many years [13].

Patients with AL or ATTR amyloidosis frequently experience bilateral carpal tunnel syndrome or require multiple carpal tunnel release surgeries. Therefore, these symptoms should be regarded a red flag [12].

A study in the United States of patients with cardiac amyloidosis due to AL or ATTR amyloidosis found that carpal tunnel syndrome was a presenting symptom in 16% of patients and occurred in 40% of the overall cohort [12]. Hahn et al. reported that approximately 12% of patients over 50 years of age experience carpal tunnel syndrome. Therefore, patients undergoing surgical treatment for transverse carpal ligament issues might benefit from histological evaluation for amyloidosis.

CTS is less prevalent in patients with AL amyloidosis compared to those with ATTR amyloidosis, but it still affects a significant portion of AL amyloidosis patients. Research indicates that nearly 30% of individuals with AL amyloidosis experience CTS, often with bilateral symptoms [12, 14].

The prevalence of CTS in patients with ATTR varies depending on the presence of 9a hereditary mutation, typically ranging from 29 to 68% [12].

Spinal Stenosis

The presence of spinal claudication in patients with systemic amyloidosis was originally described by Benson and colleagues [15, 16]. Current emerging research has shown a high prevalence of amyloid deposits in surgical samples from patients undergoing surgery for lumbar spinal stenosis. Spinal stenosis is a condition characterized by compression of the spinal cord due to thickening of the ligamentum flavum, which can lead to neurological symptoms (Figs. 1 and 2). Multiple studies have indicated significant ATTR amyloid deposits in cases of spinal stenosis, as well as symptoms of systemic amyloidosis. Notably, symptomatic carpal tunnel syndrome (CTS) often appears alongside spinal stenosis proceeding the onset of cardiac amyloidosis, potentially serving as an early indicator of disease development [17].

In the largest prospective study to date of 324 patients undergoing surgical treatment for spinal stenosis, Godara et al. reported that 33–45% of these patients had ATTR amyloid deposits in the ligamentum flavum. His findings may reflect the pathologic role of ATTR amyloidosis in the development of spinal stenosis [18]. Similarly in a prospective study of 47 patients 34% of subjects undergoing clinically indicated lumbar spine surgery had amyloid detected on explanted tissue by Congo red staining [15]. Additionally, in a large prospective study of 250 patients undergoing surgical treatment for lumbar spinal stenosis, Eldhagen observed a notably high prevalence of ATTR amyloid deposits in vertebral ligament tissue, with 37% of patients over the age of 50 exhibiting these deposits [13].

Studies suggest that elderly men with spinal stenosis are at an increased risk for ATTR amyloidosis (Fig. 3). Hence, current recommendations advocate for conducting a biopsy in these patients [3].

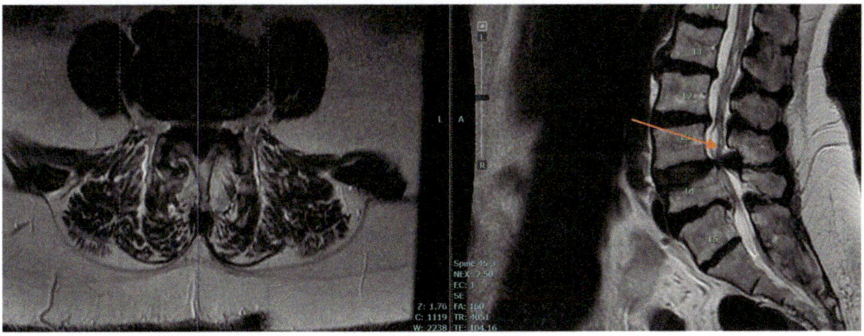

Fig. 1 In this patient with spinal stenosis and amyloidosis, we can see severe thickening of the ligmanetus flavum at the L3-4 level. On the picture on the left we can see the axial cut with severe spinal stenosis, and on the picture on the right we can see the sagittal view with the thickened ligament as indicated by the arrow

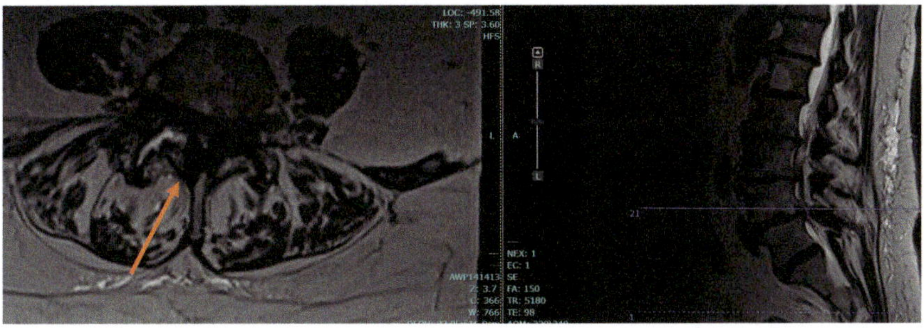

Fig. 2 In this patient with severe spinal stenosis at the L4-5 level we can see complete occlusion of the canal due to thickening of the flavum, and facet hypertrophy. On the picture on the left we can see the axial cut with severe spinal stenosis, as indicated by the arrow and on the picture on the right, we can see the sagittal view with the overall spinal stenosis

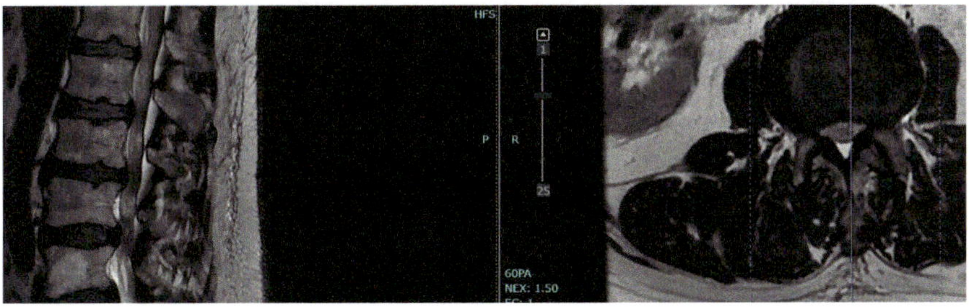

Fig. 3 This patient has over all spinal stenosis, with global thickening of the flavum, causing severe stenosis all over the spinal canal

Joints and Bone Lesions.

Literature reports indicate a correlation between systemic amyloidosis and musculoskeletal diseases. A significant proportion of patients with AL or ATTR amyloidosis develop amyloid deposits in musculoskeletal soft tissues, including ligaments, tendons, and articular cartilage [3, 7, 19, 20].

TTR and light chain amyloid deposits have been identified in synovial tissue biospecimens from patients undergoing hip and knee arthroplasties. Rubin et al. demonstrated that total hip replacements and total knee replacements were notably more common in patients with ATTR-cardiac amyloidosis compared to the general population. Additionally, the study revealed that these joint replacements were more frequent among those with ATTR-cardiac amyloidosis than those with AL-cardiac amyloidosis. Rubin et al. Proposed that his observation might indicate that total hip and knee replacements, along with carpal tunnel syndrome (CTS) and spinal stenosis, could serve as clinical markers for the future development of ATTR amyloidosis [10].

TR and light-chain amyloid deposits were found in the hip and knee synovium of patients undergoing hip and knee arthroplasties. Whether the amyloid deposition in the synovium is age associated and found by coincidence, or corresponds to a diagnosis of systemic disease, has not been elucidated [3].

Joint dysfunction linked to amyloid arthropathy arises from elevated levels of amyloid protein in the synovial fluid and/or its deposition as aggregates in the synovium, articular cartilage, and subchondral bone. The first documented case of amyloid arthropathy was described by Buch in 1873 [21].

Amyloid arthropathy is rare, comprising only 5% of all arthropathies. Most cases are linked to β2M. Following which it presents in patients with AL and ATTR amyloidosis being less common in that order. Typically, amyloid arthropathy occurs in adults aged 30 to 90, with an average onset at 55 years. The condition affects males about twice as often as females [21].

AL amyloid related to plasma cell disorders accounts for approximately 20–25% of amyloid arthropathy cases. However, the occurrence of amyloid arthropathy in patients with plasma cell proliferations is relatively rare, affecting only 2–5% of these individuals [21].

Amyloid arthropathy is often underdiagnosed due to its varied clinical presentation, which can be clinically mistaken for other rheumatoid factor-negative inflammatory arthropathies. Accurate diagnosis is crucial, as joint involvement and associated symptoms may be early indicators of a potentially life-threatening systemic disease. Furthermore, precise identification of the type of amyloid and the extent of amyloidosis is vital for assessing prognosis and planning appropriate treatment.

The clinical presentation of amyloid arthropathy varies based on the extent and amount of amyloid deposition. The initial presenting symptoms often include pain and stiffness in the shoulders, affecting about 80% of cases. This is followed by involvement of the wrists, knees, hips, and other large joints, with the metacarpophalangeal joints typically being affected later [21].

Diagnosis

To obtain accurate diagnosis of amyloidosis a biopsy of the affected organ is recommended, as this method offers the highest sensitivity and can also reveal any associated pathologies. In cases where biopsy is too invasive, such as with the kidneys or heart—where there is a risk of bleeding—a less invasive approach is preferred for suspected amyloidosis. Techniques such as subcutaneous fat aspiration or biopsies of the rectal or gastric mucosa often yield suboptimal results due to issues with misinterpretation and poor smear quality [22].

The gold standard for diagnosing all types of amyloidosis involves positive staining with Congo red and confirmation of a fibrillar appearance via electron microscopy (ELMI). Congo red staining results in apple-green birefringence under polarized light microscopy. To accurately type amyloidosis, Congo red positivity must be interpreted in conjunction with immunohistochemistry, correlating areas that test positive for amyloidosis with the Congo red staining results.

Laser microdissection combined with mass spectrometry-based proteomic analysis is a precise and valuable tool when routine immunofluorescence (IF) and/or immunohistochemical testing fail to definitively classify amyloid deposits [22].

Treatment

Early diagnosis of amyloidosis results in optimal treatment outcomes.

Treatment methods of AL amyloidosis are aimed at eliminating the production of free light chains (FLCs) to eliminate the precursor proteins forming amyloid fibrils and improve organ function. Achieving a complete response or a very good partial hematologic response is linked to the best prognosis. Severe organ dysfunction related to AL amyloidosis may prevent the use of certain medications, necessitating the use of risk-adapted and response-tailored treatment strategies. In cases of cardiac amyloidosis, the prognosis is generally poor and remains largely unaffected by current treatments [22].

Conventional treatment methods for AL amyloidosis include chemotherapy, novel drugs including proteasome inhibitors, immunomodulatory drugs and autologous stem cell transplantation.

Chemotherapy regimens for amyloidosis are adapted from those used in multiple myeloma. Treatment typically involves a combination of melphalan and prednisolone, administered for 12–24 months based on the patient's response. For patients who are ineligible for autologous stem cell transplantation, the gold tandard treatment involves a combination of melphalan and high-dose dexamethasone.

Bortezomib, a proteasome inhibitor, is now considered the frontline treatment for AL amyloidosis. It has been shown to be effective in combination with melphalan and dexamethasone. Other proteasome inhibitors are currently undergoing clinical trials [22].

Thalidomide, an immunomodulatory drug, is often used in combination with cyclophosphamide and dexamethasone, though it is associated with severe adverse effects. Lenalidomide, an additional immunomodulatory drug, has demonstrated partial hematologic response. However, doses exceeding 15 mg of lenalidomide are linked to significant side effects [22].

High-dose melphalan with autologous stem cell transplantation remains the standard of care for low-risk patients with AL amyloidosis. However, eligible patients should undergo thorough eligibility evaluation to minimize the risk of high transplant-related mortality. Recent updates on long-term survival for patients achieving complete remission after autologous stem cell transplantation suggest that the estimated probability of overall survival for these patients is as high as 86% at five years [22].

In summary AL amyloidosis remains a severe disease with poor prognosis. Recent advancement and novel treatment methods including innovative hematologic drugs and immunotherapy, offer promising prospects for improved survival in what was once considered an incurable disease [22].

Similarly, treatment therapies for ATTR amyloidosis have undergone significant advances in recent years. Until recently there were limited therapeutic options for ATTR amyloidosis. For wild-type ATTR (ATTR-wt) amyloidosis, only supportive therapy was available. In variant/hereditary ATTR (ATTR-v) amyloidosis, organ transplantation was considered. However, in the last decade tremendous progress has been made in developing therapeutics for ATTR amyloidosis [23].

Currently, therapeutic options for ATTR include: (1) "stabilizers" that attach to the thyroxine-binding site to maintain the tetrameric form of TTR, thereby reducing the monomeric form; and (2) "silencers" that target TTR mRNA for degradation, which prevents the synthesis of TTR protein. Among the available stabilizers, Diflunisal—a nonsteroidal anti-inflammatory drug (NSAID)—binds to the thyroxine binding site, thereby stabilizing the tetrameric form of transthyretin (TTR). It is FDA-approved for arthritis and has proven effective in treating ATTR amyloidosis. Another approved stabilizer, Tafamidis, has been used to treat cardiac ATTR amyloidosis and has not been associated with any significant side effects [15, 23].

Patisiran, a small interfering RNA a silences therapy, reduces circulating TTR protein levels. It is administered intravenously every three weeks and is generally well tolerated, with only minor infusion reactions reported. Inotersen, another silencing drug, is an antisense oligonucleotide that lowers TTR protein production. Administered as a weekly subcutaneous injection, it may cause thrombocytopenia and glomerulonephritis, so it should be used with caution [23].

Conclusion

Amyloidosis is a complex disease with various subtypes and can manifest as either localized or systemic. Systemic amyloidosis is linked to a worse prognosis, making early diagnosis crucial for improving outcomes. The subtype of the disease is determined by the location of the amyloid deposits. Diagnosing ATTR and AL amyloidosis can be challenging due to nonspecific symptoms, overlapping conditions, and a tendency for these diseases to be under-recognition by physicians. Since patients often exhibit musculoskeletal symptoms prior to disease diagnosis, orthopedic surgeons might play a vital role in early detection. Patients presenting with symptoms such as CTS or spinal stenosis should be assessed for amyloidosis [3].

References

1. Marchi F, Kessler C, Distefano D, Terzi di Bergamo L, Fumagalli L, Averaimo M, et al. Prevalence of amyloid in ligamentum flavum of patients with lumbar spinal stenosis. Amyloid. 2023;30(4):416–23. https://doi.org/10.1080/13506129.2023.2230516.
2. Westermark P, Westermark GT, Suhr OB, Berg S. Transthyretin-derived amyloidosis: probably a common cause of lumbar spinal stenosis. Ups J Med Sci. 2014;119(3):223–8. https://doi.org/10.3109/03009734.2014.895786.
3. Wininger AE, Phelps BM, Le JT, Harris JD, Trachtenberg BH, Liberman SR. Musculoskeletal pathology as an early warning sign of systemic amyloidosis: a systematic review of amyloid deposition and orthopedic surgery. BMC Musculoskelet Disord. 2021;22(1):51.
4. Rapezzi C, Merlini G, Quarta CC, et al. Systemic cardiac amyloidoses: disease profiles and clinical courses of the 3 main types. Circulation. 2009;120(13):1203–12.
5. Lane T, Fontana M, Martinez-Naharro A, et al. Natural history, quality of life, and outcome in cardiac Transthyretin amyloidosis. Circulation. 2019;140(1):16–26.
6. Grogan M, Dispenzieri A, Gertz MA. Light-chain cardiac amyloidosis: strategies to promote early diagnosis and cardiac response. Heart. 2017;103(14):1065–722.
7. Prokaeva T, Spencer B, Kaut M, Ozonoff A, Doros G, Connors LH, Skinner M, Seldin DC. Soft tissue, joint, and bone manifestations of AL amyloidosis: clinical presentation, molecular features, and survival. Arthritis Rheum. 2007;56(11):3858–68. https://doi.org/10.1002/art.22959.
8. Brown CR, Bergin JD, Deal DN. Amyloidosis and considerations for the hand surgeon. J Hand Surg Am. 2024;49(3):260–6. https://doi.org/10.1016/j.jhsa.2023.10.013.
9. Radmer S, Andresen JR. Carpal tunnel syndrome, spinal canal stenosis, cardiomyopathy, renal insufficiency, enteropathy, and diffuse myopathy as an expression of systemic ATTR amyloidosis—diagnostics and therapy. J Surg Case Rep. 2024;2024(3):rjae183. https://doi.org/10.1093/jscr/rjae183.
10. Rubin J, Alvarez J, Teruya S, Castano A, Lehman RA, Weidenbaum M, et al. Hip and knee arthroplasty are common among patients with transthyretin cardiac amyloidosis, occurring years before cardiac amyloid diagnosis: can we identify affected patients earlier? Amyloid. 2017;24(4):226–30. https://doi.org/10.1080/13506129.2017.1375908.
11. Kramer MR, van Dijk JM, Hadas I, Hershko C. Destructive bone lesions in primary amyloidosis. Postgrad Med J. 1986;62(733):1037–41. https://doi.org/10.1136/pgmj.62.733.1037.
12. Donnelly JP, Hanna M, Sperry BW, Seitz WH Jr. Carpal tunnel syndrome: a potential early, red-flag sign of amyloidosis. J Hand Surg Am. 2019;44(10):868–76. https://doi.org/10.1016/j.jhsa.2019.06.016.

13. Eldhagen P, Berg S, Lund LH, Sörensson P, Suhr OB, Westermark P. Transthyretin amyloid deposits in lumbar spinal stenosis and assessment of signs of systemic amyloidosis. J Intern Med. 2021;289(6):895–905. https://doi.org/10.1111/joim.13222.
14. Dubrey SW, Cha K, Anderson J, Chamarthi B, Reisinger J, Skinner M, et al. The clinical features of immunoglobulin light-chain (AL) amyloidosis with heart involvement. QJM. 1998;91(2):141–57. https://doi.org/10.1093/qjmed/91.2.141. PMID: 9578896.
15. Maurer MS, Smiley D, Simsolo E, Remotti F, Bustamante A, Teruya S, et al. Analysis of lumbar spine stenosis specimens for identification of amyloid. J Am Geriatr Soc. 2022;70(12):3538–48.
16. Harats N, Worth R, Benson MD. Spinal claudication in systemic amyloidosis. J Rheumatol. 1989;16:1003–6.
17. Aus dem Siepen F, Hein S, Prestel S, Baumgärtner C, Schönland S, Hegenbart U, Röcken C, et al. Carpal tunnel syndrome and spinal canal stenosis: harbingers of transthyretin amyloid cardiomyopathy? Clin Res Cardiol. 20190.
18. Godara A, Riesenburger RI, Zhang DX, Varga C, Fogaren T, Siddiqui NS, et al. Association between spinal stenosis and wild-type ATTR amyloidosis. Amyloid. 2021;28(4):226–33.
19. Sueyoshi T, Ueda M, Jono H, et al. Wild-type transthyretin-derived amyloidosis in various ligaments and tendons. Hum Pathol. 2011;42(9):1259–64.
20. Rubin J, Alvarez J, Teruya S, Castano A, Lehman RA, Weidenbaum M, et al. Hip and knee arthroplasty are common among patients with transthyretin cardiac amyloidosis, occurring years before cardiac amyloid diagnosis: can we identify affected patients earlier? Amyloid. 2017;24(4):226–30.
21. Diaz-Perez JA, Conway SA, Zuo Y, Nielsen GP, Selig M, Rosenberg AE. Amyloid arthropathy: a review. Adv Anat Pathol. 2021;28(6):415–25.
22. Ryšavá R. AL amyloidosis: advances in diagnostics and treatment. Nephrol Dial Transplant. 2019;34(9):1460–6.
23. Campbell CM, Zhang K, Lenihan DJ, Witteles R. Developing therapy for transthyretin amyloidosis. Am J Med. 2022;135(Suppl 1):S44–8.

Gastrointestinal and Hepatic Manifestations of Systemic Amyloidosis

Yuval Ishay and Tiberiu Hershcovici

Abstract Amyloidosis of the gastrointestinal tract is an uncommon disorder characterized by the deposition of amyloid in its different segments. Due to its rarity and protean manifestations the diagnosis and treatment are difficult. Herein we expound on the various aspects of diagnosis (pathological, endoscopic, and clinical), the unique characteristics of each clinical gastrointestinal manifestation and its therapeutic implications. We aim to give a bird's eye view of this oft-neglected area and make it accessible to the scientist and physician.

Keywords Systemic amyloidosis · Gastrointestinal amyloidosis

Background

As the general principles of amyloidosis have been greatly expounded upon in this book by other authors, we shall attempt to provide a focused review of the gastrointestinal manifestations of amyloidosis. Gastrointestinal manifestations of amyloidosis are often non-specific and can easily be attributed to other more common etiologies such as inflammation, infection, primary motility disorders or functional gastrointestinal disorders. A high index of suspicion should thus be maintained, especially in individuals with pre-disposing or related conditions.

When endoscopy is undertaken in patients with amyloidosis, both endoscopic and pathologic findings (excluding specific stains) may be non-specific. Mucosal involvement by amyloidosis may manifest on endoscopy as mucosal atrophy, a somewhat subtle endoscopic finding. Other changes may include a friable mucosa with a bleeding tendency, possibly related to the deposition of amyloid in the submucosa and endothelial spaces. In certain cases, pathology shows profound amyloid infiltration of the tissue, producing thick amyloid band at the submucosal level, or even

Y. Ishay · T. Hershcovici (✉)
Department of Gastroenterology and Hepatology, Hadassah University Medical Center, Hebrew University, Jerusalem, Israel
e-mail: tiberiu.hershcovici@gmail.com

E. Herzog (ed.), *Cardiac Amyloidosis*, https://doi.org/10.1007/978-3-031-88342-2_19

complete alteration of normal tissue architecture by amyloid. At times, an inflammatory picture predominates, with stricturing and ulcerating disease seen at endoscopy. These cases in particular may prove a diagnostic and therapeutic challenge [1].

When examined through the lens of histopathology, biopsy-confirmed gastrointestinal amyloidosis seems to be more common in elderly males, with ATTR amyloidosis patients tending to be older than those with other types. Pathology-confirming gastrointestinal amyloidosis is often obtained from the colon (especially rectum), and stomach, likely reflecting to some extent the relative endoscopic accessibility of these organs. The mucosal and submucosal layers often yield positive results in cases of amyloidosis, underlining the fact that deep tissue biopsies are usually not required for the diagnosis [2]. In gastrointestinal AA amyloidosis, a sequential involvement was hypothesized, with amyloid accumulation progressing from the vasculature to the GI muscle layer and to the interstitial cells of Cajar (with their pacemaker action) [3].

AL, AA and ATTRv amyloidosis have all been described as causing gastrointestinal amyloidosis. It appears that wild-type ATTR patients have no gastrointestinal manifestations [4]. Still, a vexing truth of gastrointestinal amyloidosis is that it is hard to assess with any degree of certainty which forms of amyloidosis most commonly cause gastrointestinal manifestations and if any manifestation occurs more commonly in one form or the other. The relative rarity of this condition and the lack of studies makes our ability to gain high-quality insight limited, and any data needs to be interpreted with caution.

Mucosal Manifestations of Amyloidosis

Gastrointestinal amyloidosis has been characterized as the cause of diarrhea in many case series and case reports. While these changes may be attributed at least partially to neural changes and motility effects of the disease, mucosal inflammation and malabsorption are likely contributors in many cases.

In a study of 19 patients with confirmed amyloidosis, weight loss was seen in all patients, and steatorrhea—fat-containing stools indicating malabsorption—in nearly all patients [5]. Protein-losing enteropathy is another manifestation of gastrointestinal amyloidosis, and is another possible cause of diarrhea and malabsorption [6].

Malabsorption due to mucosal involvement by amyloidosis may occur through a variety of mechanisms.

Mucosal inflammation, sometimes associated with ulceration, luminal stenosis, and bleeding, likely occurs in the setting of ischemic changes due to deposition of amyloid in blood vessels. This is probably best exemplified in the catastrophic—and thankfully rare—cases of intestinal perforation due to amyloidosis, where blood supply is sufficiently compromised as to cause complete loss of organ integrity [7].

Amyloidoma—a rare finding of accumulated amyloid protein in tissue—has been described as arising in various locations in the gastrointestinal tract. These may be found in every gastrointestinal organ but are most common in the colon and small bowel. They may cause mass effects on both the tissue and the lumen, causing inflammation and bleeding or obstructive symptoms, respectively. On endoscopy, they resemble malignancy, and thus need to be thoroughly biopsied to allow for the correct diagnosis [8].

Small intestinal bacterial overgrowth—a disorder characterized by an abnormal increase in the number of small intestine bacteria—has not been well studied and described in the context of intestinal amyloidosis. However, this disorder is recognized as associated with motility disorders, and it is likely that its prevalence is increased in amyloidosis patients. It is also known to cause intestinal inflammation and malabsorption [9]. Recently, changes in gut microbiota in amyloidosis patients have been demonstrated in a study, with future studies possibly further elucidating microbiome changes in amyloidosis [10].

Hepatic Manifestations of Amyloidosis

AL amyloidosis has been the type most frequently associated with hepatic involvement and subsequent dysfunction, while AA amyloidosis less frequently causes hepatic abnormalities.

Hepatic abnormalities include a high prevalence of hepatomegaly, and cholestatic type liver enzyme abnormalities with marked elevation of alkaline phosphatase level.

Deposition of amyloid in the liver parenchyma, in the vascular wall and in the liver sinusoidal spaces, can cause portal hypertension in some patients. Signs of portal hypertension and hepatic dysfunction, including low platelet counts and elevated bilirubin, have been associated with reduced survival in patients with hepatic amyloidosis [11]. Unfortunately, diagnosis of hepatic amyloidosis may be challenging without a biopsy, especially considering the often-non-specific findings on imaging studies.

Dysmotility Due to Amyloidosis

Bowel dysmotility is axiomatic in amyloidosis patients. In hereditary ATTR dysmotility symptoms have been described in 56–69% of patients [4], and while robust number do not exist separately for all amyloidosis types, dysmotility is often experienced in patients with all types of amyloidosis.

Bowel dysmotility is likely multi-factorial in nature, owing to neurological dysfunction, mucosal dysfunction and tissue changes due to amyloid infiltration.

Broadly, changes in bowel motility can be classified to those affecting the upper gastrointestinal tract—esophagus, stomach, and small bowel—and those affecting the lower gastrointestinal tract, i.e. the colon.

Autonomic (vagal) denervation causing impaired esophageal and gastric motility may be a major contributor to at least some of the upper gastrointestinal manifestation of amyloidosis such as early satiety, heartburn, and dyspepsia type pain. This has been demonstrated by changes in Vagus nerve cross-sectional area as imaged by ultrasound in cases of transthyretin familial autonomic neuropathy [12].

Gastric and small bowel motility have been further studied in ATTRv amyloidosis, demonstrating delayed gastric emptying by scintigraphy in one-third of patients, and neuromyopathic small bowel changes in 58% of patients in another cohort [13, 14]. Notably, both these studies suggested multi-factorial (i.e. not purely neurogenic) causes for these changes, further stressing the combined etiology of these findings.

Dilation of the colon—or, less commonly, the small intestine—to the extent where severe distention and discomfort are caused, sometimes progressing to a state of compromising intestinal wall integrity and perforation, is known as intestinal pseudo-obstruction. Intestinal pseudo-obstruction has long been associated with amyloidosis, with clear descriptions of this association dating as early as 1970 [15]. This disorder may be thought of as the culmination of dysmotility, and may be especially exacerbated by opiate treatment, electrolyte disturbances, and immobilization. This underlines the need for a high index of suspicion for diagnosis in hospitalized and medicated amyloidosis patients.

Pancreatic Insufficiency Due to Amyloidosis

While amyloid deposition in pancreatic parenchyma has been described, systematic studies are lacking and usually confined to case reports. However, a general picture may be drawn from the accumulated reported cases. Deposition of amyloid protein in islet cells has been demonstrated in type 2 diabetes, and associated with reduced β-cell mass [16]. These findings, however, are usually seen in patients without systemic amyloidosis.

In systemic amyloidosis, amyloid deposition in pancreatic islets have been demonstrated, but appear to be sparser, and their association with pancreatic endocrine insufficiency less robustly demonstrated [17, 18].

While exocrine pancreatic insufficiency may have been expected in amyloidosis, few studies have demonstrated this, and no robust evidence exists to support this manifestation.

Amyloidosis Caused by Gastrointestinal Inflammation

An under-recognized interface of amyloidosis and the gastrointestinal tract is the role of inflammatory bowel disease as a recognized, albeit rare, cause of AA amyloidosis. Amyloidosis is generally reported as present in 0.5% of IBD patients [19]. This rare cause of amyloidosis appears to be more common in colonic Crohn's disease than in ulcerative colitis and is usually accompanied by proteinuria due to concomitant renal involvement [20, 21]. Clinically, hospitalized patients with amyloidosis complicating IBD appear to have a worse clinical course. Poorly controlled IBD may be a significant factor in their worse outcomes, as active IBD is widely accepted to increase the risk of amyloidosis, likely due to increased elaboration of inflammation-related substances [22]. Amyloidosis as a manifestation of IBD is generally agreed to occur in the setting of long-standing disease, with cases of simultaneous diagnosis usually attributed to a delay in the diagnosis and treatment of IBD.

Therapeutic Implications of Gastrointestinal Amyloidosis

There are several biomarkers for assessment of amyloidosis severity and prognostication. Biomarkers signifying end-organ damage such as pro-BNP and cardiac troponin in cardiac amyloidosis are correlated with worse outcomes. In response to therapy, reduction in elevated biomarkers of the damaged organ has been correlated with improved outcomes, including overall survival [23, 24].

No robust, reproducible biomarkers for diagnosis, prediction of severity or response to treatment have been found in amyloidosis of the gastrointestinal tract or the liver. Due to lack of specific treatment for amyloidosis, we think that is reasonable to treat amyloidosis-related end-organ damage to achieve improvement in gastrointestinal symptoms. As there is a relative paucity of high-quality trials, treatment must for the time be guided by clinical judgement and experience.

Notably, one form of disease-specific therapy for ATTRv has been liver transplantation, providing a significant crossroads between amyloidosis and the gastrointestinal system. In this case, the liver is the source of the mutated protein, and liver transplantation provides de-facto gene therapy. While results of liver transplant in ATTRv patients have been encouraging, results vary according to co-morbidities, disease length, and concurrent transplantation of other organs [25]. The overall benefit of this therapy compared with anti-amyloid drugs bears further assessment, and likely depends on patient selection and center experience [26].

Therapy directed at dysbiosis: Rifaximin, a well-studied oral antibiotic, has shown efficacy in SIBO, and can be expected to be beneficial for symptoms of distention, diarrhea and malabsorption caused by SIBO in amyloidosis patients. Dietary changes and probiotic supplementation have also been studied in SIBO, to much less robust results. These may be considered as adjunctive treatment in non or partial responders.

Therapy directed at malabsorption: Patients manifesting symptoms of malabsorption, such as fatty stools, diarrhea, weight loss or markers of malnutrition, should receive nutritional support. If the cause of malabsorption cannot be treated, then supportive strategies including nutritional support should be started. Severe malabsorption, especially if combined with underlying dysmotility, may need to be more aggressively managed via percutaneous feeding strategies (such as feeding gastrostomy or jejunostomy), and in some cases with parenteral nutrition. In such cases the value of a multidisciplinary management team including physicians and dieticians cannot be overstated.

Management of dysmotility: The cornerstone of constipation management should always be lifestyle changes. Patients should be encouraged to ambulate and engage in physical activity, increase fiber and water intake, and be taught toilet hygiene including timed evacuations. Laxatives are the next step, with osmotic and stimulant laxatives gradually titrated according to patient response. Other types of laxatives and enemas may be judiciously used, if required. In patients with severe constipation suspected or proven to stem from prolonged intestinal transit, use of acetylcholine esterase inhibitors (e.g. oral pyridostigmine), metoclopramide, and domperidone have been used to varying degrees of success.

Prucalopride, a 5-HT_4 agonist that increases colonic motility, has shown benefit in chronic intestinal pseudo-obstruction, and is thus likely to exert benefit also in cases that are amyloid related [27].

Other novel therapies used for constipation, such as Chloride channel activators and Guanylate cyclase C agonists, may provide benefit but have not been widely used in this setting.

Sacral nerve stimulation has shown benefit in some cases of intractable constipation, as have various modalities of transcutaneous neural stimulation. However, they have not been studied in chronic intestinal pseudo-obstruction due to amyloidosis.

Though surgery is a tenuous prospect in some of these patients, surgical treatment may provide great symptomatic relief in a subset of patients. In rare cases, where constipation becomes debilitating and refractory to therapy, ileostomy or colostomy with scheduled external irrigation may be required.

In patients with predominant diarrhea**,** therapy is best directed at its presumptive cause.

Osmotic diarrhea due to malabsorption of specific nutrients may be improved by reducing dietary lactose or by usage of specific medical nutrition containing partially or completely hydrolyzed amino acids.

Judicious use of anti-motility agents, such as loperamide, may be required, and results are sometimes seen only when higher doses are reached. In more refractory cases, use of somatostatin analogues to reduce colonic motility or of bile-acid sequestrants to treat diarrhea due to bile acid malabsorption may be useful, but should be individualized and discussed with physicians with experience in treating these conditions [28].

Management of pancreatic insufficiency: Severe endocrine pancreatic insufficiency may need to be addressed with subcutaneous insulin. In milder cases, other oral and parenteral medications can be used, as in other cases of diabetes.

Management of Liver disease: Unfortunately, severe liver dysfunction accompanying amyloidosis is unlikely to be significantly improved via supportive measures and should be managed, similar to cases of cirrhosis, in the setting of a multidisciplinary team. Liver transplantation for treatment of hepatic amyloidosis may be considered, and has been described in small-scale studies, but long-term results are unclear, especially when compared with therapy for the primary disease, where possible [29, 30]. When cholestasis is the predominant manifestation, use of ursodeoxycholic acid, along with judicious use of interventions aimed at improving bile drainage, may be considered as an adjunctive measure.

In conclusion, amyloidosis of the gastrointestinal tract may manifest in a host of ways, and may pose a diagnostic challenge, especially if gastrointestinal manifestations precede more classic signs. As few findings are pathognomonic, a high index of suspicion must be maintained in appropriate patients. Therapeutically, there are few disease-specific therapies, and a patient-oriented, multi-modal approach administered by a multi-disciplinary team is likely to yield the best results.

References

1. Latorre G, Vargas JI, Espino A. Endoscopic features of gastrointestinal amyloid light-chain amyloidosis. Lancet Gastroenterol Hepatol. 2021;6:874.
2. Freudenthaler S, Hegenbart U, Schönland S, et al. Amyloid in biopsies of the gastrointestinal tract-a retrospective observational study on 542 patients. Virchows Arch. 2016;468:569–77.
3. den Braber-Ymker M, Heijker S, Lammens M, et al. Intestinal involvement in amyloidosis is a sequential process. Neurogastroenterol Motil. 2018;30: e13469.
4. Wixner J, Mundayat R, Karayal ON, et al. THAOS: gastrointestinal manifestations of transthyretin amyloidosis—common complications of a rare disease. Orphanet J Rare Dis. 2014;9:61.
5. Hayman SR, Lacy MQ, Kyle RA, et al. Primary systemic amyloidosis: a cause of malabsorption syndrome. Am J Med. 2001;111:535–40.
6. Fushimi T, Takahashi Y, Kashima Y, et al. Severe protein losing enteropathy with intractable diarrhea due to systemic AA amyloidosis, successfully treated with corticosteroid and octreotide. Amyloid. 2005;12:48–53.
7. Harada K, Ichikawa D, Konishi H, et al. Perforation of the sigmoid colon and massive ischemia of the small intestine caused by amyloidosis associated with multiple myeloma: a case report. Int Surg. 2014;99:685–90.
8. Talar-Wojnarowska R, Jamroziak K. Intestinal amyloidosis: clinical manifestations and diagnostic challenge. Adv Clin Exp Med. 2021;30:563–70.
9. Bushyhead D, Quigley EMM. Small intestinal bacterial overgrowth—pathophysiology and its implications for definition and management. Gastroenterology. 2022;163:593–607.
10. Chen C-C, Tseng P-H, Hsueh H-W, et al. Altered gut microbiota in Taiwanese A97S predominant transthyretin amyloidosis with polyneuropathy. Sci Rep. 2024;14:6195.
11. Park MA, Mueller PS, Kyle RA, et al. Primary (AL) hepatic amyloidosis: clinical features and natural history in 98 patients. Medicine. 2003;82:291–8.
12. Du K, Xu K, Chu X, et al. Vagus nerve ultrasound in transthyretin familial amyloid polyneuropathy: a pilot study. J Neuroimaging. 2022;32:285–91.
13. Wixner J, Karling P, Rydh A, et al. Gastric emptying in hereditary transthyretin amyloidosis: the impact of autonomic neuropathy. Neurogastroenterol Motil. 2012;24:1111-e568.
14. Wixner J, Törnblom H, Karling P, et al. Abnormal small bowel motility in patients with hereditary transthyretin amyloidosis. Neurogastroenterol Motil. 2018;30: e13354.
15. Legge DA, Wollaeger EE, Carlson HC. Intestinal pseudo-obstruction in systemic amyloidosis. Gut. 1970;11:764–7.
16. Hull RL, Westermark GT, Westermark P, et al. Islet amyloid: a critical entity in the pathogenesis of type 2 diabetes. J Clin Endocrinol Metab. 2004;89:3629–43.
17. Tomita T. Amyloidosis of pancreatic islets in primary amyloidosis (AL type). Pathol Int. 2005;55:223–7.

18. Ozdemir DMD, Dagdelen SMD, Erbas TMD. Endocrine involvement in systemic amyloidosis. Endocr Pract. 2010;16:1056–63.
19. Tosca Cuquerella J, Bosca-Watts MM, Anton Ausejo R, et al. Amyloidosis in inflammatory bowel disease: a systematic review of epidemiology, clinical features, and treatment. J Crohns Colitis. 2016;10:1245–53.
20. Greenstein AJ, Sachar DB, Panday AK, et al. Amyloidosis and inflammatory bowel disease. A 50-year experience with 25 patients. Medicine (Baltimore) 1992;71:261–70.
21. Sattianayagam PT, Gillmore JD, Pinney JH, et al. Inflammatory bowel disease and systemic AA amyloidosis. Dig Dis Sci. 2013;58:1689–97.
22. Sharma P, Aguilar R, Siddiqui OA, et al. Secondary systemic amyloidosis in inflammatory bowel disease: a nationwide analysis. Ann Gastroenterol. 2017;30:504–11.
23. Dittrich T, Kimmich C, Hegenbart U, et al. Prognosis and staging of AL amyloidosis. Acta Haematol. 2020;143:388–400.
24. Griffin JM, Rosenthal JL, Grodin JL, et al. ATTR amyloidosis: current and emerging management strategies. JACC: CardioOncology 2021;3:488–505.
25. Ericzon B-G, Wilczek HE, Larsson M, et al. Liver transplantation for hereditary transthyretin amyloidosis: after 20 years still the best therapeutic alternative? Transplantation. 2015;99:1847–54.
26. Socie P, Benmalek A, Cauquil C, et al. Comparison between tafamidis and liver transplantation as first-line therapy for hereditary transthyretin amyloidosis. Amyloid. 2023;30:303–12.
27. Mutalib M, Kammermeier J, Vora R, et al. Prucalopride in intestinal pseudo obstruction, paediatric experience and systematic review. Acta Gastroenterol Belg. 2021;84:429–34.
28. Sattianayagam PT, Hawkins PN, Gillmore JD. Systemic amyloidosis and the gastrointestinal tract. Nat Rev Gastroenterol Hepatol. 2009;6:608–17.
29. Elnegouly M, Specht K, Zoller H, et al. Liver transplantation followed by autologous stem cell transplantation for acute liver failure caused by AL amyloidosis. Case report and review of the literature. Ann Hepatol. 2016;15:592–7.
30. Riveiro-Barciela M, Gironella M, Senín A, et al. Decompensated liver disease due to primary hepatic amyloidosis: is liver transplantation still mandatory? Hepatology. 2019;69:2701–3.

Follow up and Prognosis of Patients with Cardiac Amyloidosis

Jean Marc Weinstein

Abstract Cardiac amyloidosis (CA) is a slowly progressive disease, causing myriad presentations in affected patients, including heart failure (the predominant problem), conduction system defects and arrhythmias (especially atrial fibrillation). Symptoms and signs appear over a long timeframe and result in significant limitation in functional capacity, deteriorating quality of life and often lead to recurrent cardiac and heart failure hospitalizations. Involvement of other organ systems, leading to neurological, orthopaedic, renal, gastrointestinal or haematological pathology is widespread and add to the patients' burden of morbidity. Close follow-up by multidisciplinary teams specializing in cardiac CA is the optimal method of monitoring, with emphasis on clinical and functional assessment, follow-up of various biomarkers and other laboratory parameters, and monitoring using electrocardiography and imaging techniques (specifically echocardiography). The prognosis in this disease has always been considered dismal, as no specific treatment was available. Over the past few years, however, new drugs have improved the outlook both in ATTR (transthyretin) and AL (light chain) cardiac amyloidosis.

Keywords Cardiac amyloidosis · Follow-up · Symptoms · Biomarkers · Electrocardiography · Imaging · Prognosis

Introduction

This chapter will suggest recommendations for follow-up and monitoring of patients who have already been diagnosed with cardiac amyloidosis (CA), and delve into the present knowledge on prognosis. It should be stressed that amyloidosis is a multi-system disorder, often with concomitant involvement of the neurological, musculoskeletal, nephrological, haematological and gastrointestinal systems to varying extents. Patients remain under clinical surveillance by the appropriate teams, but

---

J. M. Weinstein (✉)
Regional Heart Failure Service, Cardiology Department, Soroka University Medical Centre, Clalit Health Services, Southern Region, Beer Sheva, Israel
e-mail: jmwein@bgu.ac.il

E. Herzog (ed.), *Cardiac Amyloidosis*, https://doi.org/10.1007/978-3-031-88342-2_20

below we shall detail the recommendations solely regarding cardiology follow-up and monitoring.

Follow-up

Cardiac amyloidosis (CA) is a progressive disease usually with a slow, gradual deterioration in the clinical state of the patient, punctuated by occasional acute episodes often requiring hospitalization. Modes and frequency of follow-up have been proposed in several recent documents [1–4]. In this chapter, a summary of the recommendations will be made.

Setting of Follow-up

It is recommended that all patients with a diagnosis of CA should be referred to a multispecialty CA centre [1, 4], although not all medical organizations have this facility available. In the absence of an accessible CA centre, telemedicine with CA experts could be considered [4].

Clinical Follow-up

Lifelong follow-up is essential to ensure clinical stability, to detect worsening symptoms or new disease-related cardiac complications such as arrhythmias or conduction disorders, or complications involving other organs or systems.

A recent consensus document [2] proposed a comprehensive scheme for monitoring the course of patients with CA based on a set of 11 measurable features across three domains: clinical and functional endpoints, biomarkers and laboratory markers, and electrocardiographic and imaging parameters. The authors recommend that one marker from each of the three domains provides the minimum requirements for assessing disease progression (Fig. 1).

Clinical and Functional Monitoring

Regarding follow-up of clinical and functional endpoints, the panel of experts [2] propose delving into the medical history, with an emphasis on cardiovascular (in particular heart failure [HF]) admissions, New York Heart Association (NYHA) classification, and assessing quality of life, utilizing tools such as the Kansas City

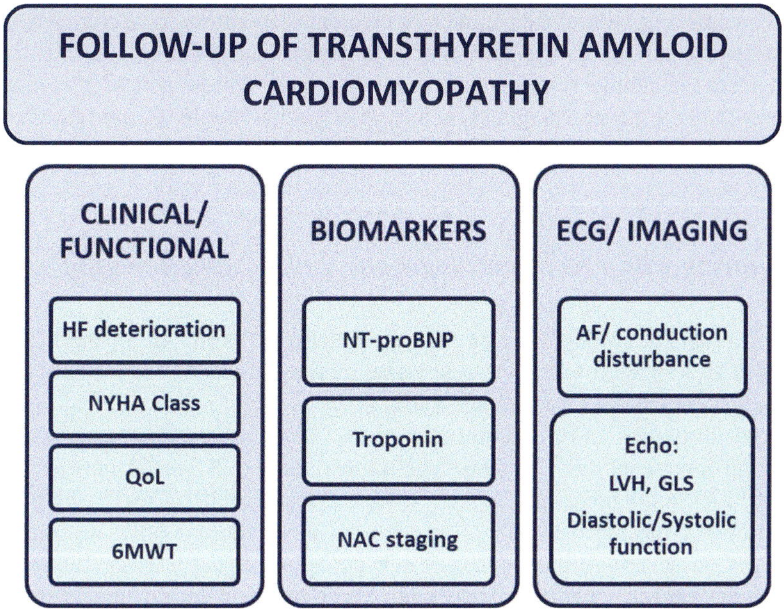

Fig. 1 AF: atrial fibrillation; ECG: electrocardiogram; Echo: echocardiogram; GLS: global longitudinal strain; HF: heart failure; LVH: left ventricular hypertrophy; NAC: UK National Amyloidosis Centre; NYHA: New York Heart Association; NT-proBNP: N-terminal pro-B type natriuretic peptide; QoL: quality of life; 6MWT: Six-minute walk test. [2] Adapted from Garcia-Pavia et al.

Cardiomyopathy Questionnaire (KCCQ). The six-minute walk test (6MWT) is also suggested as an appropriate objective method for assessing functional capacity.

Most patients with CA will have some degree of heart failure (HF), usually presenting with fluid overload. Careful clinical assessment is essential, with the initiation of loop diuretics but exercising caution to avoid excessive diuresis which may lead to symptomatic hypotension or orthostatic hypotension, to which these patients are prone [3, 5]. Similarly, drugs commonly administered for HF or for underlying hypertension, such as beta blockers, angiotensin converting enzyme inhibitors (ACEIs), angiotensin receptor blockers (ARBs) or angiotensin receptor/neprilysin inhibitor (ARNI) may require doses reduced, or be stopped, because of bradycardia or hypotension [3, 5], often with improvement in symptoms after discontinuation.

Monitoring of Biomarker and Laboratory Markers

In the consensus document [2], the use of biomarkers and other laboratory markers in follow-up is emphasized, and assessment of disease stability/progression by measuring levels of N-terminal proBNP [NT-proBNP] (typically strikingly elevated in CA) and troponin (generally elevated but not markedly so). These two biomarkers may be combined with other parameters including laboratory measurements, such as glomerular filtration rate (GFR), or dose of diuretic and NYHA class, and utilized to calculate the clinical staging of a patient during the disease course, and monitor changes [4, 6–9]. Several staging schemes exist, such as the NAC, the UK National Amyloidosis Centre staging system.

Monitoring with Electrocardiography and Cardiac Imaging

The third domain proposed for monitoring patients [2] is the use of the ECG and Holter ECG, looking for the appearance of atrial fibrillation (AF) or various types of conduction defects, all of which are common in CA.

Atrial fibrillation (AF) and embolic events are frequent complications during follow-up of patients with CA. The reported prevalence of AF in CA may be as high as 56% in AL amyloidosis and 70% in ATTR amyloidosis [10]. The risk for intracardiac thrombus may reach 33% in CA and may be present even in fully anticoagulated patients. Consequently, transesophageal echocardiography (TEE) is recommended to exclude the presence of left atrial appendage thrombus even if the patient is anticoagulated [11]. The CHA_2DS_2-VASc score did not correlate well with clinical outcome in a recent study [12] and it is recommended not be used to assess thromboembolic risk in CA, and prophylactic anticoagulation is advised in all patients with CA and AF [1, 3].

Close monitoring for conduction defects is warranted, as these are common in CA [10], necessitating implantation of a permanent pacemaker. Cardiac resynchronization therapy (CRT) may be considered, and could be preferable to standard pacing in terms of efficacy [13], although not assessed in a controlled fashion.

In addition, monitoring by cardiac imaging particularly with serial echocardiography follow-up is an excellent tool for detecting changes in the degree of left ventricular hypertrophy (LVH)—one of the hallmarks of CA, change in the diastolic properties of the LV, change in global longitudinal strain (GLS) or change in systolic function. MRI is an essential tool in the initial diagnosis of CA, but has not been adequately assessed as a tool for routine follow-up, and in addition is expensive, not widely available and its use may be limited in patients with pacemakers. Cardiac scintigraphy with bone avid tracers such as ^{99m}Tc-pyrophosphate (PYP) is also a crucial investigation in the preliminary diagnosis of ATTR CA, but has not been evaluated as an appropriate method in the follow-up of the patients.

Frequency of Follow-up

No studies have specifically addressed the optimal follow up protocol for patients with CA, but based on proposals by the ESC Working Group on Myocardial and Pericardial Diseases [1] and an expert consensus document [2], a reasonable scheme would involve 3- to 6-month visits with ECG and complete blood tests (including NT- proBNP and troponin), and annual echocardiography and 24-h Holter ECG. Quality of life and functional capacity are suggested to be assessed every 6 months with the KCCQ or similar tool, and 6MWT [1, 2]. Obviously, if any interim clinical deterioration occurs, follow-up will need to be intensified accordingly.

Prognosis

Cardiac amyloidosis is a relentlessly progressive disease, with a poor prognosis if not identified and treated as early as possible.

ATTR Amyloid

In ATTR CA, several parameters influence the prognosis of patients affected. These include the variant involved (better prognosis in the wild-type variant [$ATTR_{wt}$] than in a genetic mutation [$ATTR_m$], particularly the V122I variant [14]), the degree of cardiac involvement, and the neurological phenotype [6–8]. Staging systems have been developed, as mentioned above, which may be utilized to assess a patient's prognosis [4, 6–9]. These staging systems may be specific for the wild-type, or for both the wild-type and the genetic variant mutations.

The main goals of treatment for ATTR CA are to stabilize the transthyretin or to halt its production. The landmark ATTR-ACT study [15] demonstrated a reduction in all-cause mortality and in cardiovascular hospitalizations in patients randomized to receive tafamidis, a stabilizer of transthyretin. The greatest impact was achieved in those in NYHA class I or II, but recently even patients in NYHA III showed a survival benefit in long-term follow-up [16] and also in octogenarians, similar to younger patients [17]. Tafamidis is presently the mainstay of targeted therapy in ATTR CA, but new drugs- both transthyretin stabilizers and drugs to diminish its production—are in various stages of development and early clinical evaluation [18]. Recently, the Helios-B trial demonstrated the efficacy of vutrisiran, a subcutaneously administered RNA interference therapeutic agent, which inhibits the production of hepatic transthyretin, in reducing the risk of death from any cause and cardiovascular events compared to placebo and also preserving functional capacity and quality of life [19].

AL Amyloid

Cardiac involvement due to light chain deposition from various haematological conditions (AL amyloid) carries a worse prognosis than amyloid deposition due to transthyretin (ATTR amyloid) and generally demonstrates a faster deterioration of HF [20]. Delay in the diagnosis of CA results in more cardiac involvement, which is the main adverse prognostic parameter in the disease. Indeed, the mortality risk in AL amyloid may reach 35–60% in the first year after diagnosis, depending on the degree of cardiac involvement [21]. Staging systems have been developed, using biomarkers and other parameters, to assess prognosis in patients with AL CA [22, 23]. Recent major advances in the treatment of the underlying haematological disorder in AL amyloidosis have significantly improved the prognosis. Chemotherapy, immunotherapy (involving targeting monoclonal antibodies), and autologous stem cell transplant may attain prolonged remission and survival in low-stage disease [21]. Precise details on the various therapies are beyond the scope of this summary, and the reader may refer to more in-depth reviews [21].

References

1. Garcia-Pavia P, Rapezzi C, Adler Y, Arad M, Basso C, Brucato A, Burazor I, Caforio ALP, Damy T, Eriksson U, Fontana M, Gillmore JD, Gonzalez-Lopez E, Grogan M, Heymans S, Imazio M, Kindermann I, Kristen AV, Maurer MS, Merlini G, Pantazis A, Pankuweit S, Rigopoulos AG, Linhart A. Diagnosis and treatment of cardiac amyloidosis: a position statement of the ESC working group on myocardial and pericardial diseases. Eur Heart J. 2021;42(16):1554–68. https://doi.org/10.1093/eurheartj/ehab072. PMID: 33825853;PMCID: PMC8060056.
2. Garcia-Pavia P, Bengel F, Brito D, Damy T, Duca F, Dorbala S, Nativi-Nicolau J, Obici L, Rapezzi C, Sekijima Y, Elliott PM. Expert consensus on the monitoring of transthyretin amyloid cardiomyopathy. Eur J Heart Fail. 2021;23(6):895–905. https://doi.org/10.1002/ejhf.2198. Epub 2021 May 24. PMID: 33915002; PMCID: PMC8239846.
3. Arbelo E, Protonotarios A, Gimeno JR, Arbustini E, Barriales-Villa R, Basso C, Bezzina CR, Biagini E, Blom NA, de Boer RA, De Winter T, Elliott PM, Flather M, Garcia-Pavia P, Haugaa KH, Ingles J, Jurcut RO, Klaassen S, Limongelli G, Loeys B, Mogensen J, Olivotto I, Pantazis A, Sharma S, Van Tintelen JP, Ware JS, Kaski JP; ESC scientific document group. 2023 ESC guidelines for the management of cardiomyopathies. Eur Heart J. 2023;44(37):3503–626. https://doi.org/10.1093/eurheartj/ehad194. PMID: 37622657.
4. Kittleson MM, Ruberg FL, Ambardekar AV, Brannagan TH, Cheng RK, Clarke JO, Dember LM, Frantz JG, Hershberger RE, Maurer MS, Nativi-Nicolau J, Sanchorawala V, Sheikh FH. ACC expert consensus decision pathway on comprehensive multidisciplinary care for the patient with cardiac amyloidosis: a report of the American College of Cardiology Solution Set Oversight Committee. J Am Coll Cardiol. 2023;81(11):1076–1126. https://doi.org/10.1016/j.jacc.2022.11.022. Epub 2023 Jan 23. Erratum in: J Am Coll Cardiol. 2023;81(11):1135. PMID: 36697326.
5. Oghina S, Bougouin W, Bézard M, Kharoubi M, Komajda M, Cohen-Solal A, Mebazaa A, Damy T, Bodez D. The impact of patients with cardiac amyloidosis in HFpEF trials. JACC Heart Fail. 2021;9(3):169–78. https://doi.org/10.1016/j.jchf.2020.12.005. Epub 2021 Feb 3 PMID: 33549560.
6. Grogan M, Scott CG, Kyle RA, Zeldenrust SR, Gertz MA, Lin G, Klarich KW, Miller WL, Maleszewski JJ, Dispenzieri A. Natural history of wild-type transthyretin cardiac amyloidosis and risk stratification using a novel staging system. J Am Coll Cardiol. 2016;68(10):1014–20. https://doi.org/10.1016/j.jacc.2016.06.033. Erratum in: J Am Coll Cardiol 2017;69(23):2882 PMID: 27585505.
7. Gillmore JD, Damy T, Fontana M, Hutchinson M, Lachmann HJ, Martinez-Naharro A, Quarta CC, Rezk T, Whelan CJ, Gonzalez-Lopez E, Lane T, Gilbertson JA, Rowczenio D, Petrie

A, Hawkins PN. A new staging system for cardiac transthyretin amyloidosis. Eur Heart J. 2018;39(30):2799–806. https://doi.org/10.1093/eurheartj/ehx589. PMID: 29048471.

8. Cheng RK, Levy WC, Vasbinder A, Teruya S, De Los Santos J, Leedy D, Maurer MS. Diuretic dose and NYHA functional class are independent predictors of mortality in patients with transthyretin cardiac amyloidosis. JACC CardioOncol. 2020;2(3):414–24. https://doi.org/10.1016/j.jaccao.2020.06.007. Epub 2020 Sep 15. PMID: 33073249; PMCID: PMC7561022.
9. Law S, Petrie A, Chacko L, Cohen OC, Ravichandran S, Gilbertson JA, Rowczenio D, Wechalekar A, Martinez-Naharro A, Lachmann HJ, Whelan CJ, Hutt DF, Hawkins PN, Fontana M, Gillmore JD. Disease progression in cardiac transthyretin amyloidosis is indicated by serial calculation of National Amyloidosis Centre transthyretin amyloidosis stage. ESC Heart Fail. 2020;7(6):3942–49. https://doi.org/10.1002/ehf2.12989. Epub 2020 Sep 13. PMID: 32924285; PMCID: PMC7755026.
10. Giancaterino S, Urey MA, Darden D, Hsu JC. Management of arrhythmias in cardiac amyloidosis. JACC Clin Electrophysiol. 2020;6(4):351–61. https://doi.org/10.1016/j.jacep.2020.01.004. PMID: 32327068.
11. El-Am EA, Dispenzieri A, Melduni RM, Ammash NM, White RD, Hodge DO, Noseworthy PA, Lin G, Pislaru SV, Egbe AC, Grogan M, Nkomo VT. Direct current cardioversion of atrial arrhythmias in adults with cardiac amyloidosis. J Am Coll Cardiol. 2019;73(5):589–97. https://doi.org/10.1016/j.jacc.2018.10.079. PMID: 30732713; PMCID: PMC6378685.
12. Vilches S, Fontana M, Gonzalez-Lopez E, Mitrani L, Saturi G, Renju M, Griffin JM, Caponetti A, Gnanasampanthan S, De Los Santos J, Gagliardi C, Rivas A, Dominguez F, Longhi S, Rapezzi C, Maurer MS, Gillmore J, Garcia-Pavia P. Systemic embolism in amyloid transthyretin cardiomyopathy. Eur J Heart Fail. 2022;24(8):1387–96. https://doi.org/10.1002/ejhf.2566. Epub 2022 Jul 11. PMID: 35650018; PMCID: PMC9542906.
13. Donnellan E, Wazni OM, Saliba WI, Baranowski B, Hanna M, Martyn M, Patel D, Trulock K, Menon V, Hussein A, Aagaard P, Jaber W, Kanj M. Cardiac devices in patients with transthyretin amyloidosis: Impact on functional class, left ventricular function, mitral regurgitation, and mortality. J Cardiovasc Electrophysiol. 2019;30(11):2427–32. https://doi.org/10.1111/jce.14180. Epub 2019 Sep 25 PMID: 31515942.
14. Ruberg FL, Maurer MS, Judge DP, Zeldenrust S, Skinner M, Kim AY, Falk RH, Cheung KN, Patel AR, Pano A, Packman J, Grogan DR. Prospective evaluation of the morbidity and mortality of wild-type and V122I mutant transthyretin amyloid cardiomyopathy: the transthyretin amyloidosis cardiac study (TRACS). Am Heart J. 2012;164(2):222-228.e1. https://doi.org/10.1016/j.ahj.2012.04.015. PMID: 22877808.
15. Maurer MS, Schwartz JH, Gundapaneni B, Elliott PM, Merlini G, Waddington-Cruz M, Kristen AV, Grogan M, Witteles R, Damy T, Drachman BM, Shah SJ, Hanna M, Judge DP, Barsdorf AI, Huber P, Patterson TA, Riley S, Schumacher J, Stewart M, Sultan MB, Rapezzi C; ATTR-ACT Study Investigators. Tafamidis treatment for patients with transthyretin amyloid cardiomyopathy. N Engl J Med. 2018;379(11):1007–16. https://doi.org/10.1056/NEJMoa1805689. Epub 2018 Aug 27. PMID: 30145929.
16. Elliott P, Gundapaneni B, Sultan MB, Ines M, Garcia-Pavia P. Improved long-term survival with tafamidis treatment in patients with transthyretin amyloid cardiomyopathy and severe heart failure symptoms. Eur J Heart Fail. 2023;25(11):2060–4. https://doi.org/10.1002/ejhf.2974. Epub 2023 Jul 26 PMID: 37434378.
17. Garcia-Pavia P, Sultan MB, Gundapaneni B, Sekijima Y, Perfetto F, Hanna M, Witteles R. Tafamidis efficacy among octogenarian patients in the phase 3 ATTR-ACT and ongoing long-term extension study. JACC Heart Fail. 2024;12(1):150–60. https://doi.org/10.1016/j.jchf.2023.08.032. Epub 2023 Nov 8 PMID: 37943223.
18. Garcia-Pavia P, Aus dem Siepen F, Donal E, Lairez O, van der Meer P, Kristen AV, Mercuri MF, Michalon A, Frost RJA, Grimm J, Nitsch RM, Hock C, Kahr PC, Damy T. Phase 1 trial of antibody NI006 for depletion of cardiac transthyretin amyloid. N Engl J Med. 2023;389(3):239–250. https://doi.org/10.1056/NEJMoa2303765. Epub 2023 May 20. PMID: 37212440.
19. Fontana M, Berk JL, Gillmore JD, Witteles RM, Grogan M, Drachman B, Damy T, Garcia-Pavia P, Taubel J, Solomon SD, Sheikh FH, Tahara N, González-Costello J, Tsujita K, Morbach

C, Pozsonyi Z, Petrie MC, Delgado D, Van der Meer P, Jabbour A, Bondue A, Kim D, Azevedo O, Hvitfeldt Poulsen S, Yilmaz A, Jankowska EA, Algalarrondo V, Slugg A, Garg PP, Boyle KL, Yureneva E, Silliman N, Yang L, Chen J, Eraly SA, Vest J, Maurer MS; HELIOS-B Trial Investigators. Vutrisiran in patients with transthyretin amyloidosis with cardiomyopathy. N Engl J Med. 2024. https://doi.org/10.1056/NEJMoa2409134. Epub ahead of print. PMID: 39213194.

20. Rapezzi C, Merlini G, Quarta CC, Riva L, Longhi S, Leone O, Salvi F, Ciliberti P, Pastorelli F, Biagini E, Coccolo F, Cooke RM, Bacchi-Reggiani L, Sangiorgi D, Ferlini A, Cavo M, Zamagni E, Fonte ML, Palladini G, Salinaro F, Musca F, Obici L, Branzi A, Perlini S. Systemic cardiac amyloidoses: disease profiles and clinical courses of the 3 main types. Circulation. 2009;120(13):1203–12. https://doi.org/10.1161/CIRCULATIONAHA.108.843334. Epub 2009 PMID: 19752327.
21. Bianchi G, Zhang Y, Comenzo RL. AL amyloidosis: current chemotherapy and immune therapy treatment strategies. JACC CardioOncol. 2021;3(4):467–87. https://doi.org/10.1016/j.jaccao.2021.09.003. PMID: 34729520; PMCID: PMC8543128.
22. Kumar S, Dispenzieri A, Lacy MQ, Hayman SR, Buadi FK, Colby C, Laumann K, Zeldenrust SR, Leung N, Dingli D, Greipp PR, Lust JA, Russell SJ, Kyle RA, Rajkumar SV, Gertz MA. Revised prognostic staging system for light chain amyloidosis incorporating cardiac biomarkers and serum free light chain measurements. J Clin Oncol. 2012;30(9):989–95. https://doi.org/10.1200/JCO.2011.38.5724. Epub 2012. PMID: 22331953; PMCID: PMC3675680.
23. Lilleness B, Ruberg FL, Mussinelli R, Doros G, Sanchorawala V. Development and validation of a survival staging system incorporating BNP in patients with light chain amyloidosis. Blood. 2019;133(3):215–23. https://doi.org/10.1182/blood-2018-06-858951. Epub 2018 Oct 17 PMID: 30333122.

Clinical Cases of Patients Using the "Cardiac Amyloidosis" Pathway

Case Presentation of Patients Using the Cardiac Amyloidosis Pathway

Batel Nissan, Elchanan Parnasa, Yonatan Rashi, Mutaz Karameh, Karen Meir, David Leibowitz, Eyal Herzog, and Arthur Pollak

Abstract Our team developed and published in late 2023 a novel and simple pathway to help health care providers diagnose and treat patients with cardiac amyloidosis. In the book of "Cardiac Amyloidosis" we have updated and modified this pathway. The pathway starts with a section titled "suspicion" in which we provide simple clues or "red flags" that are associated with the cardiac amyloidosis phenotype. It is followed by a section titled "diagnosis," where we present in a simplified 2 × 2 format the laboratory and imaging tests that must be performed for an accurate diagnosis. In the section titled "treatment," we describe the 4 pillars in the management of patients with cardiac amyloidosis, which include: heart failure treatments, management of arrhythmias, treatment of significant aortic stenosis, and appropriate selection of disease modifying therapies. Our algorithm ends with our simplified recommendation for follow-up. In this chapter we present the same pathway with 14 steps to guide health care providers in managing patients with cardiac amyloidosis. We present 6 cases of patients diagnosed with cardiac amyloidosis. These cases illustrate clinical application of the cardiac amyloidosis pathway, and illustrate the process of suspicion, diagnosis, treatment and follow up of patients with cardiac amyloidosis.

Keywords Cardiac amyloidosis · Heart failure · Tafamidis · Transthyretin protein · Pathway · Clinical cases

---

B. Nissan (✉) · M. Karameh · D. Leibowitz · E. Herzog · A. Pollak
Department of Cardiology, Hadassah Medical Center, Hebrew University of Jerusalem, Jerusalem, Israel
e-mail: Batelni@hadassah.org.il

E. Parnasa · Y. Rashi
Department of Medicine, Hadassah Medical Center, Hebrew University of Jerusalem, Jerusalem, Israel

K. Meir
Department of Pathology, Hadassah Medical Center, Hebrew University of Jerusalem, Jerusalem, Israel

E. Herzog (ed.), *Cardiac Amyloidosis*, https://doi.org/10.1007/978-3-031-88342-2_21

Introduction

Our team developed and published in late 2023 a novel and simple pathway to help health care providers diagnose and treat patients with cardiac amyloidosis [1]. In this book of "Cardiac Amyloidosis" we have updated and modified our pathway and outlined it in details in Chap. 1.

The pathway starts with a section titled "suspicion" in which we provide simple clues or "red flags" that are associated with the cardiac amyloidosis phenotype. It is followed by a section titled "diagnosis," where we present in a simplified 2×2 format the laboratory and imaging tests that must be performed for an accurate diagnosis. In the section titled "treatment," we describe the 4 pillars in the management of patients with cardiac amyloidosis, which include: heart failure treatments, management of arrhythmias, treatment of significant aortic stenosis, and appropriate selection of disease modifying therapies. Our algorithm ends with our simplified recommendation for follow-up.

In this chapter we present the same pathway with 14 steps to guide health care provider in managing patients with cardiac amyloidosis. The revised algorithm is seen in Fig. 1.

We present 6 cases of patients diagnosed with cardiac amyloidosis. These cases illustrate clinical application of the cardiac amyloidosis pathway, and illustrate the process of suspicion, diagnosis, treatment and follow up of patients with cardiac amyloidosis.

Case 1

81 year old male with medical history of hypertension, hyperlipidemia, diagnosis of cervical and lumbar spine discopathy and history of carpal tunnel surgery on the left side (Fig. 1, step 5).

For the past two years, he has complained of shortness of breath upon exertion, particularly when walking uphill and when climbing three flights of stairs. There is no chest discomfort during exertion, and his condition was classified as New York Heart Association (NYHA) class II (Fig. 1, step 1).

Evidence of concentric thickening of the left ventricular heart muscle was found on the echocardiogram (Fig. 1, step 2), (Fig. 2) along with diastolic dysfunction (Fig. 3). However, the ECG showed relatively small QRS complexes (Fig. 1, step 3), (Fig. 4).

Hematologic tests showed kappa and lambda within the normal limits, negative electrophoresis and no evidence of urine monoclonal bence jones protein thereby excluding plasma cell disease (Fig. 1, step 7). Additional laboratory results supporting the diagnosis of cardiac amyloidosis (Fig. 1, step 9) included, Pro-BNP 1815 pg/ml (0–450 pg/ml) and stage IIIa of chronic kidney disease with eGFR of 47 mL/min/1.73 m^2, with creatinine level of 1.48 mg/dl.

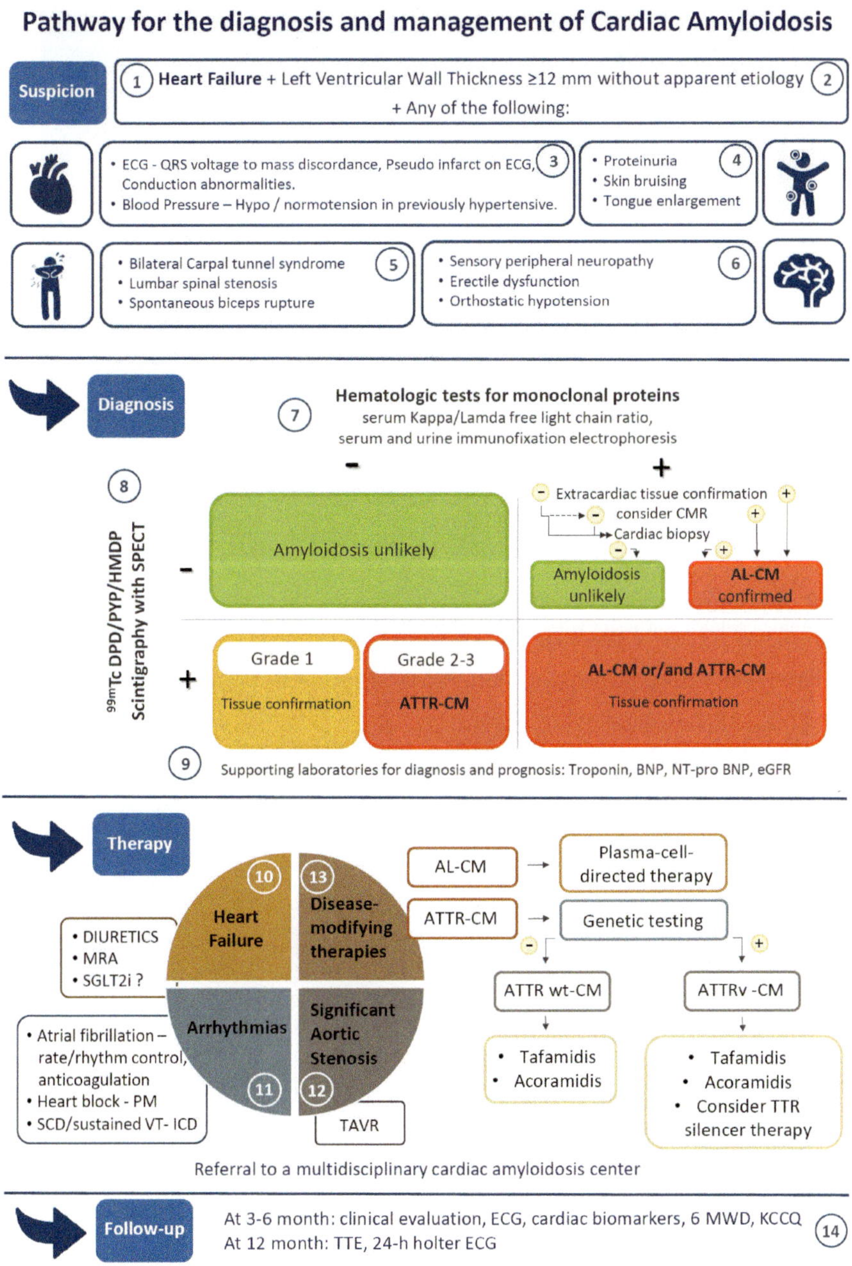

Fig. 1 Pathway for the diagnosis and management of cardiac amyloidosis

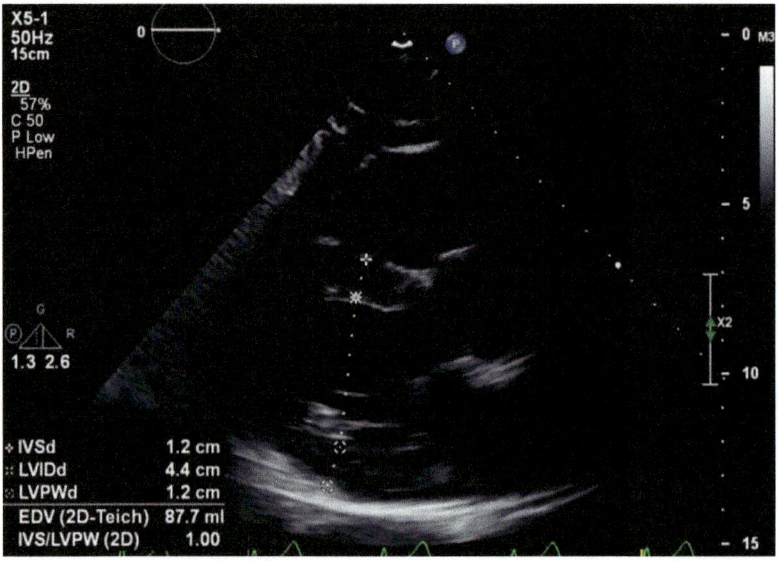

Fig. 2 Echocardiogram, case 1. Parasternal long axis view showing left ventricular wall thickening of 12 mm, a pattern consistent with cardiac amyloidosis

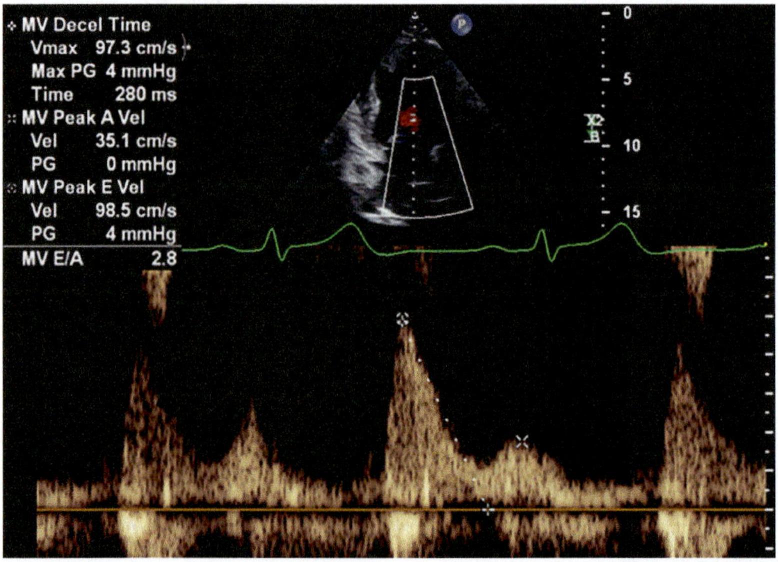

Fig. 3 Echocardiogram, case 1. Diastolic dysfunction with restrictive pattern as demonstrated at the mitral valve inflow with increased peak E velocity (measured 98.5 cm/s, white circle), reduced peak A velocity (measured 35 cm/s, white x-mark) and E/A ratio of 2.8

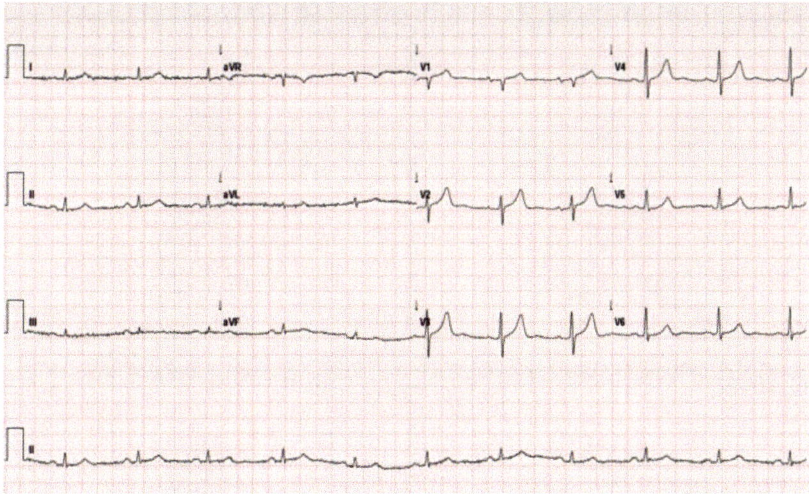

Fig. 4 Electrocardiogram, case 1. Typical finding of low voltage in a patient with cardiac amyloidosis

The patient underwent a 99mTc-PYP scan, which demonstrated cardiomyocyte uptake greater than rib uptake, (Perugini grade 3), as well as an H/CL uptake ratio of 1.7. (Fig. 1, step 8), (Fig. 5).

Following the diagnosis, the patient began treatment with diuresis (Fig. 1, step 10) and disease modifying therapy with tafamidis (Fig. 1, step 13) with clinical improvement. The patient continues follow-up for cardiac amyloidosis at a specialized clinic (Fig. 1, step 14). Over time, the patient developed an incomplete RBBB (Right Bundle Branch Block) and symptomatic bradycardia with a heart rate of 42. As a result, he underwent dual-chamber pacemaker implantation (Fig. 1, step 11).

Case 2

87 year old female with medical history of myelodysplastic disorder, hypertension, and dyslipidemia. She underwent Transcatheter Aortic Valve Replacement (TAVR) for symptomatic severe aortic stenosis, which led to a marked improvement in her symptoms (Fig. 1, step 12). Two years later, she experienced shortness of breath with effort and sought medical advice.

The patient presented with symptoms and signs of heart failure (Fig. 1, Step 1). She reported shortness of breath during exertion, particularly when climbing two flights of stairs. An echocardiogram (Fig. 6) showed left ventricular hypertrophy and diastolic dysfunction (Fig. 1, Step 1). However, her ECG did not reveal signs of hypertrophy showing normal-to-low QRS voltage (Fig. 1, Step 3). Additionally, she

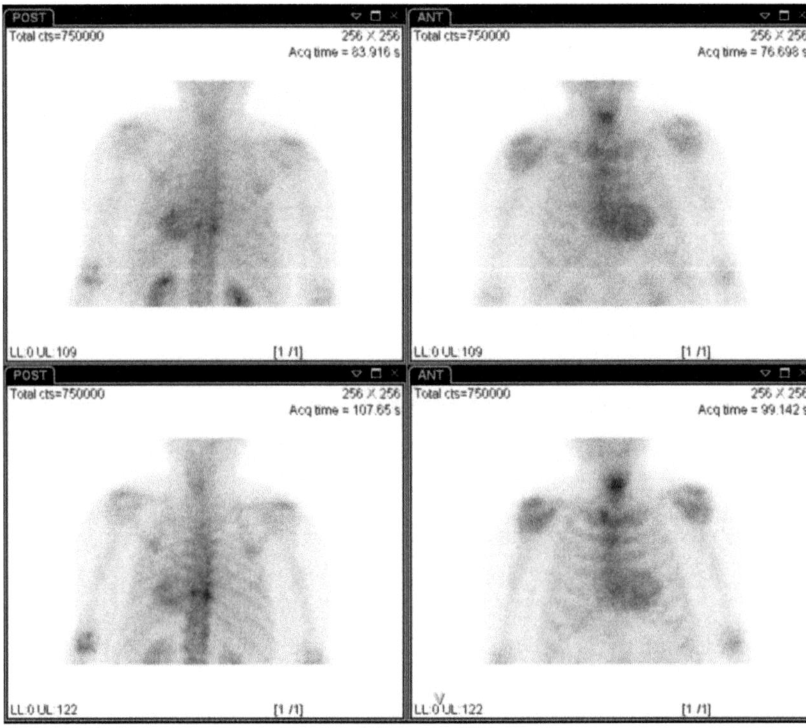

Fig. 5 99mTc-PYP scan, case 1. Typical test for ATTR amyloidosis with cardiomyocyte uptake greater than rib uptake, (Perugini grade 3), as well as an H/CL uptake ratio of 1.7

was diagnosed with carpal tunnel syndrome, which required surgery to alleviate her symptoms (Fig. 1, Step 3).

The patient underwent a 99mTc-DPD scan (Fig. 1, Step 8), which demonstrated Perugini grade 1 uptake (Fig. 7a) which is not diagnostic for ATTR amyloidosis. The patient continued follow up in the heart failure clinic. A few years later she complained of clinical deterioration and repeat echocardiogram revealed increased hypertrophy of the left ventricle. Repeat 99mTc-DPD scan demonstrated Perugini grade 2 (Fig. 7b). These findings, combined with negative genetic testing for hereditary ATTR cardiac amyloidosis and the absence of plasma cell disease (confirmed through blood tests) (Fig. 1, Step 5), were diagnostic of wild-type ATTR cardiac amyloidosis.

Supporting laboratory findings (Fig. 1, Step 9) included elevated Pro-BNP at 585 pg/mL (reference range: 0–450 pg/mL) and an eGFR of 39 mL/min/1.73 m^2, with creatinine level of 1.3 mg/dL.

The patient was treated for heart failure symptoms with furosemide and spironolactone (Fig. 1, Step 10). Beta-blockers were discontinued due to symptomatic bradycardia. Later with the availability of disease-modifying therapy, tafamidis treatment was initiated (Fig. 1, Step 13) with noticeable clinical improvement over six months.

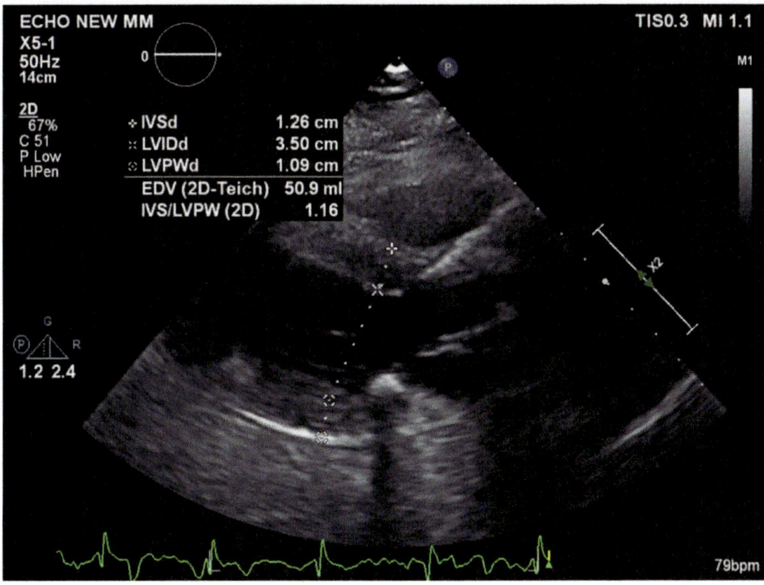

Fig. 6 Echocardiogram, case 2. Parasternal long axis view showing concentric left ventricular hypertrophy

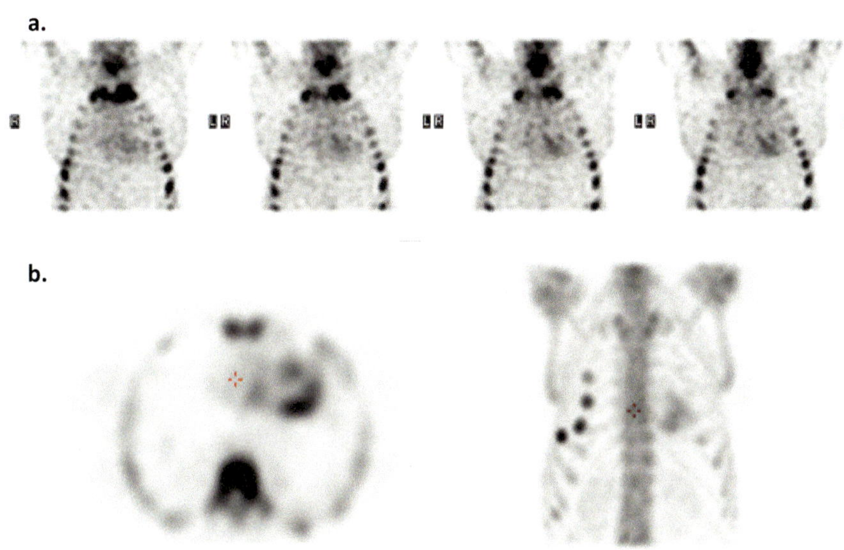

Fig. 7 99mTc-DPD scan, case 2. **a** Non-diagnostic test for ATTR amyloidosis with cardiomyocyte uptake less than rib uptake, (Perugini grade 1). **b** Repeated test a few years later demonstrating myocardial uptake equal to rib uptake (Perugini grade 2) suggestive for cardiac amyloidosis

The patient continues follow-up care for cardiac amyloidosis at a specialized clinic with a multidisciplinary team (Fig. 1, Step 14). She undergoes regular assessments, including echocardiograms, ECGs, blood tests for cardiac biomarkers, and clinical evaluations of her heart failure symptoms.

Case 3

86 year old male with medical history of hypertension and chronic renal failure (CRF) was referred to a cardiology consult due to severe dyspnea, exercise intolerance and leg edema, his condition classified as NYHA class II (Fig. 1, Step 1). In answer to targeted questions, he mentioned 2 previous surgeries for carpal tunnel syndrome (Fig. 1, Step 5).

ECG demonstrated sinus rhythm, and normal intervals, with typical findings of cardiac amyloidosis including low voltage and a pseudo infarct pattern (Q wave in III, aVF & V1) (Fig. 1, Step 3) (Fig. 8).

The echocardiogram raised the suspicions of cardiac amyloidosis due to severe concentric left ventricular thickening, with measured LVPWd (left ventricular posterior wall diastolic) of 18 mm (Fig. 1, Step 2), (Fig. 9) mildly reduced LV function, estimated LVEF 45–50% and reduced global longitudinal strain (GLS) of -6.8 with apical sparing ("Cherry on top" pattern), (Fig. 10).

Hematologic tests included FLC Kappa 80 mg/dl, Lambda 40 mg/dl, ratio of 2 with no evidence of monoclonal bence jones protein in urine. Electrophoresis was inconclusive and not typical for monoclonal gammopathy (Fig. 1, Step 7). Other

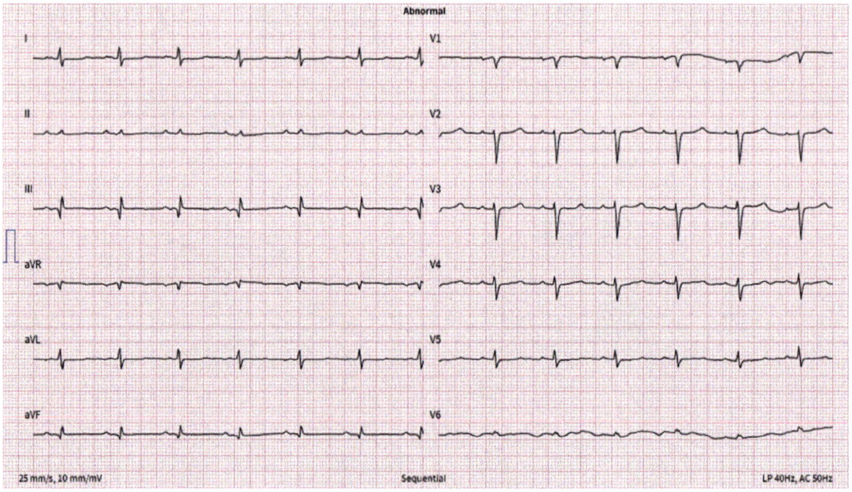

Fig. 8 Electrocardiogram, case 3. Typical finding of cardiac amyloidosis including low voltage and pseudo infarct pattern

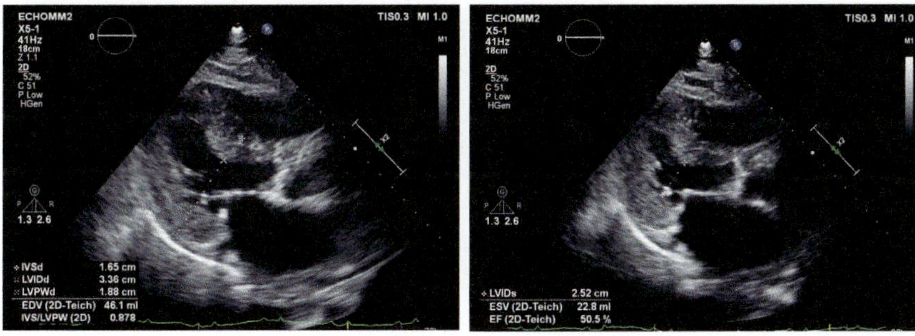

Fig. 9 Echocardiogram, case 3. Parasternal long axis view showing severe concentric left ventricular thickening, measured LVPWd of 18 mm, calculated LVEF 50.5%

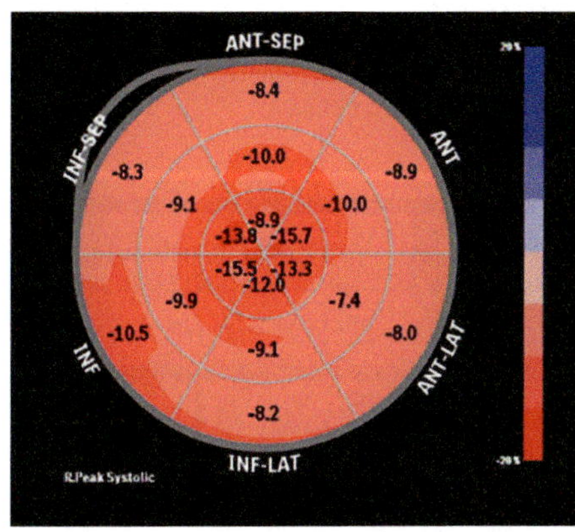

Fig. 10 Echocardiogram, case 3. Global longitudinal strain (GLS) map with reduced GLS and apical sparing ("Cherry on top" pattern)

laboratory tests included chronic renal failure with eGFR 26 mL/min/1.73 m^2, with creatinine level of 2.3 mg/dL, elevated high sensitivity troponin (hsT) 98 ng/L (reference range: 0–53 ng/L), and ProBNP 6176 pg/ml (reference range: 0–450 pg/mL), (Fig. 1, Step 9).

For confirmation of the diagnosis the patient was referred to 99mTc-PYP SPECT (Fig. 1, Step 8), he completed the test outside of our institution with a reported answer of Perugini grade 1, but heart/whole body ratio (H/WB) of 1.6.

Due to the inconclusive results of PYP scanning the patient was referred to 99mTc-DPD SPECT, that found diffuse, significant uptake in cardiomyocytes, most prominently in the left ventricle and septum, higher than rib uptake. The findings are typical for ATTR amyloidosis, Grade 3 (Fig. 11). Reassessment of the 99mTc-PYP SPECT by an amyloidosis expert revealed the misdiagnosis with cardiomyocyte uptake greater than rib, and the answer was corrected to Perugini grade 3 (Fig. 12).

Diagnosis of ATTR amyloidosis was confirmed with a recommendation for heart failure treatment including furosemide, spironolactone and dapagliflozin (Fig. 1, Step 10) with disease modifying treatment of tafamidis (Fig. 1, Step 13) with clinical improvement.

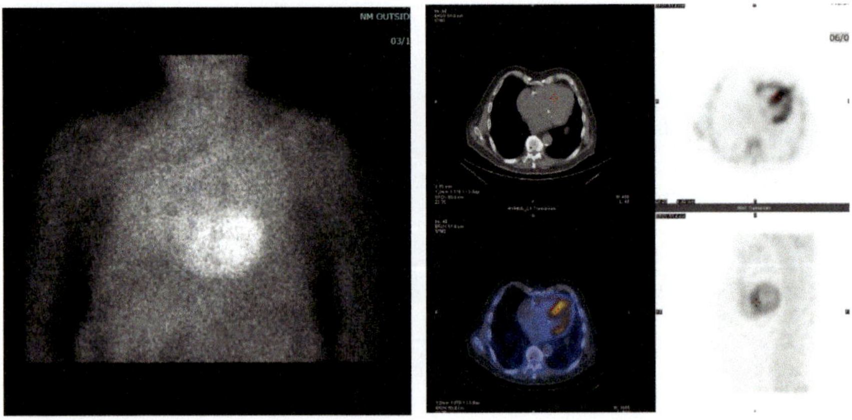

Fig. 11 SPECT-99mTc-DPD scan, case 3. Typical finding of ATTR amyloidosis with diffuse and significant uptake in cardiomyocytes, more prominent on the left ventricle and septum, higher than rib uptake. Perugini Grade 3

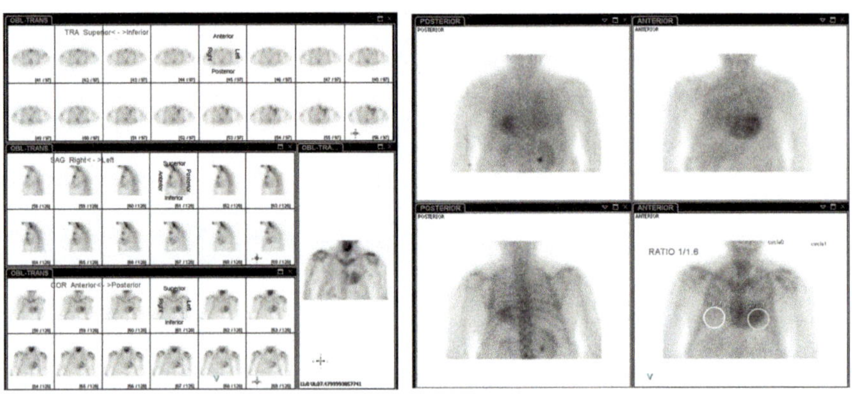

Fig. 12 SPECT-99mTc-PYP scan, case 3. Diagnostic test for ATTR amyloidosis with cardiomyocyte uptake greater than rib uptake, (Perugini grade 3) and positive Heart/whole body ratio (H/WB) of 1.6

After a few months he developed symptomatic atrial fibrillation with rapid ventricular response. He started treatment with apixaban and bisoprolol (Fig. 1, Step 11). After a month of anti-coagulation treatment, he underwent a successful electrical cardioversion and treated with amiodarone to maintain sinus rhythm.

A few months later he presented with clinical deterioration and cardiogenic shock with acute renal failure necessitating hemodialysis treatment and a component of septic shock. He passed away a year after the diagnosis of ATTR amyloidosis.

Case 4

82 year old male with medical history of ischemic heart disease and carpal tunnel syndrome in both hands (Fig. 1, Step 5), presented to the cardiology clinic due to functional deterioration and progressive exertional dyspnea, development of peripheral edema in both legs and the appearance of right-sided pleural effusion (which was aspirated, yielding 500 mL of transudative fluid) (Fig. 1, Step 1).

Electrocardiogram (ECG) revealed the presence of right bundle branch block (RBBB), atrial fibrillation and low voltage QRS complexes, (Fig. 1, Step 3), (Fig. 13). The patient underwent an echocardiogram, which revealed septal thickening (Fig. 1, Step 2), (Fig. 14) preserved systolic function, enlarged atria, moderate pulmonary hypertension, and moderate tricuspid insufficiency with elevated pulmonary pressure, findings also consistent with heart failure with preserved ejection fraction.

Given the clinical suspicion of cardiac amyloidosis, the patient was referred for 99mTc-PYP scan which demonstrated higher myocardial uptake than rib uptake, Perugini grade 3 (Fig. 1, Step 8), (Fig. 15).

For ischemic assessment he underwent stress Sestamibi radionuclide scan (MIBI), imaging which excluded a significant filling perfusion defect and reduced the suspicion for ischemic etiology (Fig. 16).

Hematological tests showed kappa 15.88 MG/L (normal range of 3.3–19.4 MG/L), lambda 15.2 MG/L (normal range: 5.7–26.3 MG/L, and a ratio of 1.04 (normal range of 0.26–1.65). Blood and urine electrophoresis was negative for monoclonal gammopathy. In the absent of plasma cell disease (Fig. 1, Step 7), these findings are diagnostic of ATTR cardiac amyloidosis.

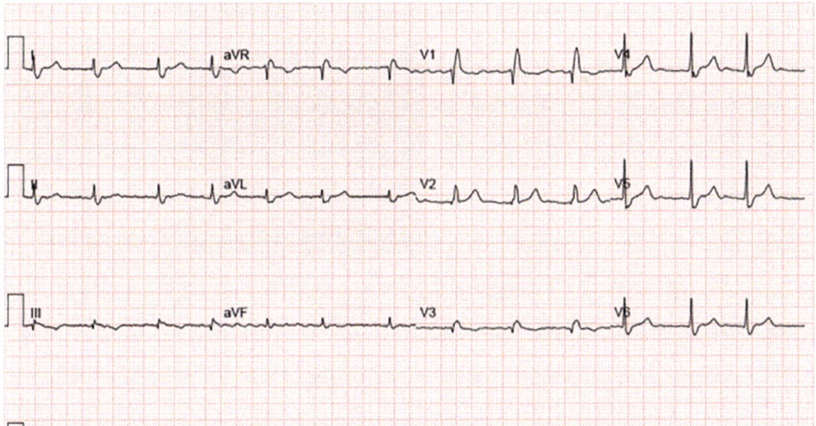

Fig. 13 Electrocardiogram, case 4. Conduction disturbance (RBBB) as well as the presence of atrial fibrillation and relatively small QRS complexes

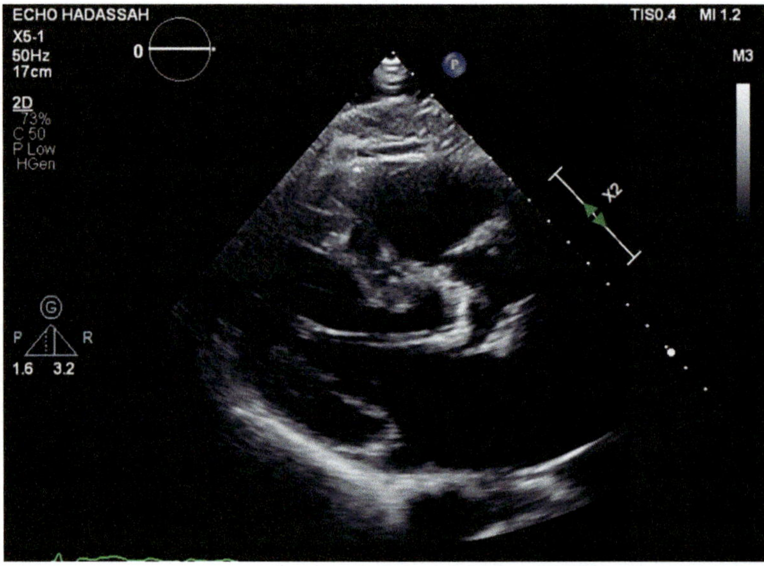

Fig. 14 Echocardiogram, case 4. Parasternal long axis view showing left ventricular hypertrophy

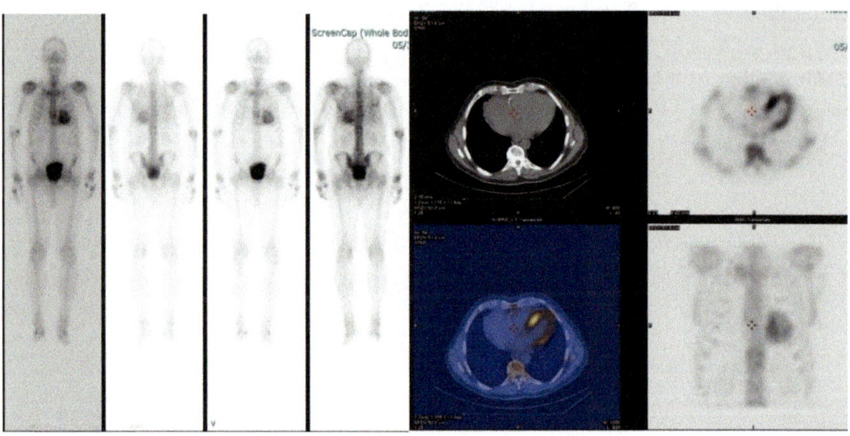

Fig. 15 SPECT-99mTc-PYP scan, case 4. Typical finding of ATTR Amyloidosis with higher myocardial uptake than rib uptake, Perugini grade 3

Additional laboratory results supporting the diagnosis of cardiac amyloidosis (Fig. 1, Step 9) included, Pro-BNP 1828 pg/ml (0–450 pg/ml), eGFR 59 ml/min/1/73 m^2 and creatinine level of 1.23 mg/dL. Troponin level of 33 NG/L (normal range 0–53 NG/L) did not contribute to the diagnosis (though it certainly did not rule it out).

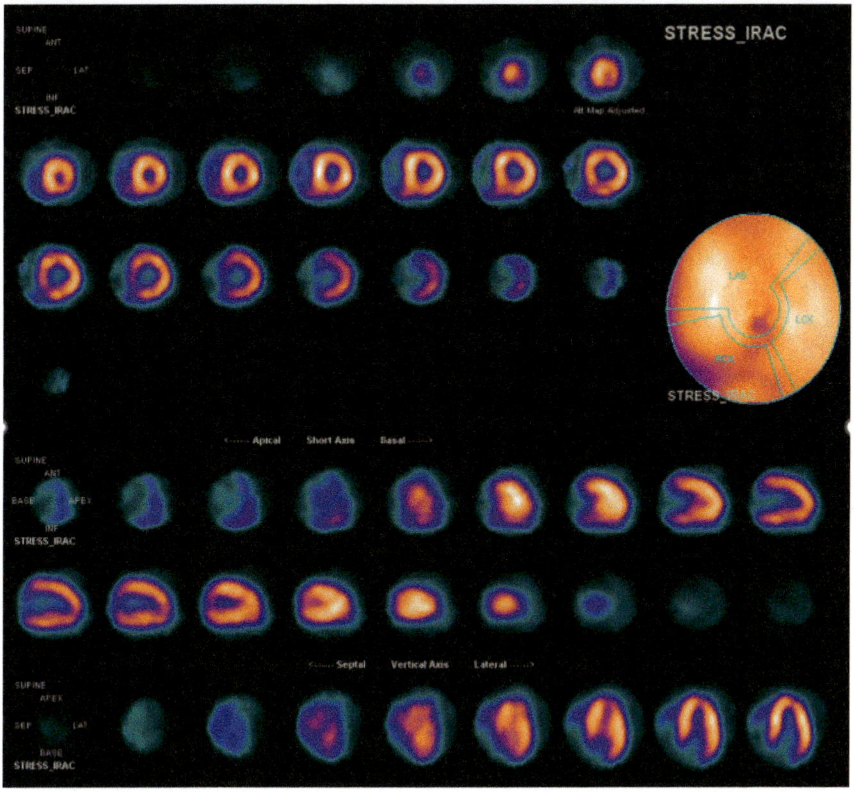

Fig. 16 Sestamibi radionuclide scan (MIBI), case 4. Stress imaging without any filling defect, not suggestive for ischemic etiology

The patient began treatment with diuretics (Fig. 1, Step 10) and received treatment for atrial fibrillation, including electrical cardioversion and catheter ablation (Fig. 1, Step 11).

Following the diagnosis of ATTR amyloidosis he received treatment with tafamidis and participated in a randomized-control study involving use of a monoclonal antibody against amyloid deposits in ATTR-CM (Fig. 1, Step 13).

The patient continues follow-up for cardiac amyloidosis at a specialized clinic in a hospital with a multidisciplinary team capable of addressing the various complications associated with cardiac amyloidosis. During the follow-up, the patient is referred annually for relevant tests: echocardiogram, ECG, cardiac biomarkers in the blood, and undergoes clinical evaluation of symptoms related to heart failure (Fig. 1, Step 14).

Case 5

68 year old male with medical history of hypertension was referred to the emergency room due to orthopnea for the past two weeks, (Fig. 1, Step 1) with no chest pain or other symptoms.

During the evaluation in the emergency room, ECG (Fig. 17) demonstrated normal sinus with right axis, low voltage in the limb leads, and T wave inversion (TWI) in the inferolateral leads. (Fig. 1, Step 3).

He had mildly elevated troponin of 100 ng/L (0–53), high levels of ProBNP 3529 pg/ml and acute renal failure (ARF) with creatinine 1.3 mg/dl (Fig. 1, Step 9). During hospitalization urine test revealed proteinuria with an albumin/creatinine ratio of 1760 mg/g (Fig. 1, Step 4). Coronary catheterization showed non-obstructive atherosclerotic disease.

Echocardiogram (Fig. 18) demonstrated mildly reduced systolic function with an LVEF of 45–50%, mild LVH (Fig. 1, Step 2), basal and septal hypokinesis with diastolic dysfunction. and mild to moderate MR, and minimal TR.

During hospitalization the patient was diagnosed with heart failure with mildly reduced ejection fraction (HFmrEF) and received treatment with Beta-blockers and ACE inhibitors. Three weeks later, he presented for follow-up in the clinic, not tolerating beta-blocker therapy due to low blood pressure with functional status of NYHA class III and a clinical suspicion of cardiac amyloidosis was suggested.

Targeted echocardiogram demonstrated reduced global longitudinal strain (GLS) of – 9.5 with apical sparing ("Cherry on top " pattern, Fig. 19).

Hematologic tests included free light chain (FLC), Kappa 17 mg/L (normal range of 3.3–19.4 MG/L), Lambda 2699 mg/L (normal range: 5.7–26.3 MG/L) with ratio

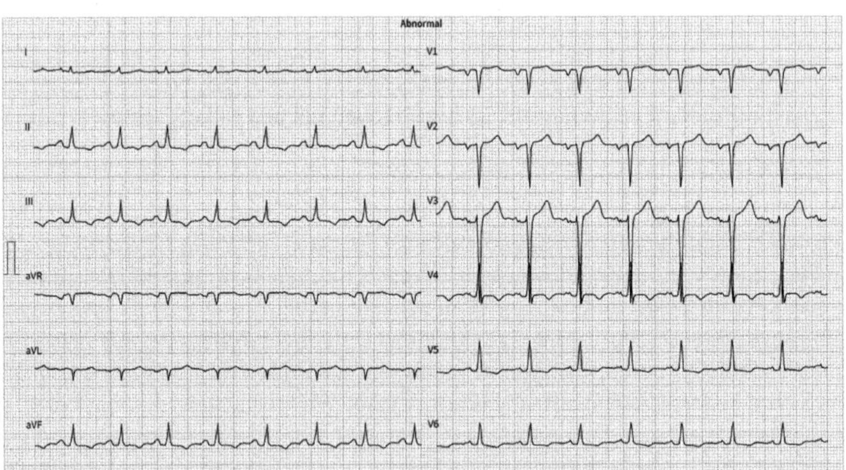

Fig. 17 Electrocardiogram, case 5. Abnormal ECG with low voltage and inferolateral TWI

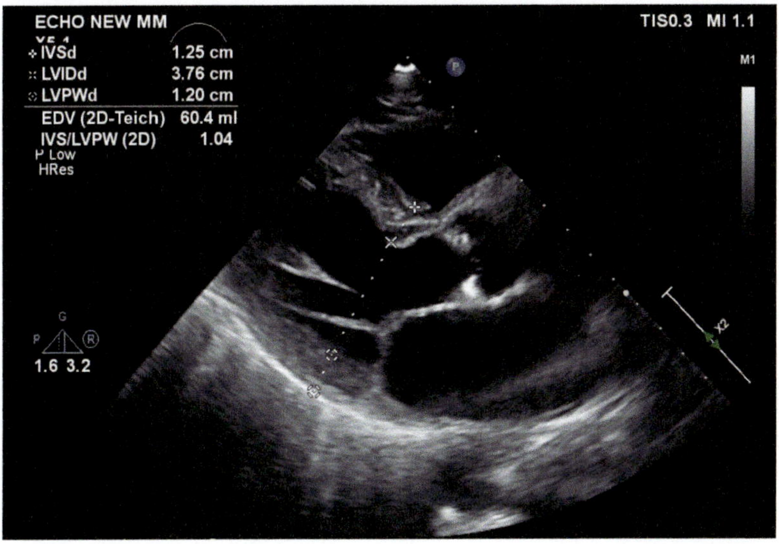

Fig. 18 Echocardiogram, case 5. Parasternal long axis view showing concentric left ventricular thickening, measuring 12 mm

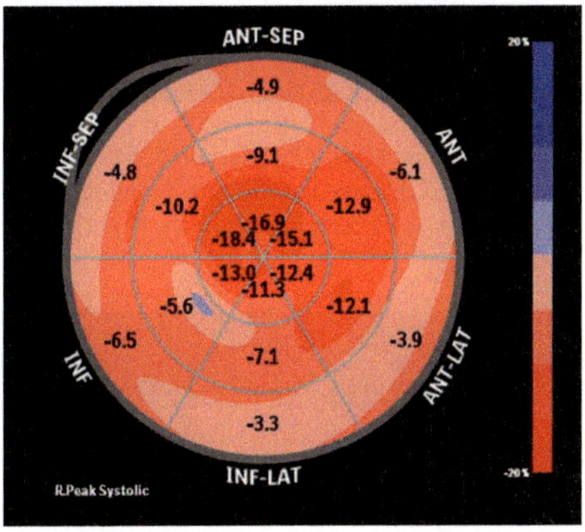

Fig. 19 Echocardiogram, case 5. Global longitudinal strain (GLS) map demonstrated reduced GLS with apical sparing ("Cherry on top" pattern)

of 0.006 (normal range of 0.26–1.65). Serum Protein Electrophoresis (SPEP) was positive and immunofixation electrophoresis (IEP) was also positive for Lambda light chain (Fig. 1, Step 7). TC99M-DPD scan was negative with Perugini grade 0 (Fig. 1, Step 8). Other laboratory tests included acute renal failure with creatinine 1.49 mg/dl, elevated high sensitivity troponin 253 ng/L, and ProBNP of 9520 pg/ml (Fig. 1, Step 9).

Given the suspicion of cardiac AL amyloidosis, biopsies were taken from bone marrow and hypodermis adipose tissue. CD138 IHC stain highlighted an increase in plasma cells (~20%); and kappa and lambda immunostaining was monotypic for lambda. Congo-red stain demonstrated amyloid deposition in periosteum, bone marrow and lower dermis.

The patient was referred to cardiac magnetic resonance (CMR) which demonstrated enlarged atria, a pleural effusion and diffuse, subendocardial Late Gadolinium Enhancement (LGE) (Fig. 20). T1 mapping reveled intermediate intensity, increased global T1 of 1167 ms (normal range 900–1100 ms) with normal native T2 (47 ms) (Fig. 21), findings consistent with cardiac amyloidosis.

Diagnosis of plasma cell myeloma, lambda light chain restricted, with cardiac AL amyloidosis were confirmed. The patient was treated with plasma cell directed therapy of daratumumab, velcade, cyclophosphamide and dexamethasone (Fig. 1,

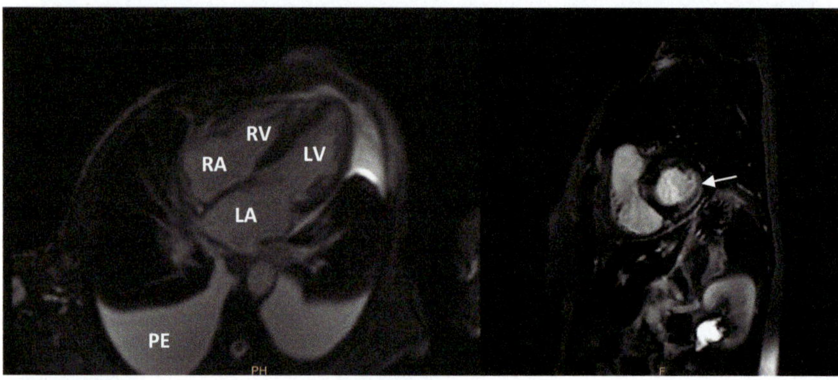

Fig. 20 Cardiac MRI (CMR), case 5. SSFP (cine) image showing large atria and pleural effusion (left panel). LGE image showing sub-endocardial LGE (right panel, arrow). Pleural effusion (PE), Right atrium (RA), Left atrium (LA), Right ventricle (RV), Left ventricle (LV)

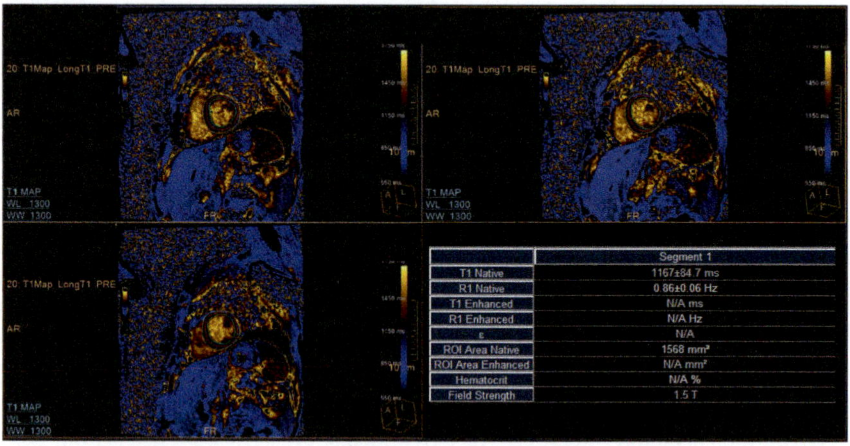

Fig. 21 Cardiac MRI (CMR), case 5. T1 mapping reveled intermediate intensity, increased global T1 of 1167 ms (normal range 900–1100 ms)

Step 13) in addition to heart failure treatment (Fig. 1, Step 10) including furosemide and spironolactone with clinical and laboratory improvement.

Six months later he had a rapid and good clinical and hematological response, He continues routine follow-up with a multidisciplinary team (Fig. 1, Step 14). One year later, the patient is currently in remission with maintenance therapy using daratumumab alone.

Case 6

68 year old male with medical history of hypertension, epilepsy and a transient ischemic attack (TIA). A year before his current presentation, he was diagnosed with multiple myeloma without targeted treatment due to smoldering disease. He presented to the emergency room due to shortness of breath with minimal exertion such as walking and when climbing upstairs for the past two months,. There was no chest discomfort during exertion, and his condition was classified as NYHA class II (Fig. 1, Step 1).

The ECG shows relatively small complexes especially in the limb leads with PR interval prolongation up to 400 ms and a pseudoinfarct pattern (q waves in inferior leads, poor R wave progression) (Fig. 1, Step 3) (Fig. 22).

Echocardiogram revealed low normal systolic function with estimated LVEF of 50–55%, and moderate concentric left ventricular hypertrophy (Fig. 1, Step 2) (Fig. 23).

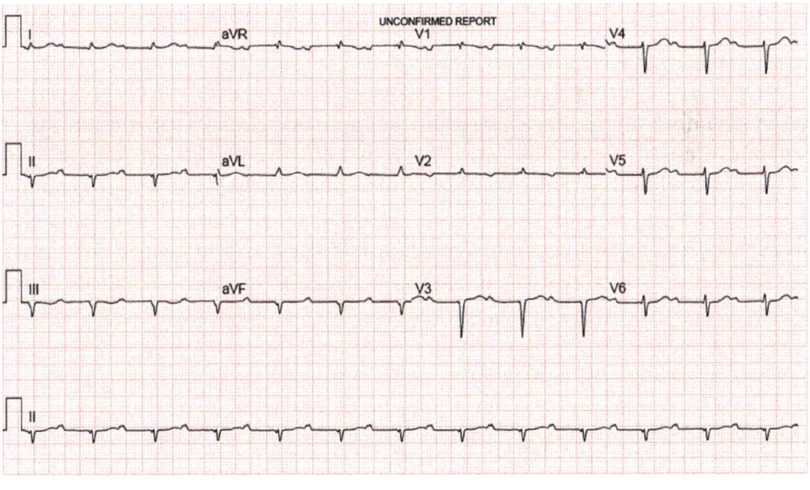

Fig. 22 Electrocardiogram, case 6. Typical finding of cardiac amyloidosis including low voltage complexes, conduction abnormalities including PR prolongation and pseudoinfarct pattern (q waves in inferior leads, poor R wave progression)

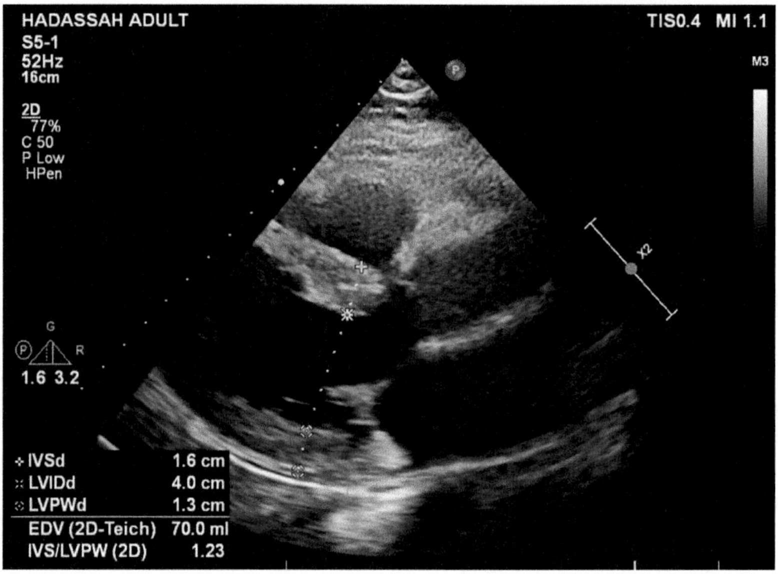

Fig. 23 Echocardiogram, case 6. Parasternal long axis view showing left ventricular hypertrophy, a pattern characteristic of cardiac amyloidosis

Hematologic tests included FLC Kappa 10.6 mg/l (normal range of 3.3–19.4 mg/l), Lambda 671 mg/l (normal range: 5.7–26.3 MG/L) with positive ratio of 0.02 (normal range of 0.26–1.65). Urine protein electrophoresis and immunofixation was positive for Lambda light chain gammopathy (Fig. 1, Step 7). Other laboratory tests included acute renal failure with creatinine up to 2.18 mg/dl, elevated high sensitivity troponin 943 ng/L (normal range 0–53), and ProBNP 1767 pg/ml (Fig. 1, Step 9).

A bone marrow biopsy was taken which demonstrated abundance of plasma cells (CD138+, lambda light chain restricted), comprising 20–30% of the marrow cell population. Congo red stain negative for amyloidosis andreticulin stain showed a mild increase in fibers (MF1). Skin biopsy was inconclusive.

Coronary catheterization showed non-obstructive atherosclerotic disease. Right heart catheterization demonstrated almost normal left and right ventricular pressures and mild pulmonary hypertension with abnormal cardiac output. An endo-myocardial biopsy was taken and using Congo red staining, microscopic tiny foci consistent with amyloid were observed. No granulomas, giant cells, eosinophils or cardiomyocyte damage were observed (Fig. 24).

A diagnosis of primary AL amyloidosis was made, with extremely severe cardiac involvement, MAYO stage 4, highly symptomatic with NYHA III, with very rapid progression over time.

Immediately after diagnosis heart failure treatment for heart failure with preserved ejection fraction (HFpEF) was initiated with spironolactone, empagliflozin and furosemide (Fig. 1, Step 10) in addition to plasma cell directed therapy of daratumumab, velcade, cyclophosphamide and dexamethasone (Fig. 1, Step 13). Due to

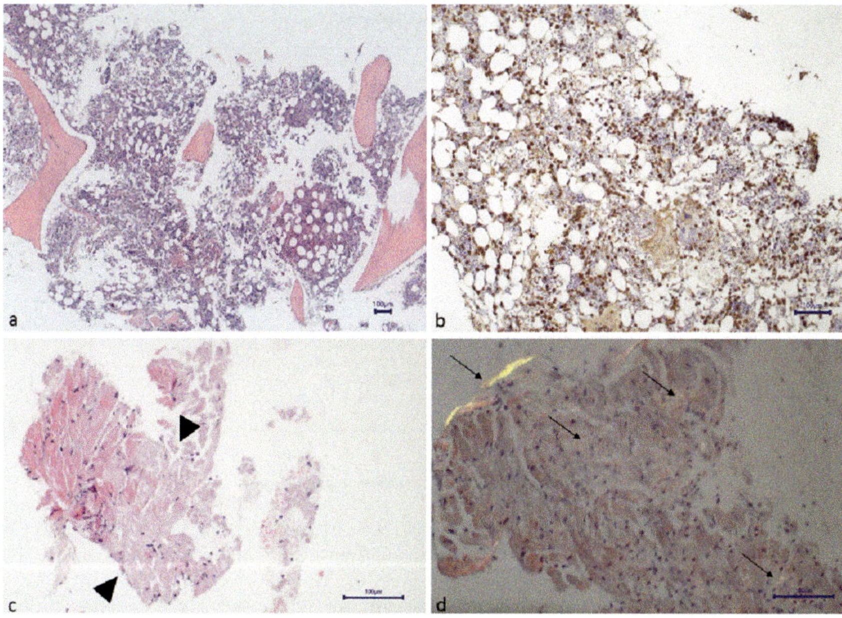

Fig. 24 Bone marrow and cardiac biopsies, case 6. Sections show hypercellular bone marrow with trilineage hematopoiesis and monotypic immunostaining for lambda light chain (**a** hematoxylin and eosin; **b** lambda light chain immunoperoxidase). Cardiac biopsy from the same patient shows amorphous pale eosinophilic extracellular material (**c** arrowheads; hematoxylin and eosin) which demonstrates "apple green" birefringence on Congo red staining examined under polarized light (arrows, **d**)

the high severity of stage 4 cardiac amyloidosis, the patient was found eligible for a randomized control trial of a monoclonal antibody against misfolded kappa and lambda light chains.

During follow-up the patient presented with fatigue and clinical deterioration with vital signs revealing low blood pressures and extreme bradycardia down to 35 beats per minute (bpm). ECG showed sinus bradycardia with isorhythmic A-V dissociation (Fig. 25). He underwent urgent pacemaker implantation due to combined conduction abnormality (Fig. 1, Step 11).

At one month follow-up, he had a good hematological response with mild clinical improvement. The patient continues follow-up with a multidisciplinary team (Fig. 1, Step 14).

Summary

We present in this Chap. 6 cases of patients with a diagnosis of cardiac amyloidosis, demonstrating the flow of patients using the cardiac amyloidosis pathway.

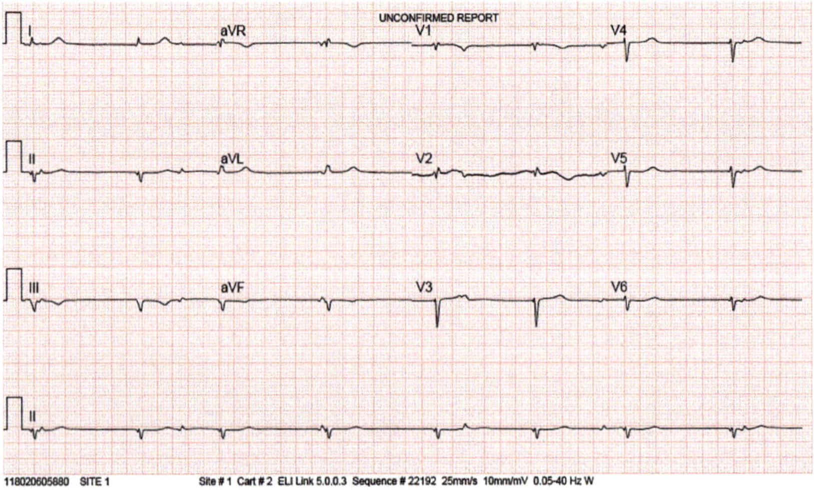

Fig. 25 Electrocardiogram, case 6. Bradycardia at 46 bpm, irregular rhythm, with the appearance of P waves at a rate of 35 bpm and escape rhythm around 45 bpm—Sinus bradycardia with isorhythmic A-V dissociation

Abbreviations for Fig. 1

AL-CM	Amyloid monoclonal immunoglobulin light chain cardiomyopathy
ATTR-CM	Amyloid transthyretin cardiomyopathy
ATTRv-CM	Variant transthyretin amyloid cardiomyopathy
ATTRwt-CM	Wild-type transthyretin amyloid cardiomyopathy
BNP	B-type natriuretic peptide
CMR	Cardiac magnetic resonance
DPD	Diphosphono-1,2-propanodicarboxylic acid
ECG	Electrocardiogram
HMDP	Hydroxymethylene diphosphonate
ICD	Implantable cardioverter defibrillator
KCCQ	Kansas City Cardiomyopathy Questionnaire
MRA	Mineralocorticoid receptor antagonists
NT-pro BNP	N-terminal pro–B-type natriuretic peptide
PPM	Permanent pacemaker
PYP	Pyrophosphate
SCD	Sudden cardiac death
SGLT2i	Sodium glucose cotransporter 2 inhibitor
SPECT	Single-photon emission computed tomography
TAVR	Transaortic valve replacement
TTE	Transthoracic echocardiography
TTR	Transthyretin
VT	Ventricular tachycardia

Reference

1. Herzog E, Leibowitz D, Gatt ME, Pollak TKA. Pathway for the diagnosis and management of cardiac amyloidosis. Crit Pathways Cardiol. 2023;22:114–9.